Practical Perimetry

Practical Perimetry

Second Edition

Editors

Shibal Bhartiya MS (Ophthalmology)
Additional Director
Department of Ophthalmology
Fortis Memorial Research Institute
Gurugram, Haryana, India

Murali Ariga MS DNB FAICO PGDMLE
Director
Swamy Eye Clinic, Chennai
Director, Academics and Research
MN Eye Hospitals and Postgraduate Institute, Chennai
Visiting Consultant
Sundaram Medical Foundation
Chennai, Tamil Nadu, India

George V Puthuran MS (Ophthalmology)
Head
Department of Glaucoma
Aravind Eye Hospital
Madurai, Tamil Nadu, India

Ronnie George DO DNB MS
Director, Glaucoma Services
Department of Glaucoma Services
Sankara Nethralaya
Chennai, Tamil Nadu, India

Foreword

Lingam Vijaya

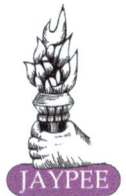

JAYPEE BROTHERS MEDICAL PUBLISHERS
The Health Sciences Publisher
New Delhi | London

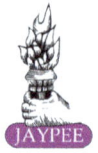 **Jaypee Brothers Medical Publishers (P) Ltd**

Headquarters

Jaypee Brothers Medical Publishers (P) Ltd
EMCA House, 23/23-B
Ansari Road, Daryaganj
New Delhi 110 002, India
Landline: +91-11-23272143, +91-11-23272703
+91-11-23282021, +91-11-23245672
Email: jaypee@jaypeebrothers.com

Corporate Office

Jaypee Brothers Medical Publishers (P) Ltd
4838/24, Ansari Road, Daryaganj
New Delhi 110 002, India
Phone: +91-11-43574357
Fax: +91-11-43574314
Email: jaypee@jaypeebrothers.com

Overseas Office

JP Medical Ltd
83 Victoria Street, London
SW1H 0HW (UK)
Phone: +44 20 3170 8910
Fax: +44 (0)20 3008 6180
Email: info@jpmedpub.com

Website: www.jaypeebrothers.com
Website: www.jaypeedigital.com

© 2024, Jaypee Brothers Medical Publishers

The views and opinions expressed in this book are solely those of the original contributor(s)/author(s) and do not necessarily represent those of editor(s) or publisher of the book.

All rights reserved. No part of this publication may be reproduced, stored or transmitted in any form or by any means, electronic, mechanical, photocopying, recording or otherwise, without the prior permission in writing of the publishers.

All brand names and product names used in this book are trade names, service marks, trademarks or registered trademarks of their respective owners. The publisher is not associated with any product or vendor mentioned in this book.

Medical knowledge and practice change constantly. This book is designed to provide accurate, authoritative information about the subject matter in question. However, readers are advised to check the most current information available on procedures included and check information from the manufacturer of each product to be administered, to verify the recommended dose, formula, method and duration of administration, adverse effects and contraindications. It is the responsibility of the practitioner to take all appropriate safety precautions. Neither the publisher nor the author(s)/editor(s) assume any liability for any injury and/or damage to persons or property arising from or related to use of material in this book.

This book is sold on the understanding that the publisher is not engaged in providing professional medical services. If such advice or services are required, the services of a competent medical professional should be sought.

Every effort has been made where necessary to contact holders of copyright to obtain permission to reproduce copyright material. If any have been inadvertently overlooked, the publisher will be pleased to make the necessary arrangements at the first opportunity.

Inquiries for bulk sales may be solicited at: jaypee@jaypeebrothers.com

Practical Perimetry

First Edition: 2016

Second Edition: 2024

ISBN: 978-93-5696-311-5

Dedicated to

All those who navigate the intricate pathways of vision, both as clinicians and researchers, this book is dedicated to your unwavering dedication to unraveling the mysteries of the visual field. May it illuminate your path as you explore the fascinating world of perimetry, ultimately leading to better understanding, diagnosis, and care for those affected by visual impairments. Your tireless pursuit of knowledge and compassion for your patients inspire us all.

Contributors

Aji Kunnath Devadas
Optometrist
Department of Optometry
Mahathma Eye Hospital (P) Limited
Tiruchirappalli, Tamil Nadu, India

Alejandra Hernandez-Oteyza
Attending Physician
Department of Glaucoma
Association to Prevent Blindness in
Mexico, IAP
Mexico City, Mexico

Ankur Sinha
Director
Department of Ophthalmology
Max Vision Eye Care Centre
Jaipur, Rajasthan, India

Ann Mary Mathews
Consultant
Department of Glaucoma Services
Aravind Eye Hospital
Madurai, Tamil Nadu, India

Chitralekha De
Consultant
Department of Vitreoretina
Prabha Eye Clinic and Research Centre
Bengaluru, Karnataka, India

Chris A Johnson
Professor
Department of Ophthalmology
and Visual Sciences
University of Iowa
Iowa City, Iowa, USA

Dewang Angmo
Associate Professor
Department of Ophthalmology
Dr RP Centre for Ophthalmic Sciences
All India Institute of Medical Sciences
New Delhi, India

Faisal TT
Associate Professor
Department of Ophthalmology
Advanced Eye Centre
Postgraduate Institute of Medical
Education and Research
Chandigarh, India

Ganesh V Raman
Head, Department of Glaucoma
Aravind Eye Hospital
Coimbatore, Tamil Nadu, India

George V Puthuran
Head, Department of Glaucoma
Aravind Eye Hospital
Madurai, Tamil Nadu, India

Gitanjali Sharma
Consultant and Head
Department of Ophthalmology
Max Vision Eye Care Centre
Nayan Jyoti Eye Care Centre
Kolkata, West Bengal, India

Gowri J Murthy
Senior Consultant and Head
Department of Glaucoma Service
Prabha Eye Clinic and Research Centre
Bengaluru, Karnataka, India

Harsha L Rao
Consultant
Department of Glaucoma
Glaucoma Clinic
Narayana Nethralaya
Bengaluru, Karnataka, India

Hennaav Dhillon
Associate Consultant
Department of Pediatric Ophthalmology
and Strabismus
Sankara Nethralaya
Chennai, Tamil Nadu, India

Jayasudha Roopesh
Consultant
Department of Ophthalmology
Swamy Eye Clinic
Chennai, Tamil Nadu, India

Mohana Sinnasamy
Consultant
Department of Ophthalmology
Swamy Eye Clinic
Chennai, Tamil Nadu, India

Monica Gandhi
Senior Consultant
Glaucoma and Anterior Segment
Director, Digital Initiatives
Department of Glaucoma
Dr Shroff's Charity Eye Hospital
Gurugram, Haryana, India

Mrunali M Dhavalikar
Consultant
Department of Glaucoma
Aravind Eye Hospital
Coimbatore, Tamil Nadu, India

Murali Ariga
Director, Swamy Eye Clinic, Chennai
Director, Academics and Research
MN Eye Hospitals and Postgraduate
Institute, Chennai
Visiting Consultant
Sundaram Medical Foundation
Chennai, Tamil Nadu, India

Najiya Sundus K Meethal
Postdoctoral Fellow
Department of Glaucoma
Sankara Nethralaya
Chennai, Tamil Nadu, India

Neiwete Lomi
Senior Resident
Postgraduate Institute of Ophthalmology
Chandigarh, India

Nikhil S Choudhari
Consultant
Glaucoma Services
LV Prasad Eye Institute
Hyderabad, Telangana, India

Niranjana Balasubramaniam
Consultant
Department of Glaucoma Services
Aravind Eye Hospital
Madurai, Tamil Nadu, India

Oscar Albis-Donado
Consultant
Department of Glaucoma
Visual Sense
Mexico City, Mexico

Contributors

Padmamalini Mahendradas
Head
Uveitis and Ocular Immunology Services
Narayana Nethralaya
Bengaluru, Karnataka, India

Palaniswamy Krishnamurthy
Consultant
Department of Glaucoma and Cataract Microsurgery
Navkiran Netralaya
Bengaluru, Karnataka, India

Parul Ichhpujani
Professor
Department of Ophthalmology
Government Medical College and Hospital
Chandigarh, India

Prasanna Venkatesh Ramesh
Head
Department of Glaucoma and Research
Mahathma Eye Hospital (P) Limited
Tiruchirappalli, Tamil Nadu, India

Preeti Gupta
Consultant
Department of Glaucoma
Aravind Eye Hospital
Madurai, Tamil Nadu, India

Priyanka Sudhakar
Consultant
Department of Glaucoma
Prabha Eye Clinic and Research Centre
Bengaluru, Karnataka, India

Rajani S Battu
Senior Consultant
Department of Ophthalmology
Aster CMI Hospital
Bengaluru, Karnataka, India

Rengaraj Venkatesh
CMO and Head
Department of Glaucoma Services
Aravind Eye Hospital
Puducherry, India

Ronnie George
Director, Glaucoma Services
Department of Glaucoma Services
Sankara Nethralaya
Chennai, Tamil Nadu, India

Sathidevi AV
Head, Department of Glaucoma Services
Narayana Nethralaya
Bengaluru, Karnataka, India

Savleen Kaur
Senior Resident
Department of Ophthalmology
Postgraduate Institute of Ophthalmology
Chandigarh, India

Shantha B
Senior Consultant
Department of Glaucoma Services
Sankara Nethralaya
Chennai, Tamil Nadu, India

Shibal Bhartiya
Additional Director
Department of Ophthalmology
Fortis Memorial Research Institute
Gurugram, Haryana, India

Shruthy Vaishali Ramesh
Consultant
Department of Cataract and Refractive Surgery
Mahathma Eye Hospital (P) Limited
Tiruchirappalli, Tamil Nadu, India

Sirisha Senthil
Head, Department of Glaucoma Services
LV Prasad Eye Institute
Hyderabad, Telangana, India

Sneha Sharma
Consultant, Department of Glaucoma
Aravind Eye Hospital
Madurai, Tamil Nadu, India

Sunada Subramaniam
Consultant, Department of Glaucoma
Aravind Eye Hospital
Coimbatore, Tamil Nadu, India

Suneeta Dubey
Director, Glaucoma Services
Department of Glaucoma
Dr Shroff's Charity Eye Hospital
New Delhi, India

Supriya Dabir
Senior Consultant
Department of Vitreoretina
Rajan Eye Care
Chennai, Tamil Nadu, India

Surinder Singh Pandav
Professor
Department of Ophthalmology
Postgraduate Institute of Ophthalmology
Chandigarh, India

Sushmita Kaushik
Professor
Department of Ophthalmology
Postgraduate Institute of Ophthalmology
Chandigarh, India

Talla Sruthi
Glaucoma Fellow
Aravind Eye Hospital
Madurai, Tamil Nadu, India

Tanuj Dada
Professor
Dr RP Centre for Ophthalmic Sciences
All India Institute of Medical Sciences
New Delhi, India

Vijaya L
Head
Department of Glaucoma Services
Sankara Nethralaya
Chennai, Tamil Nadu, India

Vinaya Kumar Konana
Consultant
Department of Vitreoretina
Vittala International Institute of Ophthalmology
Bengaluru, Karnataka, India

Vivek Velumani
Medical Officer
Department of Retina
Joseph Eye Hospital
Tiruchirappalli, Tamil Nadu, India

Yamunadevi Lakshmanan
Postdoctoral Research Associate
Department of Clinical Neuroscience
University of Cambridge
Madingley, Cambridge, UK

Zia S Pradhan
Consultant
Department of Glaucoma Services
Narayana Nethralaya
Bengaluru, Karnataka, India

Foreword

Automated perimetry plays an important role in the diagnosis and management of certain eye diseases such as glaucoma, neurological conditions and retinal diseases. For over three decades, two types of perimeters namely Humphrey Visual Field Analyzer and Octopus are widely used across the world. Both perimeters have evolved in technology and newer programs allow us to perform the test in a shorter period with more reliability. The current perimeters also provide a wealth of information for the clinicians in relation to progression and structure function correlations. In view of constant newer developments, there is a need to update the knowledge by the clinicians.

In the present era of easy access to the internet and abundant publications available, one can say that the role of textbooks has come down. However, it is important to remember that the textbooks contain collated information from the diverse material that is available. In the second edition of *Practical Perimetry*, the authors have carefully incorporated the required information and provide an easy way of understanding it. It is a collaborative effort of Shibal Bhartiya, Murali Ariga, George V Puthuran and Ronnie George. All four editors have immense experience and are well-known glaucoma specialists from the country. The team should be congratulated for the excellent effort they have put in making this book extremely readable and informative. It is well-structured with good examples of visual field charts and color pictures with imaging. It is interesting to note that they also have included some chapters that have a very high practical value such as integrating technologies, virtual reality perimeters, care and maintenance of perimeters. I recommend this edition of *Practical Perimetry* for updating the newer information for all the clinicians and I do believe it is a valuable book for all the postgraduates, fellows and budding ophthalmologists to know the nuances of perimetry.

I deem it a great honor to have been asked to write this foreword for an important contribution to the ophthalmic literature in the field of perimetry.

Best regards,

Lingam Vijaya MBBS MS FRCS Ed FNAMS
Distinguished Senior Consultant
Smt Jadhavabai Nathmal Singhvee Glaucoma Services
Sankara Nethralaya
Chennai, Tamil Nadu, India

Preface to the Second Edition

Perimetry is the cornerstone in the realm of visual field assessment for both, ophthalmology and neurology. Its pivotal role in diagnosing and monitoring various ocular and neurological disorders cannot be overstated. Not only that, perimetry remains an art form, the performance and interpretation of which continue to confound generations of ophthalmologists and optometrists alike.

The book that you hold in your hands, the second edition of *Practical Perimetry*, is a distillation of the collective efforts of clinicians and glaucomatologists from around the globe. The book aims to provide a comprehensive understanding of the principles, techniques, and applications of visual field testing.

It also endeavors to bridge the gap between theory and clinical practice, presenting a thorough exploration of perimetry's intricacies.

Practical Perimetry commences with an in-depth exposition of the fundamental principles underlying perimetry, and then delves into the various perimetric techniques, encompassing both conventional and advanced methods. Moreover, discussions on the role of perimetry in neuro-ophthalmic conditions and the assessment of neurologic field defects augment the book's practical utility.

Throughout this compilation, an emphasis on the significance of accurate data interpretation and its implications for clinical decision-making remains paramount. This book is also an attempt to keep you abreast of the latest developments in visual field charting, especially the novel platforms available for correlation of structure and function, and its place in the serial monitoring of both, glaucoma and neuro-ophthalmological diseases.

We extend our heartfelt gratitude to the contributors, whose tireless efforts have culminated in this definitive volume. We hope that this book serves as an enduring reference, inspiring future advancements in the field of perimetry, and ultimately contributing to the enhanced care and wellbeing of patients worldwide.

Shibal Bhartiya
Murali Ariga
George V Puthuran
Ronnie George

Preface to the First Edition

Medical technology in the recent years has evolved at a pace hitherto unimaginable. Despite, the cornerstones of glaucoma diagnosis and management remain intraocular pressure measurement and perimetry, that is the monitoring of visual fields. Not only that, perimetry remains an art form, the performance and interpretation of which continue to confound generations of ophthalmologists and optometrists alike.

The book that you hold in your hands, *Practical Perimetry*, is a distillation of the collective efforts of clinicians and glaucomatologists from around the globe. The book aims to help the clinician choose the appropriate diagnostic protocol, and achieve optimal results each time the visual field is performed in terms of both reliability and interpretation. The book also elucidates the key points to look out for when using visual fields in the serial monitoring of patients. It has also been our attempt to illustrate each of the complicated concepts with pertinent clinical cases, so as to elucidate the fallacies and pitfalls in interpretation.

This book is also an attempt to keep you abreast of the latest developments in visual field charting, especially the novel platforms available for correlation of structure and function, and its place in the serial monitoring of both, glaucoma and neuro-ophthalmological diseases.

It should suffice to say that it is our earnest endeavor to help you take care of your patients better, and we hope you find reading this book as enjoyable and fruitful as we found putting it together.

Shibal Bhartiya
Murali Ariga
George V Puthuran
Ronnie George

Contents

Section 1 — Basics of Automated Perimetry

1. **Normal Visual Field** 3
   Talla Sruthi, Murali Ariga, Preeti Gupta, Sneha Sharma, George V Puthuran
   - Normal Visual Field   3
   - Principles of Visual Field Testing   4
   - Choosing Test Pattern   6

2. **Choice of Perimeters—A Comparison** 13
   Monica Gandhi, Suneeta Dubey, Shibal Bhartiya
   - Humphrey Field Analyzer   13
   - Octopus   13
   - Correlation of Fields Between the Two Perimeters   24
   - Networking and Compatibility   24
   - Merits and Demerits   24
   - Oculus Perimeters   24

Section 2 — Visual Field Interpretation

3. **Single Visual Field Analysis** 29
   Alejandra Hernandez-Oteyza, Oscar Albis-Donado
   - Identifying Information   29
   - Reliability Indices   31
   - Raw Numeric Graph   36
   - Grayscale Graph   36
   - Deviation Maps   37
   - Global Indices   39
   - Glaucoma Hemifield Test   40

4. **Octopus Perimetry: Analyzing the Single Field Report** 42
   Ann Mary Mathews, Mohana Sinnasamy, Murali Ariga
   - Plots In Single Visual Field Reports of Octopus Perimeter   42
   - Approach to Interpret the Single Visual Field Report   47

5. **Pearls and Pitfalls in Perimetry** 49
   Parul Ichhpujani, Neiwete Lomi, Savleen Kaur, Surinder Singh Pandav, Sushmita Kaushik
   - Practical Pearls in Recording Fields   49
   - Practical Pearls in Assessment of Fields   51
   - Pitfalls in Automated Perimetry   51

6. **Visual Field Progression** 62
   Yamunadevi Lakshmanan, Najiya Sundus K Meethal, Ronnie George, Shantha B, Vijaya L
   - Challenges in Assessing the Visual Field Progression   62
   - Visual Field Progression on 10-2 Protocol   83

7. **Visual Field Progression Analysis with Octopus Perimetry** 86
   Mohana Sinnasamy, Murali Ariga, Jayasudha Roopesh, Niranjana Balasubramaniam
   - Selection of Adequate Visual Fields for Progression Analysis   86
   - Progression Analysis Functions Offered by the Octopus EyeSuite Software   86
   - Summary of the Clinical Utility of Different Progression Analysis Methods   90

8. **Visual Fields—An Overview** 91
   Ankur Sinha, Gitanjali Sharma
   - Definition   91
   - Assessment and Measurement of Visual Field   91
   - Methods of Assessment of Visual Field   92
   - Automated Static Threshold Perimetry   93
   - Interpretation of A Humphrey Field Analyzer Test Report   93
   - Examples of Visual Field Defects   96

Section 3 Special Situations

9. **Structural and Functional Correlation in Glaucoma** 105
   Ganesh V Raman, Mrunali M Dhavalikar, Sunada Subramaniam

10. **Role of Perimetry in Diagnosis and Management of Neuro-ophthalmic Disorders** 119
    Nikhil S Choudhari, Sirisha Senthil
    - How Visual Field Interpretation is Different in Neuro-ophthalmology than that in Glaucoma?   119
    - Selection of an Automated Visual Field Test in Neuro-ophthalmology   121
    - Stepping into the Future   127

11. **Role of Perimetry in Diagnosis and Management of Retinal or Macular Disorders** 132
    Sathidevi AV, Gowri J Murthy, Rajani S Battu, Vinaya Kumar Konana, Supriya Dabir,
    Padmamalini Mahendradas, Chitralekha De, Priyanka Sudhakar
    - Types of Perimetry   132
    - Choosing the Test   132
    - Perimetry in Specific Retinal Diseases   133
    - Cases   135

12. **Frequency Doubling Perimetry** 159
    Parul Ichhpujani, Shibal Bhartiya, Dewang Angmo, Tanuj Dada
    - Concerns with Standard Automated Perimetry   159
    - Frequency Doubling Principle   159
    - Frequency Doubling Illusion   159
    - Frequency Doubling Perimetry Devices   160
    - Newer Strategies   162
    - Scientific Evidence   165
    - Clinical Relevance in Current Glaucoma Practice   166

13. **Short-wavelength Automated Perimetry** 169
    Rengaraj Venkatesh, Palaniswamy Krishnamurthy
    - Two-color Increment Threshold   169
    - Role of SWAP in Glaucoma   170
    - Role of SWAP in Diabetic Retinopathy   170
    - SWAP—Other Clinical Applications   171

14. **Integrating Technologies: Current Status** 173
    Shibal Bhartiya, Parul Ichhpujani, Oscar Albis-Donado, Faisal TT
    - Integration of Technology in Patient Care   173
    - Glaucoma Management Paradigm   174
    - Visual Field Progression   175
    - Challenges and the Future   178

15A. Recent Advances in Perimetry 180
Parul Ichhpujani, Hennaav Dhillon
- Virtual Reality Perimetry 180
- Procedure for Virtual Reality Perimetry 180
- Comparison of VR Perimetry with SAP (Humphrey Visual Field) 180

15B. Brief Overview of Various Types of Head-mounted Virtual Reality Perimeters 185
Prasanna Venkatesh Ramesh, Shruthy Vaishali Ramesh, Vivek Velumani, Aji Kunnath Devadas
- Introduction—The Inception of Head-Mounted Perimeter 185
- Pros of Head-mounted Devices 185
- Cons of Head-mounted Devices 185
- Types of Head-mounted Virtual Reality Perimeters 185
- Undue Advantage During COVID-19 188

16. Care and Maintenance of Perimeters 190
Shibal Bhartiya, Parul Ichhpujani
- General Instructions 190
- Humphrey's Visual Field Analyzer 190
- Octopus Perimeter 191
- Medmont Automated Perimeter 192
- Perimeter Bowl Disinfection during COVID-19 Pandemic 192

17. History of Perimetry 194
Harsha L Rao, Zia S Pradhan, Chris A Johnson
- Development of Perimetry 194

Index *197*

SECTION 1

Basics of Automated Perimetry

1. **Normal Visual Field**
   Talla Sruthi, Murali Ariga, Preeti Gupta, Sneha Sharma, George V Puthuran

2. **Choice of Perimeters—A Comparison**
   Monica Gandhi, Suneeta Dubey, Shibal Bhartiya

CHAPTER 1

Normal Visual Field

Talla Sruthi, Murali Ariga, Preeti Gupta, Sneha Sharma, George V Puthuran

INTRODUCTION

Perimetry is a vital part of the armamentarium available to the ophthalmologist for the diagnosis and monitoring of glaucoma. It is important to be thorough with the basic principles of perimetry, not only to interpret any visual field but also to order the correct test for an individual patient.

The user-friendly interface provided by automated perimeters has made them immensely popular for diagnosis and monitoring of the visual field. Advantages of automated perimetry include reproducibility, progression monitoring, standardized test formats, and facility for data storage. In this chapter, we will cover the essential aspects of Humphrey field analyzer (HFA), which is the most widely used machine worldwide.

NORMAL VISUAL FIELD

Traquair described the normal visual field as an island of vision in sea of darkness.[1] In the normal visual field examination, the fovea is the most sensitive point tested and represents the peak. The island of vision extends roughly 60° superiorly and nasally, 75° inferiorly, and 100° temporally[2] **(Fig. 1)**.

Anatomy

The hallmark of glaucoma is the nerve fiber bundle defect that results from damage at the optic nerve head (ONH). The visual field defect is seen in the areas subserved by the damaged nerve fiber bundle corresponding to the ONH damage. The superior and inferior poles of the optic nerve are more susceptible to glaucomatous damage. However, damage to small-scattered bundles of optic nerve axons also occur, resulting in generalized decrease in sensitivity.

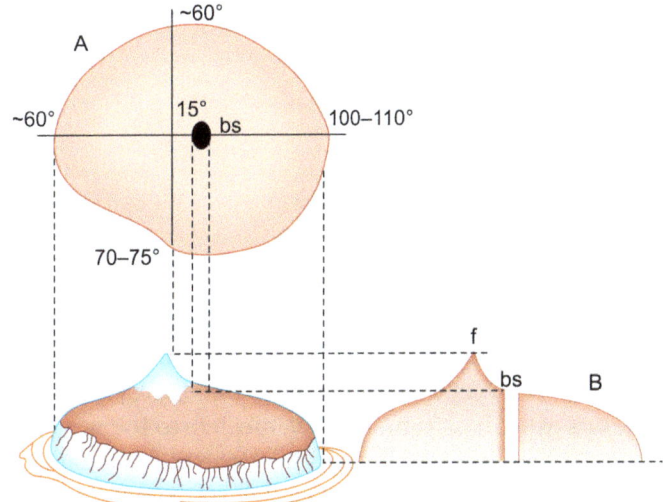

Fig. 1: Traquair's normal visual field as an island of vision in a sea of darkness. (f: fixation corresponds to foveola; bs: corresponds to blind spot)

The typical pattern of glaucomatous visual field loss at the superior and inferior poles may be attributed to following. The neuroretinal rim is physiologically broader at the inferior and superior poles than at the nasal and temporal poles.[3] The lamina cribrosa shows larger pores and a higher ratio of pore to interpore connective tissue area in the inferior and superior regions as compared with the temporal and nasal regions. A high ratio of pore area to total area is considered to predispose to glaucomatous nerve fiber loss.[4-7] Glaucomatous backward bowing of the lamina cribrosa to the outside, mainly in the inferior and superior regions, has been shown on scanning electron microscopic photographs of glaucomatous eyes.[8] The lamina cribrosa is thicker in the disc periphery, where the nerve fiber bundles have a slightly more bent course through the lamina cribrosa[9] and where they are lost earlier than in the center of the optic disc **(Fig. 2)**.

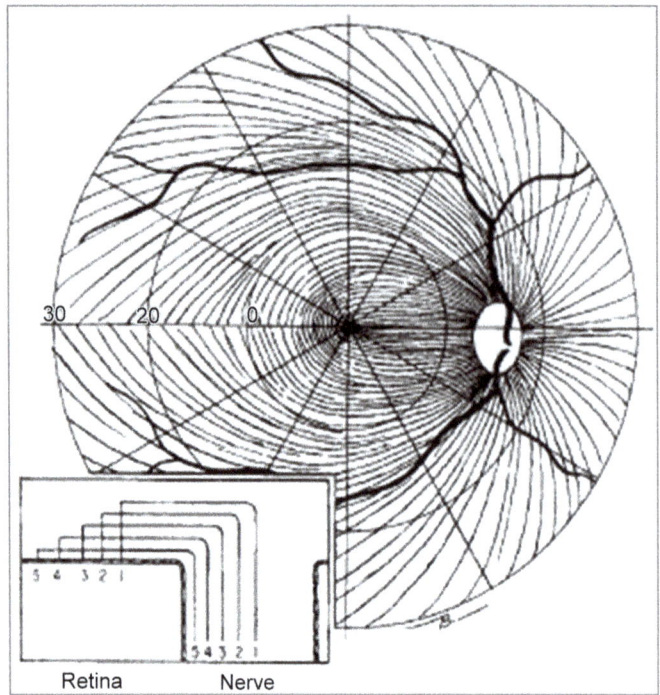

Fig. 2: Arrangement of retinal nerve fibers into the optic nerve.

Cellular Basis for the Field of Vision

Detection of visual stimuli relies on an intact neural pathway, beginning with retinal photoreceptors and then proceeding through bipolar cells. Retinal ganglion cells (RGC) and brain neurons extending from lateral geniculate to the occipital cortex. Visual field loss in glaucoma is the result of damage to RGCs. Bipolar cells synapse with several different types of RGCS, and it is believed that each type of RGC completely covers the field of vision. Some RGC types may be more damaged in glaucoma than other types, leading to the idea that visual stimuli preferentially detected by RGC types which are most likely to be damaged in glaucoma would be able to detect glaucoma at its earliest stages. The three types of ganglion cells are parvocellular, magnocellular, and koniocellular. Of these, the parvocellular or p cells are the most abundant and transmit information about color and form. The magnocellular cells transmit information about flicker and motion. The koniocellular cells are involved with transmission of short or blue wavelength. This redundancy in ganglion cells is responsible for nonselective nature of standard automated perimetry (SAP), and histological studies have shown that a significant number of ganglion cells may be lost before visual field deficits are manifested on SAP. This rationale has led to development of new perimetric tests such as short-wavelength automated perimetry (SWAP) and frequency doubling technology (FDT), which may be able to enhance earlier detection of functional loss by targeting a specific subset of ganglion cells that have sparse distribution.

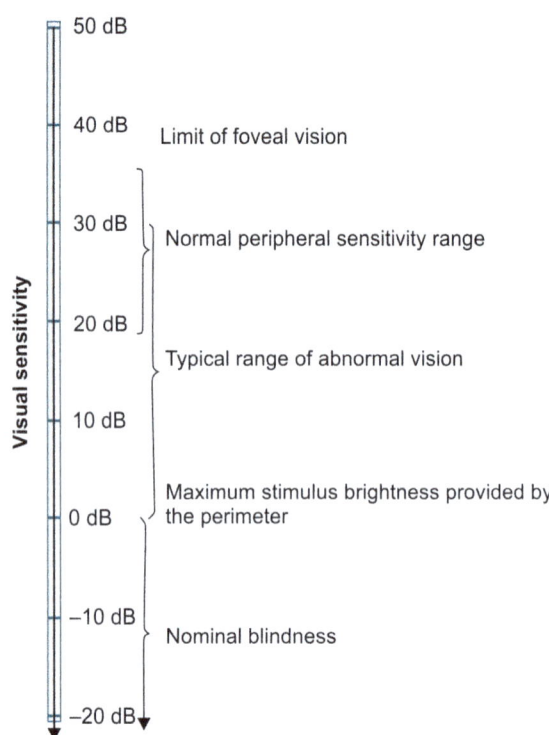

Fig. 3: Visual field testing explores differential light sensitivity throughout field of vision.

PRINCIPLES OF VISUAL FIELD TESTING

The human visual system is more adapted to perceive contrast rather than absolute magnitude of light. Estimating differential light sensitivity of stimulus against a constant illuminated background is the central essence of static perimetry.[10] Visual field testing explores differential light sensitivity throughout field of vision. Visibility of a stimulus depends on its intensity, duration, size and color, background intensity, attentiveness of patient, and refractive status of eye.[11]

Threshold

Threshold is defined as the stimulus intensity at which 50% of the presented stimuli are perceived by the patient. Suprathreshold stimuli are seen >50% of the time whereas infrathreshold or subthreshold stimuli are seen <50% of the time. Plotting the probability of seeing a stimulus against the range of stimulus intensity gives the frequency of seeing curve (**Figs. 3 and 4**).

Light intensity and its units:
　　Asb = unit of luminance (absolute unit)
　　1 asb = 0.1 miliambert = 1 lumen of total emittance/m^2
　1 candela = 1 lumen/steradian
　　1 asb = 1 pi cd/m^2

The attenuation of light is expressed in 1/10th of log units and represents change relative to maximal stimulus intensity.

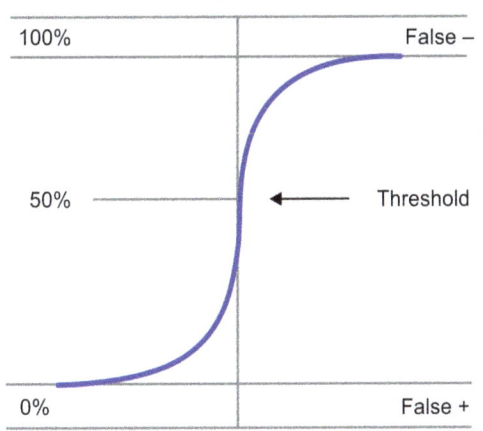

Fig. 4: Frequency of seeing curve (FOS curve).

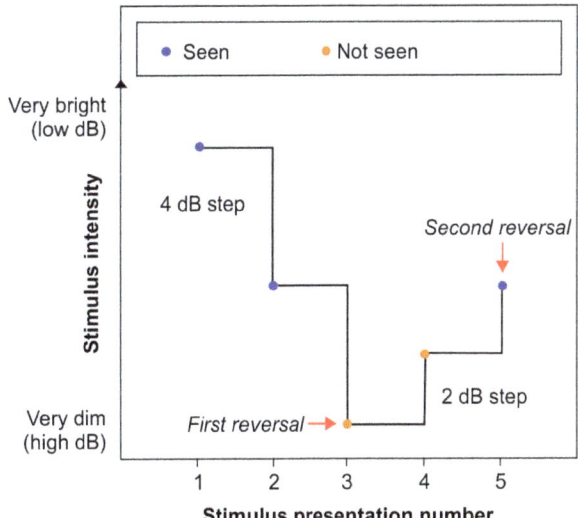

Fig. 5: Threshold estimation by bracketing.

Hence decibel (dB) is a relative unit and different on different instruments. The dB value refers to the retinal sensitivity rather than the stimulus intensity, with 0 dB corresponding to maximum brightness. A 3 dB change is equivalent to doubling of intensity, and when judging visual field loss, represents a significant change in visual field sensitivity. The maximum brightness that the Humphrey perimeter can produce is 10,000 asb. Weakest stimulus which can be perceived in healthy young patients is 40 dB, i.e., 1/10,000th of maximal stimulus. Perception of even weak stimuli, i.e., in range of 40–50 dB should alert the glaucomatologist of false positive responses.

The geographic pattern of visual field loss is more important to diagnose glaucoma rather than threshold determination.

The salient points which require attention for choosing correct test include the test strategy (supra/threshold), test pattern (30-2, 24-2, 10-2, macular program,-1 strategies), and threshold determination (bracketing).

Bracketing

Estimating threshold using full threshold strategy requires the threshold to be crossed twice. If the initial stimulus is not perceived by the patient (subthreshold stimulus), intensity of stimulus is increased by 4 dB until the patient perceives it (first crossing of threshold). The stimulus intensity is then decreased in steps of 2 dB until the patient stops perceiving the stimuli. At this point, the visual threshold is crossed again. The Humphrey Visual Field Analyzer reports threshold values as the last seen stimulus using the 4-2 strategy. If the initial stimulus is suprathreshold, stimulus intensity is decreased by 4-dB steps until the threshold is crossed, then increased in 2-dB steps (the threshold again is doubly crossed). Threshold estimation requires approximately five stimuli per test location in full threshold strategy. Patients should be told that they will miss 50% of stimuli and many of the stimuli will be too dim **(Fig. 5)**.

TABLE 1: Time taken by each program for visual field testing.

Test	Test algorithm	Time taken per eye
Humphrey full threshold	30–2	14 minutes
SITA Standard	30–2	8 minutes
FASTPAC	30–2	9 minutes
SITA Fast	30–2	5.5 minutes
SITA Standard	24–2	4 minutes
SITA Fast	24–2	3 minutes

Initial Point of Threshold Estimation

The strategies used to estimate threshold are continuously evolving in the search of a method which would give accurate threshold estimation in shortest time. Time interval for threshold estimation may be decreased if starting intensity is close to the actual threshold. Starting intensity can be adjusted according to age expected normal, from threshold. The initial presentation may be determined in part from an expected normal visual sensitivity, from threshold estimate at nearby test point, or from the threshold recorded on a previous test on that patient. But this estimation may bias the final outcome.

The approximate time taken for each program of visual field testing is represented in **Table 1**.

Swedish Interactive Threshold Algorithm

The Swedish interactive threshold algorithm (SITA) has largely replaced full threshold testing. Two SITA algorithms are currently available, SITA Standard and SITA Fast, which are analogous to the full threshold and FASTPAC algorithms, respectively. SITA uses visual field modeling based on frequency-of-seeing curves of glaucoma and normal patients. The test procedure starts by measuring threshold values at four primary points, one in each quadrant of the field at 9° from the fixation. Starting from initial stimulus intensity of 25 dB, stimuli are altered in 4–2 dB step size. Threshold values obtained at these primary points are then used to calculate starting levels at adjacent points. As the test continues, last seen stimulus intensities in neighboring points are used to calculate starting values in new points not previously opened for testing. Stimuli are presented in pseudorandom order. Stimulus used in SITA is always size III. Patient response time is taken into account to decide the interval between the successive stimuli.

FASTPAC

An alternative threshold algorithm for the HFA, the FASTPAC strategy, uses a single crossing of threshold with a constant 3 dB step size, and threshold is designated as the last-seen stimulus luminance. The examination duration of the FASTPAC algorithm is approximately 35% of that of the full threshold algorithm but is at the expense of an approximate 25% increase in the intratest variability [short-term fluctuation (SF)] and an underestimation of focal loss in glaucoma.

Short-term Fluctuation

By definition, SF at a point is standard deviation around the mean of replicate measurements. Global index of SF is estimated by retesting ten preselected sample of locations **(Fig. 6)**.

Threshold fluctuation may be seen with eccentricity from fixation, reduced retinal sensitivity, due to learning effects, reliability, pupil size, age, and mode of stimulus presentation.[11] SF as a global index was abandoned in some recent strategies when it became obvious that the SF estimate depended on whether the sampled areas were normal or abnormal and therefore SF is different at various locations.[12]

Long-term Fluctuation

Long-term fluctuation is the actual variation of threshold sensitivity due to physiological factors, irrespective of state of alertness. It should be taken into account when interpreting visual field progression and field must be retested twice before confirming progression.

■ CHOOSING TEST PATTERN

Commonly used test patterns in Humphrey field analysis include 24-2, 30-2, 10-2, and macular function test (*see* **Table 1**).

The 30-2 algorithm samples 76 test points with a uniform 6° paraxial grid within 30° from fixation which is offset from

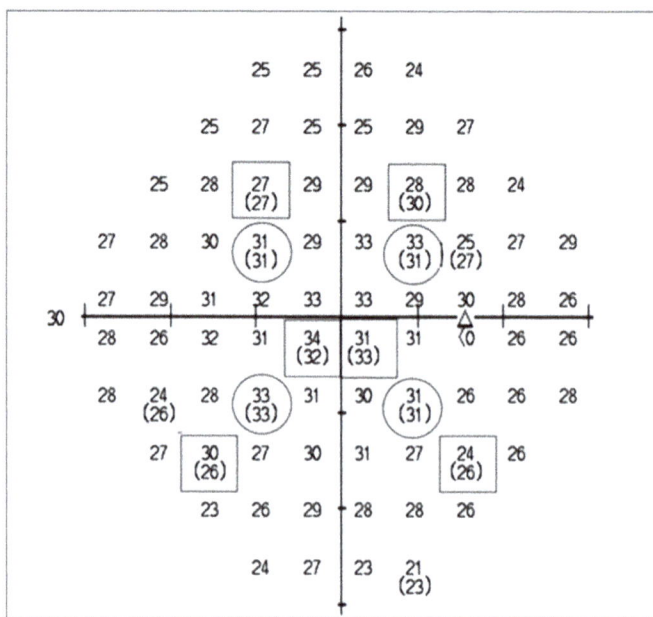

Fig. 6: Short-term fluctuation.

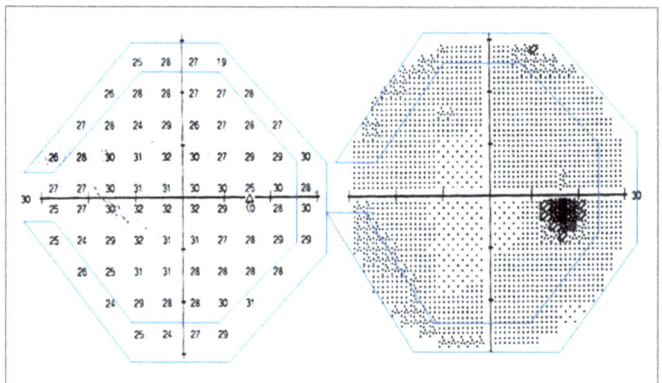

Fig. 7: 30-2 versus 24-2.

horizontal and vertical meridian. All Humphrey programs ending with-2 are paraxial. The 30° limitation is appropriate because this area is affected in almost all cases of visual field disturbance. The central 30° area also represents about 60% of all nerve fibers. The pattern of 30-1 is axial whereas pattern of 30-2 and 24-2 is paraxial. The -1 algorithm is no longer used clinically.

24-2 algorithm tests 54 locations (excludes outer outlined locations of 30-2 as shown in **Figure 7**) extending to 21° superiorly, inferiorly, and temporally but tests to 27° nasally to involve the nasal locations of 30-2. It thus decreases the test time considerably without compromising much on the data accuracy.

10-2 pattern tests 68 points in central 10° with a 2° grid offset 1° from the vertical and horizontal meridian. They are useful in defining central and paracentral scotomas, and are commonly used in advanced glaucoma **(Fig. 8)**.

Macular test tests retinal sensitivity in central 5°. 16 points are tested, and threshold is estimated thrice at each location to estimate SF **(Figs. 9A and B)**.

More recently, a new test grid has been proposed, the 24-2c, which incorporates a selection of 10 asymmetrically distributed test points, derived from 10-2 in to the 24-2 grid, and so clinicians are presented with the options of deploying the 24-2c as a catch-all method for examining the central and peripheral field, or more comprehensive assessment using the 10-2.

Monocular versus Binocular Testing

Most perimetric tests require separate testing of right and left eyes. A few tests, however, have been designed to test the binocular visual field. The Esterman test available on the HFA is a suprathreshold test for bilateral visual field loss. Points are not evenly spaced, with more points displayed near the horizontal midline. Methods have also been developed to combine the left and right eye visual field results into a simulated integrated visual field. To date, however, no evidence exists that true binocular visual fields or integrated visual fields are more predictive of important negative outcomes such as falls or motor vehicle accidents.

Stimulus Size

Stimulus size doubles in diameter and increases in area by a factor of four progressively with increasing Goldmann size as shown in **Table 2**. Doubling the stimulus diameter has roughly the same effect as increasing intensity by 5 dB. In automated static perimetry, size III (4 mm^2) is selected to permit visibility determinations at diseased areas. Size I stimulus was originally used by Goldmann for threshold determination in healthy eyes. Size I stimuli require sharp focusing of retinal image. Larger sizes up to size V (64 mm^2) can be selected in patients with central scotoma or macular disease.

Stimulus Duration

The principle of temporal summation states that visibility of stimulus increases with duration of exposure up to a critical

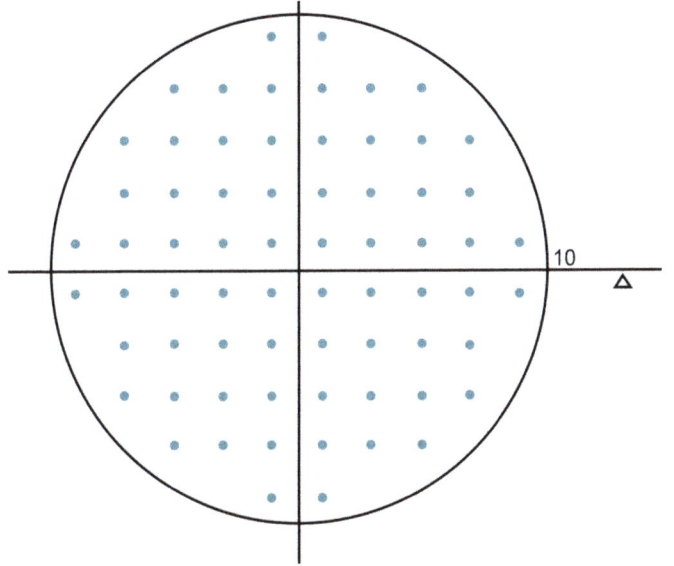

Fig. 8: 10-2 algorithm.

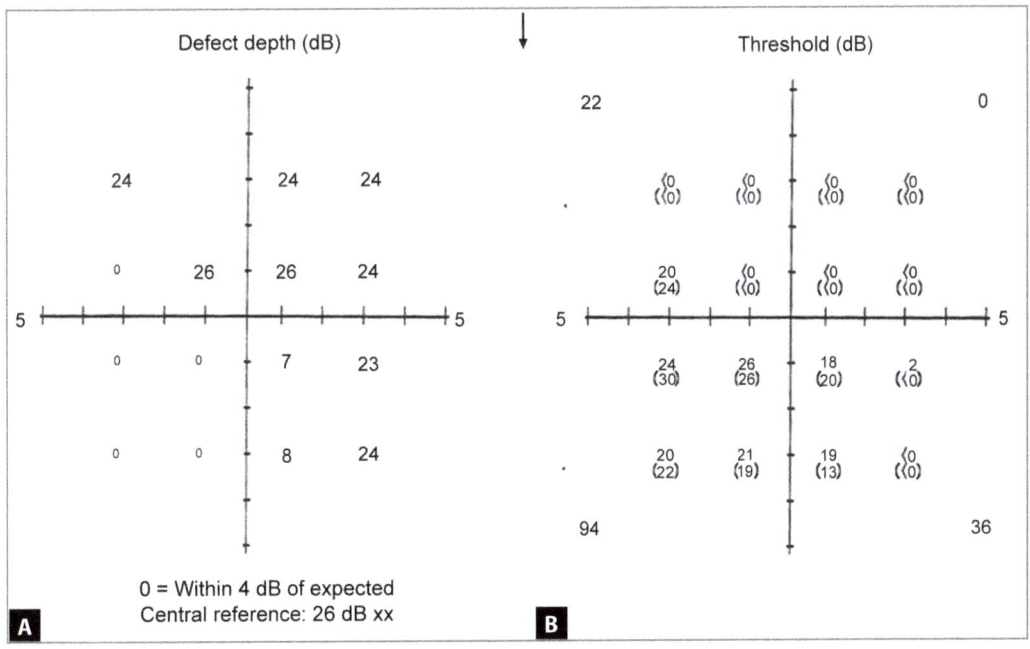

Figs. 9A and B: Macular threshold testing.

SECTION 1: Basics of Automated Perimetry

TABLE 2: Size of stimulus in Goldmann perimetry.

Goldmann stimulus size	Area on 30 cm bowl (mm²)	Angle subtended (°)
0	1/16	0.05
I	¼	0.11
II	1	0.22
III	4	0.43
IV	16	0.86
V	64	1.72

time period, usually 100 ms. Beyond this time, there is no further increase in stimulus visibility irrespective of stimulus duration. Humphrey perimeter uses a stimulus duration of 200 ms which is long enough for visibility to be affected by small variations in duration, but still shorter than the latency for voluntary eye movements (about 250 ms).[10]

Background Illumination

As differential light is measured, i.e., white stimulus of given intensity is less visible against background of similar intensity than against a dark one. Under photopic conditions, visibility depends on contrast (Weber's law).

Background intensity also determines light adaptation of retina which influences visibility. The illumination of background is kept in low photopic range, i.e., 31.5 asb commonly, because dimmer illumination tends to flatten and depress the retinal sensitivity curve centrally.[13] Profound dark adaptation may cause relative physiologic central scotoma due to poor response from cones.

Gaze Tracker

Measures gaze direction with a precision of about one degree and records a measurement each time a stimulus is presented. The gaze tracking results are shown on the video screen during testing and are printed at the bottom of the results printout. On the gaze printout, lines extending upward indicate the amount of gaze error at each stimulus presentation, with full scale indicating gaze errors of 10° or more. Lines extending downward indicate that the instrument was unsuccessful in measuring gaze direction during that particular stimulus presentation, e.g., blink.

Confounding Factors and Artifacts

- *Pupil size:* Pupil size <3 mm if combined with lens opacity produces diffuse depression of visual fields **(Figs. 10A and B)**. Hence, pupil size should be recorded on each

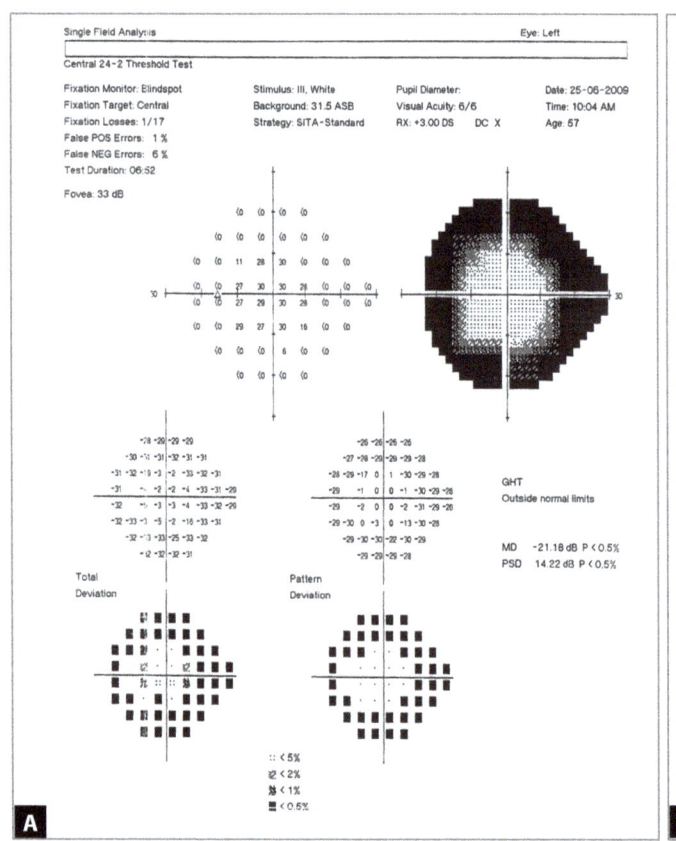
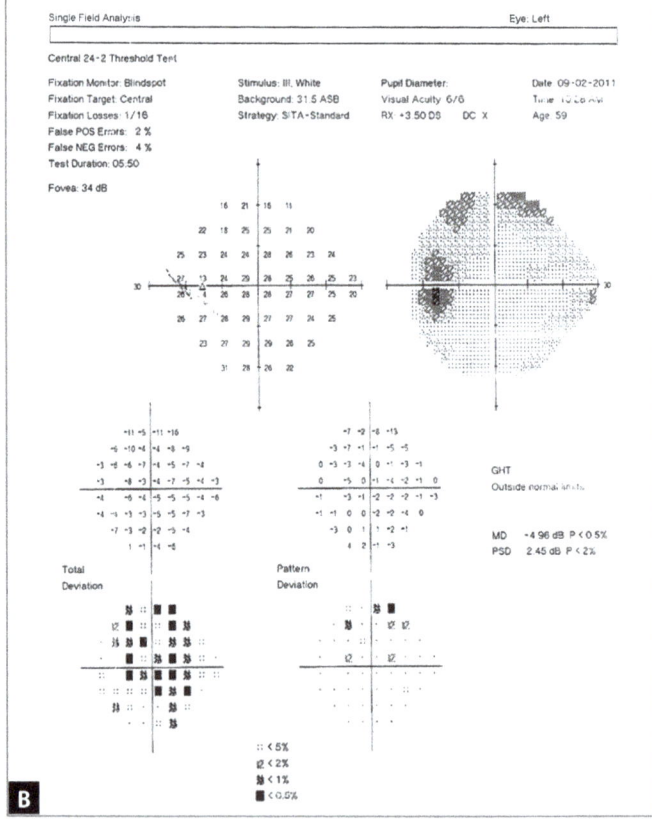

Figs. 10A and B: Effect of miosis on visual field.

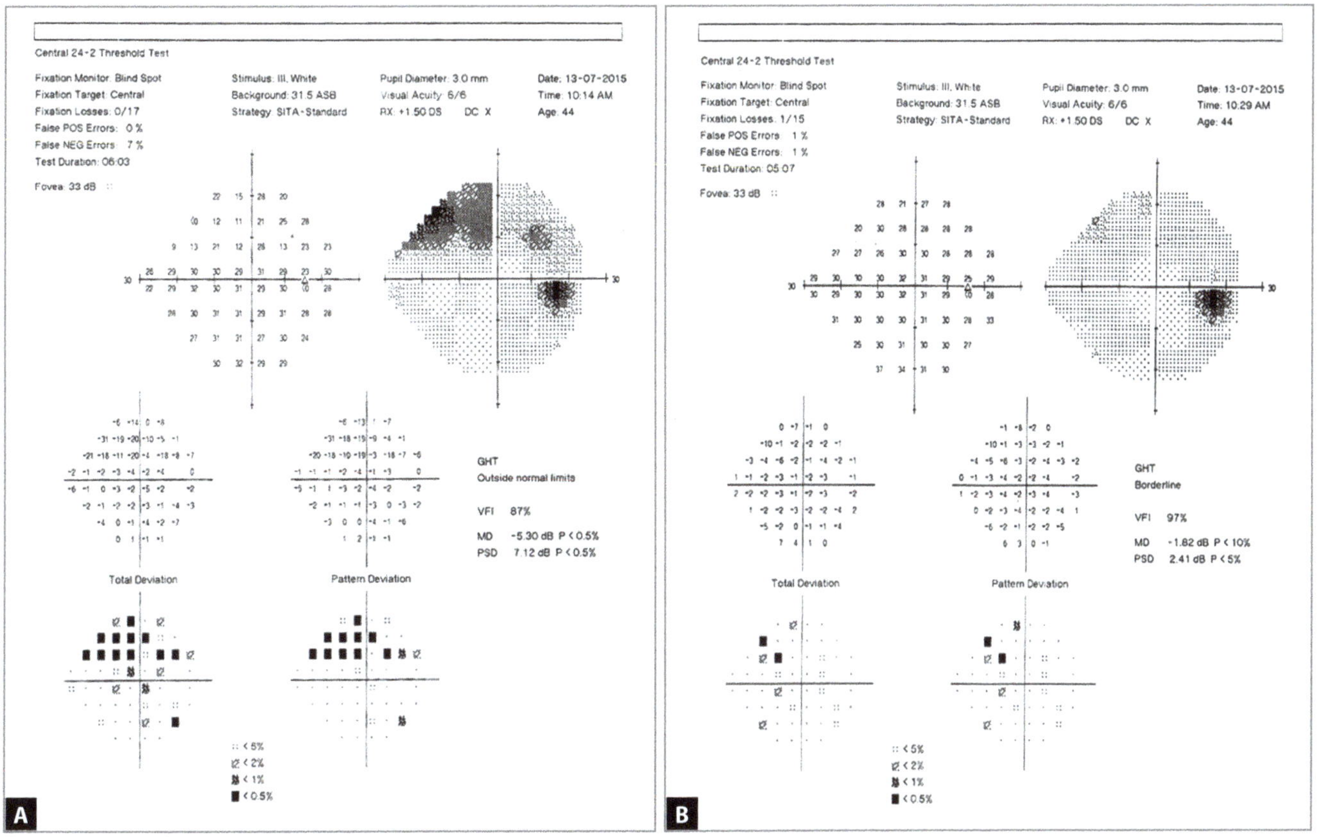

Figs. 11A and B: Learning effect.

test, when considering any change in field test result. Patient having miosis due to neuro-ophthalmic diseases, senile miosis, or miosis due to use of regular miotics should be dilated prior to testing.

- *Contrast sensitivity and glare:* Any opacity in the media may cause scattering of light and decreased contrast which may result in reduction of stimulus visibility.
- *Refractive status of the eye:* One diopter of refractive blur in an undilated patient will produce a little more than one decibel of depression of hill of vision when testing with a Goldmann size 3 stimulus.[14] The nominal testing distance of the Humphrey HFA II perimeter is 30 cm and fully presbyopic patient is provided with 3.25 diopter near additions relative to their distance refraction. Patients who are less than fully presbyopic are given smaller additions. Usually, all refractive corrections are accomplished using standard 37 mm trial lenses held in place by a trial lens holder attached the perimeter, but correction may be done with the patients' own spectacles as long as they are single lenses or contact lenses. Larger stimuli are less affected than smaller stimuli by refractive errors.
- *Learning effects:* Learning effects are more in periphery, more in fields with moderate loss, and more in points with borderline sensitivity **(Figs. 11A and B)**. Learning effects are also task specific, i.e., familiarity to SAP doesn't eliminate learning effect in SWAP.
- *Fatigue:* Longer test duration and ill health can lead to fatigue during test which may manifest as high false negatives (FNs) and clover leaf pattern on grayscale **(Fig. 12)**.

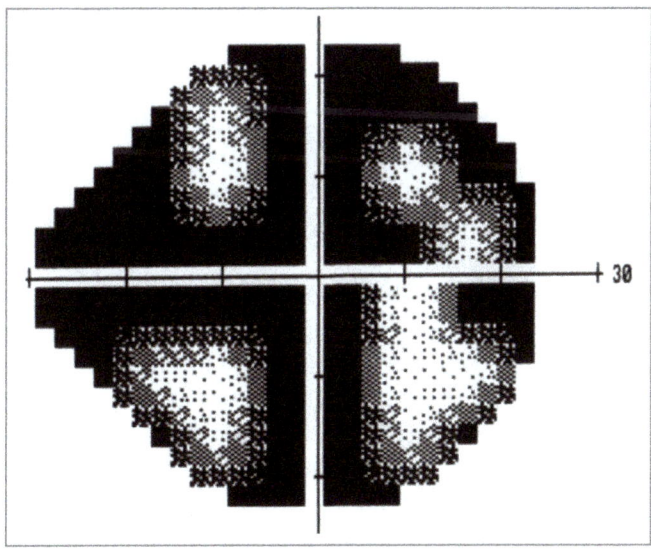

Fig. 12: Clover leaf pattern on grayscale.

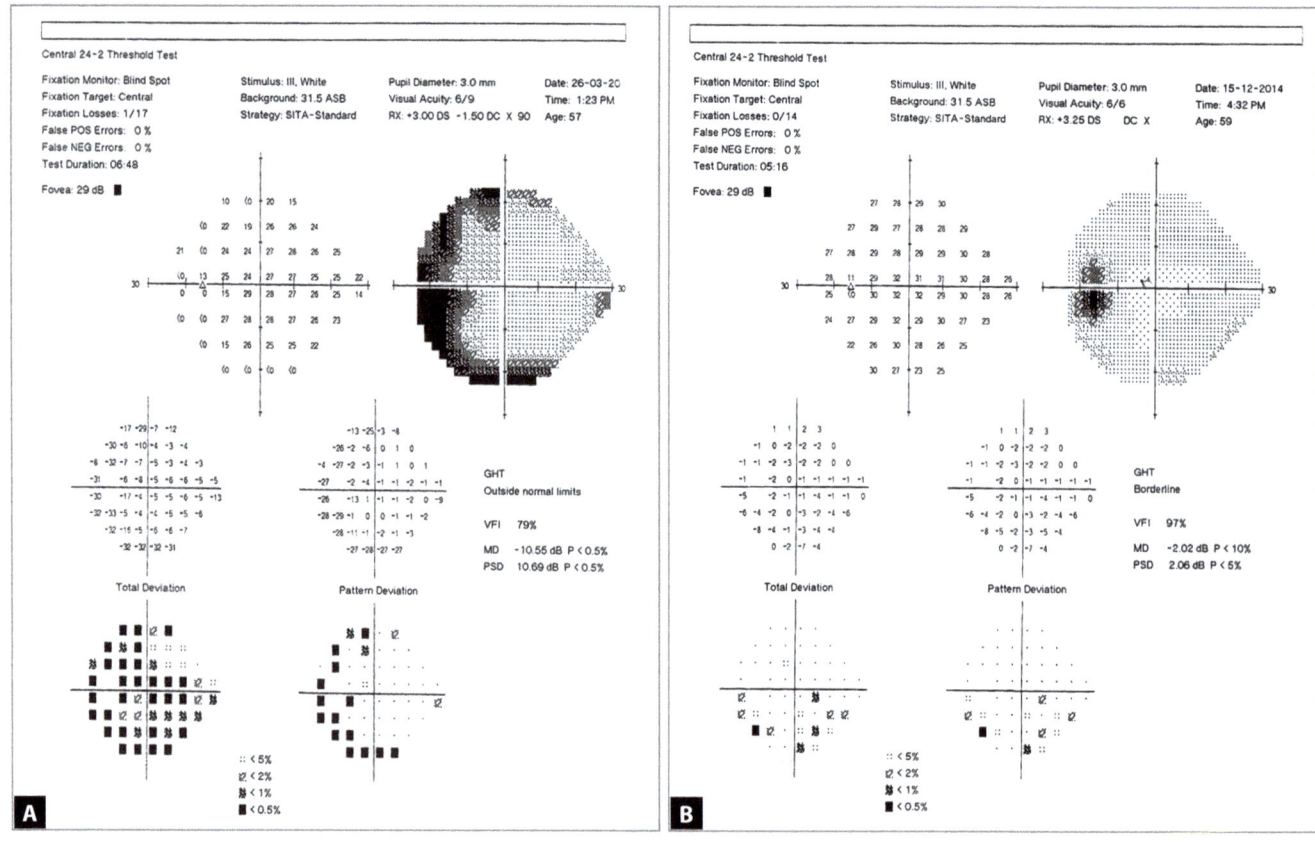

Figs. 13A and B: Rim artifact.

- *Lens artifact:* Lens with rim kept away from the eye may result in ring scotoma **(Figs. 13A and B)**. Decentered lens can cause arcuate scotoma. This can be avoided by using contact lens or rimless lenses, and correct centration and positioning of lens.
- *Lid artifact:* Drooping of upper lids may cause superior arcuate defects or superior nasal step, and can be avoided by taping the upper lid before performing the test.
- *False positives:* Occasionally, there are intervals during which the machine makes a soft click but shows no target. This error happens when an anxious subject presses the button during this interval. Grayscale of subject with high false positive appears abnormally white seen as "white scotomas". In SITA strategy, the number of these anticipatory responses is counted which are made too soon after a flash to be a response to the light.
- *False negatives:* A fairly bright suprathreshold target is flashed in a region previously tested with fainter targets. If the patient fails to indicate its presence, this is an FN error. A high FN rate usually implies inattention or fatigue and will be accompanied by a field with scattered factitious elevations of threshold.

False positive and FN error ≥33% are a warning of poor reliability and are indicated by an "xx" beside the aberrant value and a printed statement of "low patient reliability", in the upper left corner, above the glaucoma hemifield test (GHT).

Figures 14A and B show a field with high false positive and FN error showing an abnormal field which became normal in the subsequent field once reliability indices improved.

Common Causes of Visual Field Artifact

Common causes of visual field artifact are given in **Table 3**.

■ CONCLUSION

Vision is a combination of several distinct quantifiable functions including visual acuity, color vision, vernier (alignment) acuity, the perception of movement, and change in luminous intensity (flicker) or differences in luminous intensity (contrast). Visual fields are a composite of all these attributes. From the time that hemianopsias were first recognized by Hippocrates, >2,000 years ago, perimetry has evolved from confrontation visual field evaluation to the current state of the art perimeters which even offer structural and functional correlates. The wealth of information thus made available from visual field testing has revolutionized

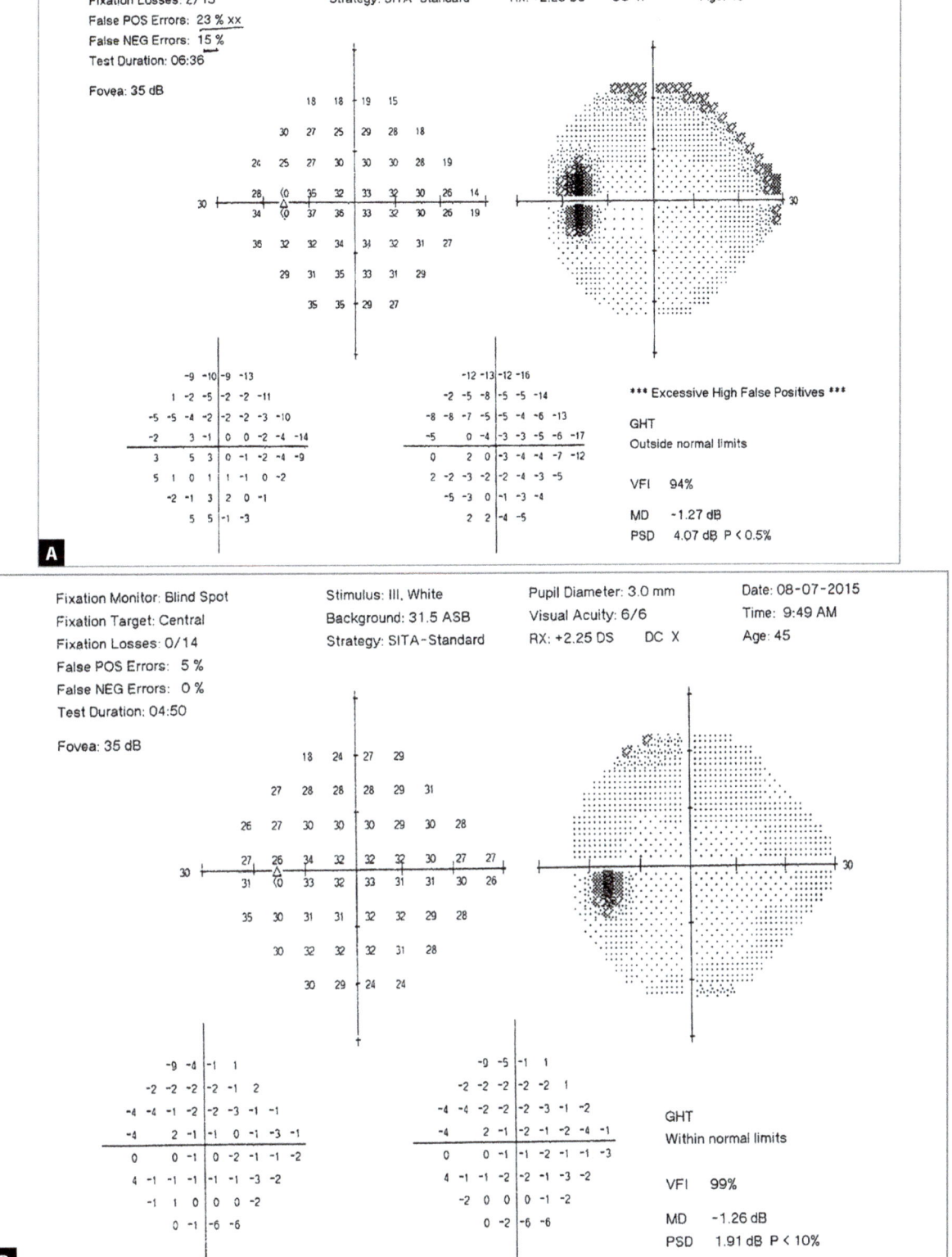

Figs. 14A and B: Improvement in visual field after decrease in false positive and false negative.

TABLE 3: Common causes of visual field artifact.

Source	Comment
Refractive error	Check refraction
Improper near correction	Always use full correction according to perimeter manual for patients with pseudophakia, aphakia, and after cycloplegia
Lens rim artifact	Reposition patients or corrective lens
Fatigue or stress	Patient reassurance, rest between visual fields, use SITA FAST or FASTPAC algorithms, only perform testing in one eye per visit
Patient movement	Reposition the patient
Miotic pupil	Dilate pupil before testing
Cognitive decline or impairment	Frequent reminders during testing, may require testing, using manual perimetry

current glaucoma practice, and has provided new dimensions to the management of neurological disease as well.

ACKNOWLEDGMENTS

The authors gratefully acknowledge Anuj Ponnappa and Muazzam Ali Akbar for their contribution to this chapter.

REFERENCES

1. Traquair HM. Clinical detection of early changes in the visual field. Trans Am Ophthalmol Soc. 1939;37:158-79.
2. Allingham R, Damji KF, Freedman S, Moroi SE, Shafranov G. Shields' Textbook of Glaucoma, 5th edition. Lippincott Williams and Wilkins; 2004.
3. Jonas JB, Gusek GC, Naumann GOH. Optic disk, cup and neuroretinal rim size, configuration, and correlations in normal eyes. Invest Ophthalmol Vis Sci. 1988;29:1151-8.
4. Jonas JB, Mardin CY, Schlötzer-Schrehardt U, Naumann GOH. Morphometry of the human lamina cribrosa surface. Invest Ophthalmol Vis Sci. 1991;32:401-5.
5. Minckler DS, McLean IW, Tso MOM. Distribution of axonal and glial elements in the rhesus optic nerve head studied by electron microscopy. Am J Ophthalmol. 1976;82:179-87.
6. Minckler DS. The organization of nerve fiber bundles in the primate optic nerve head. Arch Ophthalmol. 1980;98:1630-6.
7. Radius RL. Regional specificity in anatomy at the lamina cribrosa. Arch Ophthalmol. 1981;99:478-80.
8. Quigley HA, Addicks EM, Green WR, Maumenee AE. Optic nerve damage in human glaucoma: II. The site of injury and susceptibility to damage. Arch Ophthalmol. 1981;99:635-49.
9. Dichtl A, Jonas JB, Naumann GOH. Course of the nerve fiber bundles through the lamina cribrosa. Graefes Arch Clin Exp Ophthalmol. 1996;234:581-5.
10. Anderson DR, Patella VM. Automated static perimetry, 2nd edition. United States: Mosby; 1999.
11. Stewart CW, Hunt HH. Threshold variation in automated perimetry. Surv Ophthalmol. 1993;37(5):P353-61.
12. Anderson/Ophthalmol Clin N Am. 2003;16:205-12.
13. Kramer SG, Survey of Ophthalmology. 1991;36(1).
14. Weinreb RN, Perlman JP. The effect of refractive correction on automated perimetric thresholds. Am J Ophthalmol. 1986;101:706-9.

CHAPTER 2

Choice of Perimeters—A Comparison

Monica Gandhi, Suneeta Dubey, Shibal Bhartiya

■ INTRODUCTION

Evaluation of the visual field is the cornerstone for management of glaucoma, and is an important tool in the assessment of patients with ocular and neurological diseases. Automated static perimeters are the most commonly used for this purpose and common perimeters in use today include the Humphrey field analyzer (HFA), Octopus perimeter, Oculus, Opto, Dicon, and many others.[1-12]

■ HUMPHREY FIELD ANALYZER

The HFA is probably the most commonly used perimeter and has been in use for >25 years in research, and clinics alike. Most of the large-scale glaucoma clinical trials, including Advanced Glaucoma Intervention Study (AGIS), Early Manifest Glaucoma Trial (EMGT), Normal Tension Glaucoma Study (NTGS), and Ocular Hypertension Treatment Study (OHTS), have used the HFA for perimetry for both diagnosis and progression analysis. The GPA, or the Glaucoma Progression Analysis software is the only FDA-approved perimetry progression software, and is compatible with electronic medical record (EMR) systems **(Fig. 1)**.[1,2,5-7]

Humphrey perimeters have different models available which are designed depending on the kind of practice one has. The Humphrey 740*i* is the basic model but caters to comprehensive testing. The 720*i* is designed for low volume practices. The Humphrey 754*i* has all the features of 740*i* with additional Swedish interactive testing algorithm–short-wavelength automated perimetry (SITA-SWAP) software. The Humphrey 750*i* has all the advanced features. Newer models now available are 830, 840, 850, and 860, with additional features which are enumerated in the **Table 1**.

■ OCTOPUS

The Octopus **(Figs. 2A to C)** was the world's first automated perimeter which has gained popularity because it

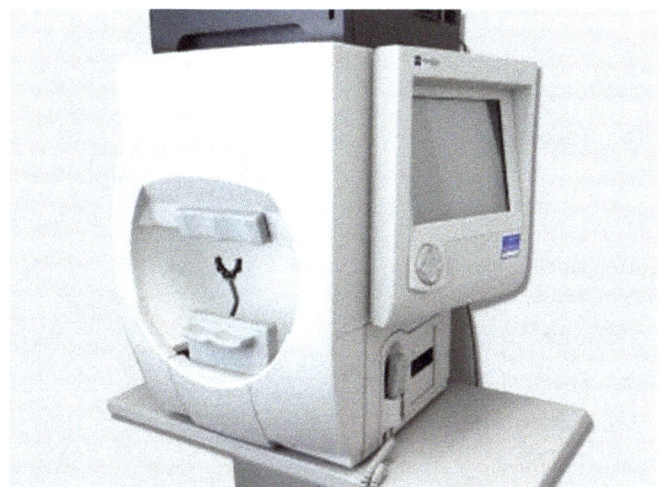

Fig. 1: Humphrey's field analyzer
Source: https://www.zeiss.com/content/dam/Meditec

incorporates all three important glaucoma perimetry standards, namely, (1) standard perimetry, (2) SWAP, and (3) flicker testing. It does not require a dark room for optimal test results and has a fast strategy that reduces the time for visual field testing to as less as two and a half minutes. The perimeter also provides fixation control and automated gaze tracking, making the test easier and more reliable. The networkability of the octopus involves both, an ethernet connection and EMR interface.[1-3,5-7]

This chapter aims to provide a comparison of each of the attributes of the two perimeters **(Tables 1 and 2)**.[1-12] The main differences are elucidated below.

Measuring Range and Scale of Sensitivities

In Humphrey perimeters, the background illumination is the same as Octopus but the maximum stimulus luminance is higher. In Humphrey visual field (HVF), 40 dB corresponds to 1 abs and 0 dB to 10,000. As a result, the normal values in HVF

TABLE 1: Comparison of characteristics of different models of Humphrey.

Technical specifications	HFA 720i	HFA 740i	HFA 745i	HFA 750i	HFA3 830	HFA3 840	HFA3 850	HFA3 860
Maximum temporal range (degrees)	89	89	89	89	90	90	90	90
Stimulus duration	200 ms	200 ms	200 ms	200 ms	200 ms	200 ms	200 ms	200 ms
Visual field-testing distance	30 cm	30 cm	30 cm	30 cm	30 cm	30 cm	30 cm	30 cm
Background illumination	31.5 asb	31.5 asb	31.5 asb	31.5 asb	31.5 asb	31.5 asb	31.5 asb	31.5 asb
Stimulus size	Goldmann III	Goldmann I–V	Goldmann I–V	Goldmann I–V	Goldman I-V	Goldmann I–V	Goldmann I–V	Goldmann I–V
Foveal threshold testing	No	Yes	Yes	Yes	No	Yes	Yes	Yes
Automatic pupil measurement	No	No	No	No	No	Yes	Yes	Yes
Threshold test library								
24-2, 30-2, 10-2	Yes	Yes	Yes	Yes	Yes	Yes	Yes	Yes
Macula	Yes	Yes	Yes	Yes	Yes	Yes	Yes	Yes
60-4, Nasal step	Yes	Yes	Yes	Yes	Yes	Yes	Yes	Yes
Test methods								
SAP	Yes	Yes	Yes	Yes	Yes	Yes	Yes	Yes
SWAP	No	No	Yes	Yes	No	No	Yes	Yes
SITA Standard, Fast, Full threshold	Yes	Yes	Yes	Yes	Yes	Yes	Yes	Yes
SITA SWAP			Yes	Yes			Yes	Yes
Fixation control								
Heijl–Krakau method	Yes	Yes	Yes	Yes	Yes	Yes	Yes	Yes
Video eye monitor	Yes	Yes	Yes	Yes	Yes	Yes	Yes	Yes
Gaze tracking		Yes	Yes	Yes		Yes	Yes	Yes
Head tracking				Yes		Yes	Yes	Yes
Vertex monitoring				Yes			Yes	Yes
Remote video eye monitor capability	Yes	Yes	Yes	Yes				
Liquid Trial Lens								Yes
Automatic pupil measurement						Yes	Yes	Yes
RelEYE eye review							Yes	Yes
Software features								
Glaucoma hemifield test (GHT)	Yes	Yes	Yes	Yes	Yes	Yes	Yes	Yes
Visual field index (VFI)	Yes	Yes	Yes	Yes	Yes	Yes	Yes	Yes
Guided progression analysis (GPA)		Yes	Yes	Yes	Yes	Yes	Yes	Yes
Serial field overview		Yes	Yes	Yes	Yes	Yes	Yes	Yes
networking	Yes	Yes	Yes	Yes	Yes	Yes	Yes	Yes
FoRUM connectivity	Yes	Yes	Yes	Yes	Yes	Yes	Yes	Yes
DICoM connectivity	Yes	Yes	Yes	Yes	Yes	Yes	Yes	Yes
Easyconnect RCT/HFA-NET pro	Yes	Yes	Yes	Yes				

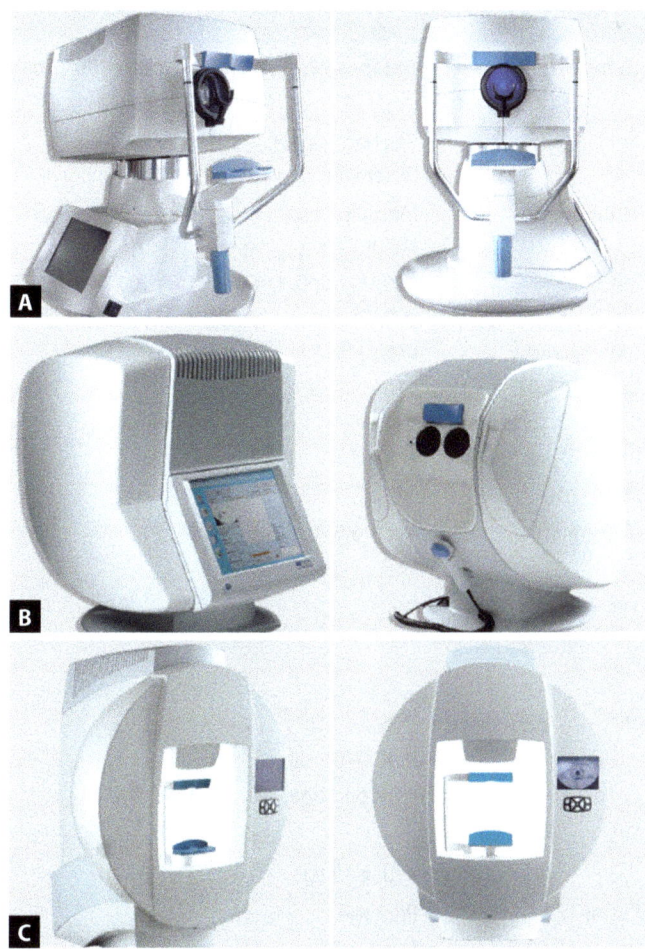

Figs. 2A to C: Octopus 300; (B) Octopus 600; (C) octopus 900
Sources:
- https://www.haag-streit.com/haag-streit-diagnostics/products/perimetry/
- http://www.haag-streit.com/products/perimetry/octopusr-600.html
- http://www.haag-streit.com/products/perimetry/octopusr-900

are 3–4 dB higher than Octopus and thus we cannot directly compare the measured sensitivities of the two instruments.

In Octopus 300, the maximum stimulus luminance and the background are brighter than Octopus 101. But the normal value expressed in decibels is the same, i.e., 40 dB corresponds to 0.1 asb and 0 dB to 1,000 abs in Octopus 300 and this has a background luminance of 31.4 abs. 40 dB corresponds to 0.48 abs and 0 dB to 4,800 abs in Octopus 101 with background luminance of 4 asb.

Octopus 101 and HVF 700 have a spherical bowl as compared to Octopus 300 which uses a direct projection system. The newer models of both are compared in the **Tables 1 and 2**.

Stimulus Size and Duration

The stimulus size Goldmann I to V are available in Octopus 101 and HVF 700 whereas Octopus 300 has size III and V.

The stimulus duration in the Octopus is 100 ms compared to 200 ms in Humphrey. This is sufficiently high to reach temporal summation yet below the reaction time of the fixation. So, the patient can see the stimulus yet not move his eyes toward it.

Measurement Strategies

Humphrey uses the 4-2 dB bracketing strategy whereas the Octopus uses the 4-2-1 dB bracketing strategy to determine the retinal sensitivity at a point. So, the threshold is crossed twice in Humphrey compared to three times in Octopus. This is applicable in full threshold strategies.

The perimetric test can be long leading to fatigue and if the procedure is prematurely stopped all data may be lost with no conclusive result. To avoid this Octopus has provision of running the examination in modular steps. In each stage, a predetermined subset of locations is tested and results saved as separate examinations. This helps to choose the critically important locations to be tested first when the patient is not fatigued. In case, the fields appear severely depressed or perfectly normal the test can be terminated after second or third stages also instead of completing all four. After each stage, the test can be restarted, continued, or saved.

The defect level indicator is available in Octopus which gives a real time display to allow the operator to judge if the fields are normal, borderline, or depressed even when the tests is in progress.

The staging and phasing concept is unique to Octopus and not available in Humphrey. It helps to make the test shorter without compromising on the information gathered. This also helps to set priorities to diagnostic relevant areas.

The newer models of HVA 3 have added features which include SITA faster and 24-C program. This machine allows mixed glaucoma progression analysis between SITA standard, SITA Fast, and SITA faster so all tests need not have been done on the same strategy.

It also has a Liquid Trial Lens so that one single lens is needed and by pressure changes in the liquid it adapts to all refractive corrections.

Individual Strategies: How to Choose

Humphrey perimeters use the full threshold strategy with the 4-2 bracketing to derive the retinal sensitivity at each test location. It also checks the short-term fluctuation where ten points are rechecked. This can be time consuming and to decrease this without compromising on the test quality other strategies like SITA were developed. SITA strategies are not only fast and accurate, but also friendly to the patient. These utilize the patient response and reaction time to pace the test timing so in a way the patient runs the perimeter rather than the machine ruling the test.

TABLE 2: Comparison of characteristics of different models of Octopus.

Technical specifications	Octopus 300 basic	Octopus 300 pro	Octopus 600 basic	Octopus 900 basic	Octopus 900 pro
Threshold test library					
Peripheral range (distance)	30° (infinite)	30° (infinite)	30° (infinite)	180° (30 cm radius Goldmann bowl)	180° (30 cm radius Goldmann bowl)
Stimulus generation	Direct projection system	Direct projection system	TFT monitor	Mirror projection system	Mirror projection system
Stimulus duration	100 ms, 200 ms, and 500 ms	100 ms, 200 ms, and 500 ms	SAP: 100; Pulsar: 500	100, 200, 500, 1,000, and infinite	100, 200, 500, 1,000, and infinite
Background illumination	31 asb	31/314	SAP: 10 cd/m^2; Pulsar: 32 cd/m^2	0/4/31/314	0/4/31/314
Stimulus size	III, V	III, V	SAP: 0.43 (Size III); Pulsar: 5	Goldmann I-V	Goldmann I-V
24-2, 30-2, 10-2	Yes	Yes	Yes	Yes	Yes
Macula	M Program	M Program	M Program	M Program	M Program
60-4, Nasal step					
General/glaucoma 30° (G1-Program, 32)	Yes	Yes	Yes	Yes	Yes
Test methods					
SAP	Yes	Yes	Yes	Yes	Yes
SWAP	With package	Yes		With package	Yes
Flicker	With package	Yes		With package	Yes
Pulsar			Yes		
Goldmann kinetic				with package	Yes
Top	Package	Yes	Pulsar	Package	Yes
Dynamic	Yes	Yes	Yes	Yes	Yes
Fixation control					
Blink control	Yes	Yes	Yes	Yes	Yes
Pupil position control	Yes	Yes	Yes	Yes	Yes
Automated eye tracking	Yes	Yes		Yes	Yes
Contact control	Yes	Yes	Yes		
Dart control			Yes		
Software features					
FoRUM connectivity					
DICoM connectivity	Yes	Yes		Yes	Yes
EMR	Yes	Yes		Yes	Yes
Ethernet	Yes	Yes	Yes	Yes	Yes
Global progression MD, sLV	Yes	Yes	Yes	Yes	Yes
Cluster trend, polar trend	Yes	Yes	Yes	Yes	Yes

Swedish interactive testing algorithm testing strategies available on the HFA II-*i*:

- *SITA Standard:* A threshold testing method which collects the same amount of information in half the time as the original Humphrey® Full Threshold standard algorithm. This is done without compromising test reproducibility.
- *SITA Fast:* A threshold testing method that collects the same amount of information in half the time as FASTPAC, without compromising test reproducibility.

Octopus perimeters have the following strategies:

- *Normal strategy:* This utilizes the 4-2-1 bracketing standard perimetry. It takes time because of thresholding

at each location and is recommended in early and shallow defects in young individuals.
- *Low vision strategy:* It uses the 4-2-1 bracketing but starts with the brightest stimulus and steps up thus reducing time to reach threshold and is recommended in end stage diseases.
- *Dynamic test strategy:* The FOSc (frequency-of-seeing curve) determines the step sizes. As the depth of defect increases the stimulus luminance can take larger decibels steps to decrease the testing time. This is indicated in early detection of field loss especially where focal defects are expected.
- *Tendency oriented perimetry:* It is a method which takes into account that threshold values of neighboring locations are correlated. It is a systematic method and not based on disease pathology so it can be extended to other perimetric methods like blue on yellow and flicker perimetry. This is useful for older patients and those with depressed fields as time taken is lesser.
- *Two level testing:* This is a qualitative test and gives a rough estimation of test being normal, relative, or absolute defect.
- *One level test:* It is used in legal testing procedures and just indicates normal or not normal qualitatively.

Special Perimetric Methods

Humphrey visual fields 30-2 program tests 76 points placed 6° apart within the central 30° region. The 24-2 program tests 54 points by omitting the outer ring points of 30-2 except the 2 nasal points. This saves time and is clinically sufficient as the edge points of 30-2 are often not considered in diagnostic criteria.

In Octopus, the program 32 is similar to the 30-2 of HVF. Due to the wide spacing of locations and no correlation with retinal topography, two different programs were introduced. Program G1 tests 59 points in central 30° and program G2 has additional 14 peripheral test locations in the 30–60° area. These test locations are specially designed for glaucoma with attention to the paracentral test locations. The macula area resolution is 2.8° compared to the 6° in program 32.

Differences while Conducting the Tests

The newer models of Humphrey like HFA II-*i* have better monitoring of the eye and head positions during the test. Earlier models had gaze tracking and used the Heijl–Krakau method to judge fixation.
- Gaze tracking records the fixation of the patient while each stimulus is presented. This is recorded at the base of the printout.
- Head tracking ensures proper alignment of the head and eye relative to the trial lens holder.
- Video eye monitoring helps to position the test eye in the center of the trial lens holder and monitor the patient during testing.
- Vertex monitoring uses the distance between two corneal reflexes to determine if the patient has moved too far back from the trial lens. The software flags the movement and asks the operator to realign the patient or reinitialize the system.

Octopus on the other hand uses the picture of the corneal reflex as the baseline and any deviation due to gaze shift makes the machine stop the test. This eliminates fixation losses altogether from the final analysis of the visual fields, making the reliability better.

Differences in Printouts

The HVF printout is a seven in one printout with demographic parameters including the test specifications. Reliability indices include fixation loss, false positive, and negative. In Octopus, these are called catch trials. There is no fixation loss in Octopus because the machine takes a picture of the corneal light reflex at the beginning of the test and any deviation is associated with pausing the test and restarting when the reflex is centered.

The raw data and grayscale of HVF is similar to values and grayscale of values in Octopus and these represent the actual retinal sensitivities in decibels.

Total deviation of HVF represents the deviation from the expected normal at each point and this is called comparisons in Octopus. Pattern deviation is called probability.

The corrected comparisons show the localized defects after discounting for the generalized depression. Similarly, the corrected probability is the statistical evaluation of the probability or significance of the defect.

Global indices in HVF are the mean deviation (MD), pattern standard deviation (PSD), short-term fluctuations, and corrected PSD. The corresponding indices in Octopus are mean defect, loss variance (LV), short-term fluctuations, and corrected LV, respectively. Additionally, a reliability factor is also calculated in the Octopus which indicates the patients' cooperation. This is calculated from the catch trials.

In HVF, there is GHT which compares five weighted zones in the superior hemisphere to their mirror images in the inferior hemisphere. In Octopus, there is the cumulative defect curve called the Bebie curve which shows the defects sorted in order of increasing depth.

Another additional feature in HVF is the visual field index which is a summary measurement of the patient's visual field status, expressed as a percentage of the normal age-adjusted visual field **(Figs. 3 and 4)**.

SECTION 1: Basics of Automated Perimetry

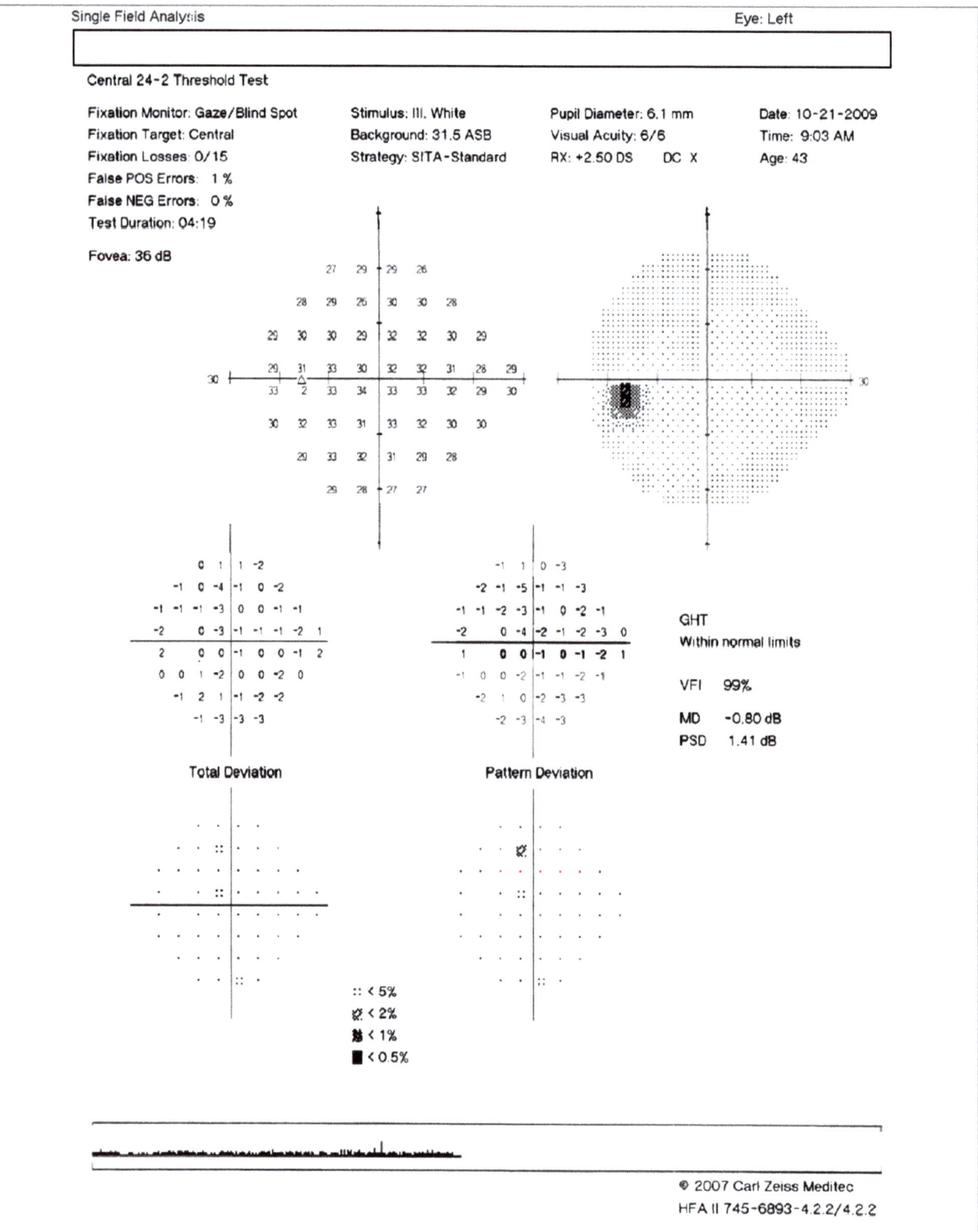

Fig. 3A
Source: Dr Shroff's charity eye hospital

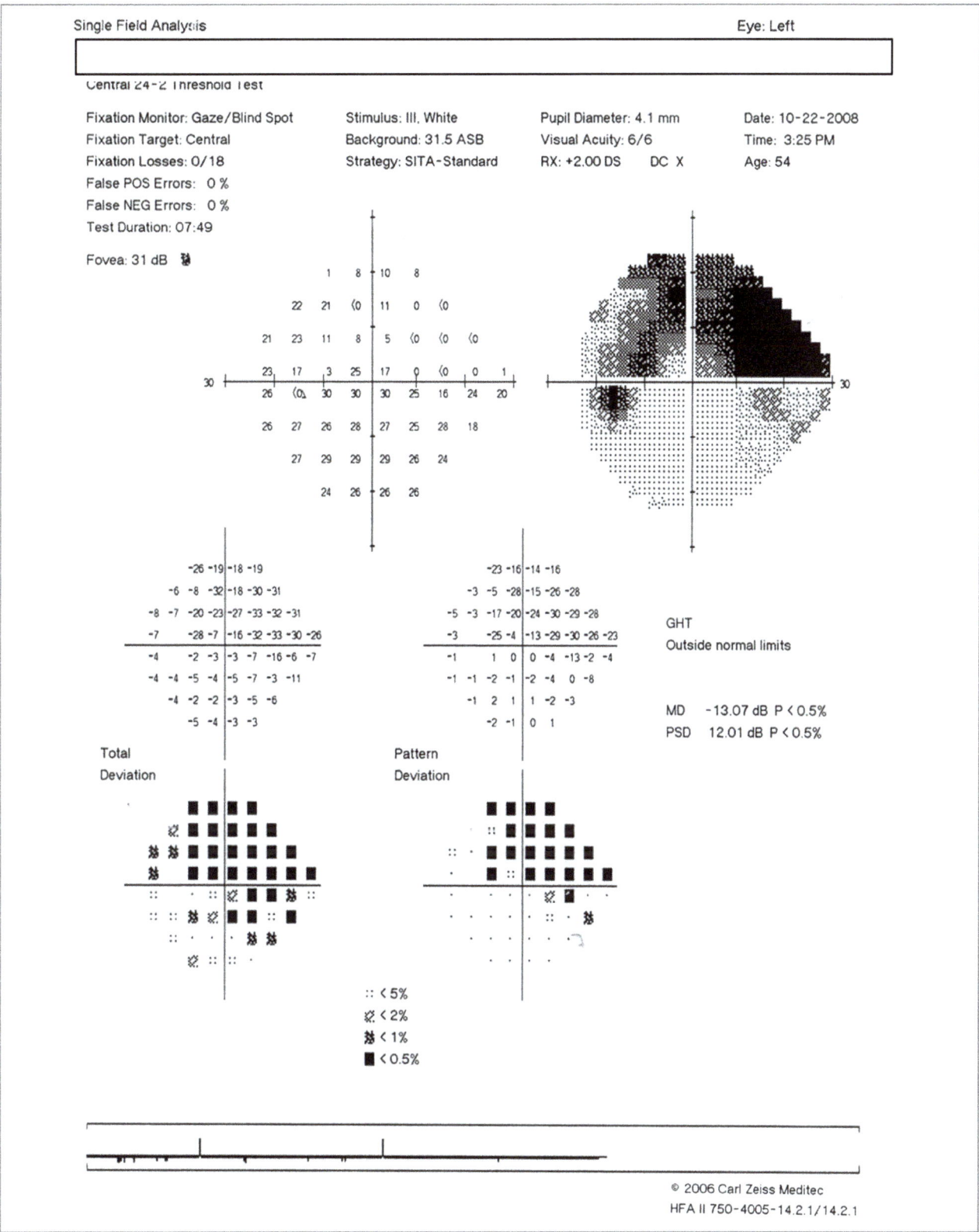

Fig. 3B
Source: Dr Shroff's charity eye hospital

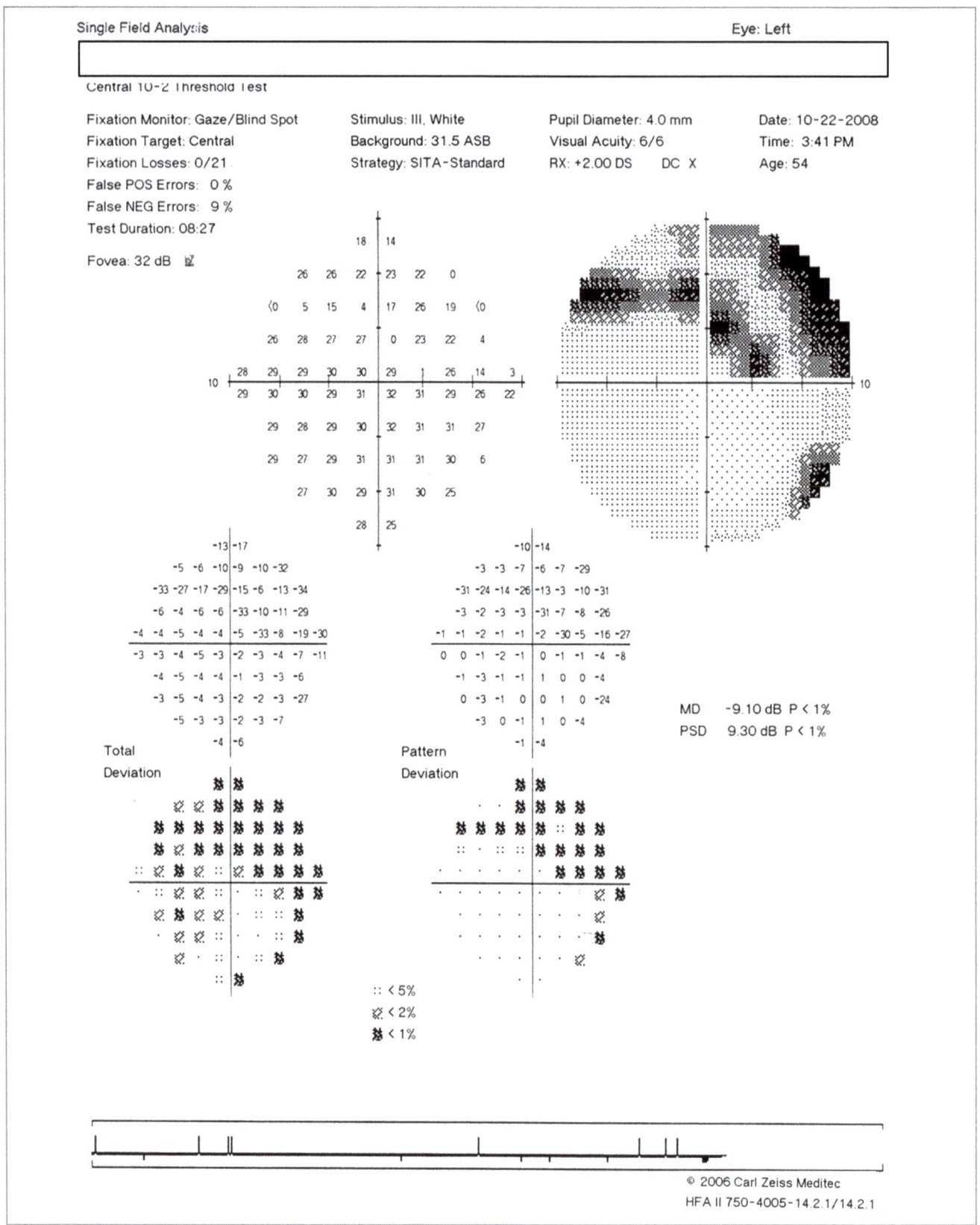

Fig. 3C

Figs. 3A to C: (A) Normal Humphreys visual field 24–2; (B) Abnormal Humphreys visual field 24–2; and (C) Abnormal Humphreys visual field 10-2 of the same patient as same patient as in **Figure 3B**. This will be more informative for follow-up of this patient.

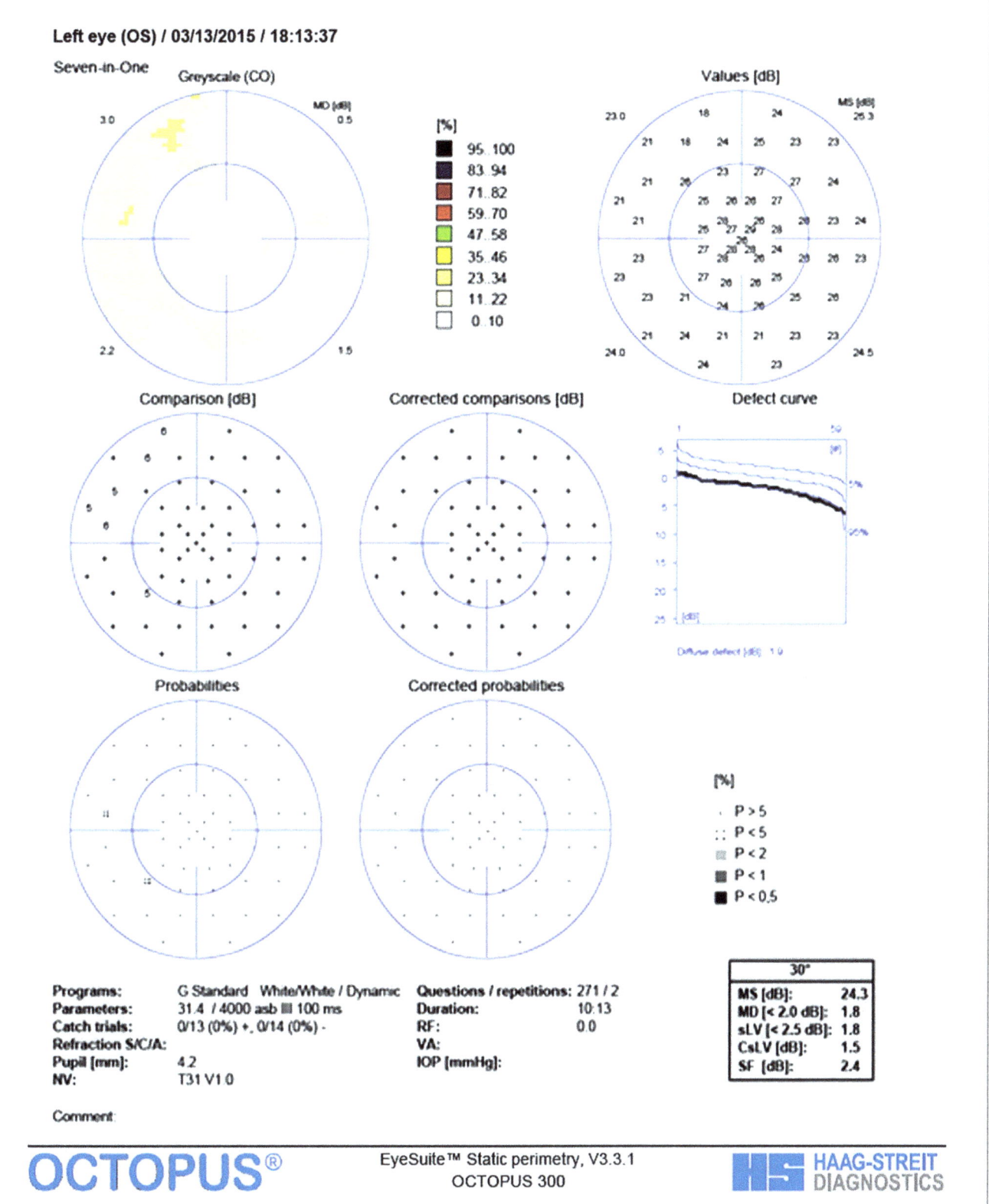

Fig. 4A

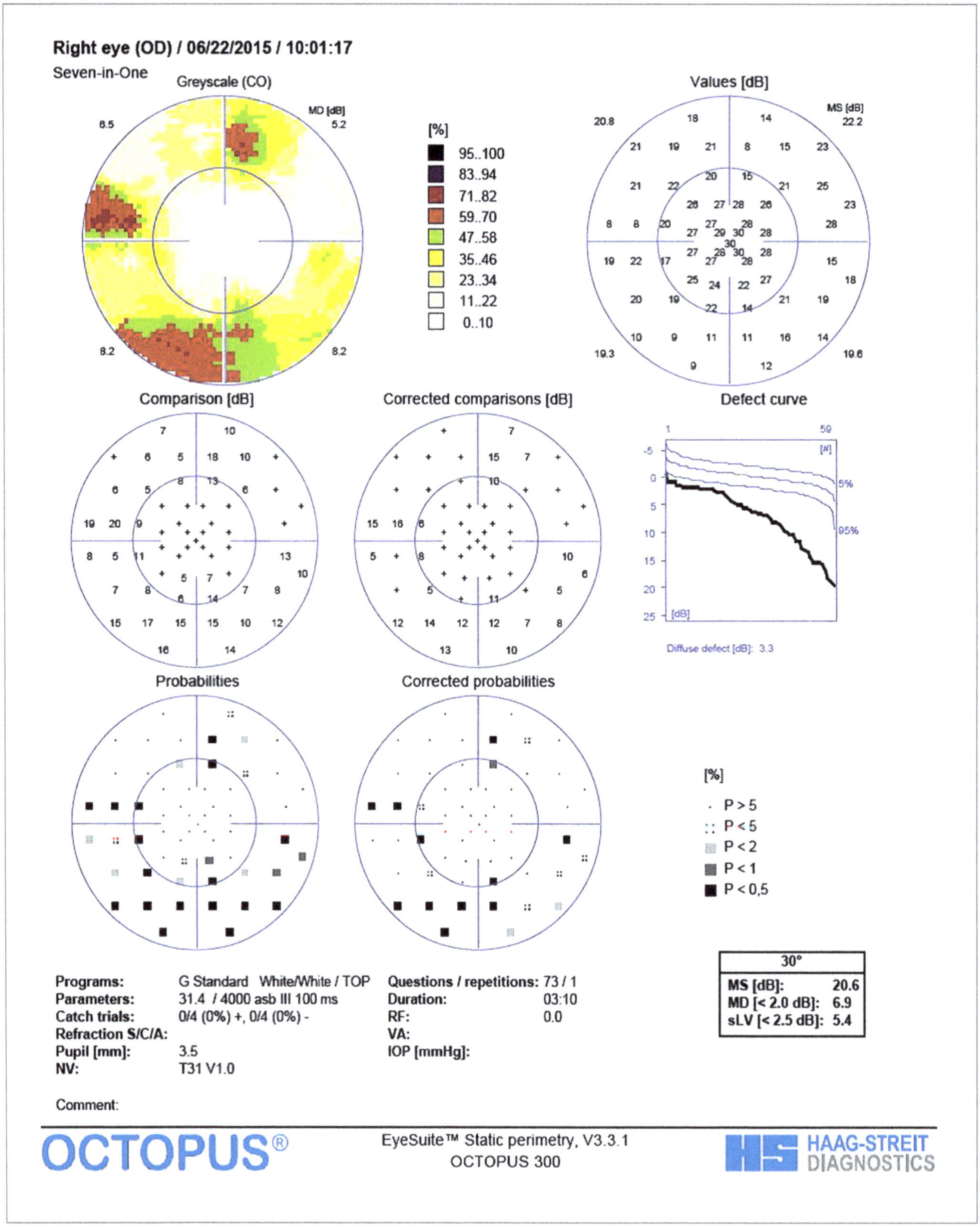
Right eye (OD) / 06/22/2015 / 10:01:17
Seven-in-One
Greyscale (CO)
Values [dB]
Comparison [dB]
Corrected comparisons [dB]
Defect curve
Diffuse defect [dB]: 3.3
Probabilities
Corrected probabilities
[%]
95..100
83..94
71..82
59..70
47..58
35..46
23..34
11..22
0..10
[%]
P > 5
P < 5
P < 2
P < 1
P < 0,5
30°
MS [dB]: 20.6
MD [< 2.0 dB]: 6.9
sLV [< 2.5 dB]: 5.4
Programs: G Standard White/White / TOP
Parameters: 31.4 / 4000 asb III 100 ms
Catch trials: 0/4 (0%) +, 0/4 (0%) -
Refraction S/C/A:
Pupil [mm]: 3.5
NV: T31 V1.0
Questions / repetitions: 73 / 1
Duration: 03:10
RF: 0.0
VA:
IOP [mmHg]:
Comment:
OCTOPUS®
EyeSuite™ Static perimetry, V3.3.1
OCTOPUS 300
HAAG-STREIT DIAGNOSTICS

Fig. 4B

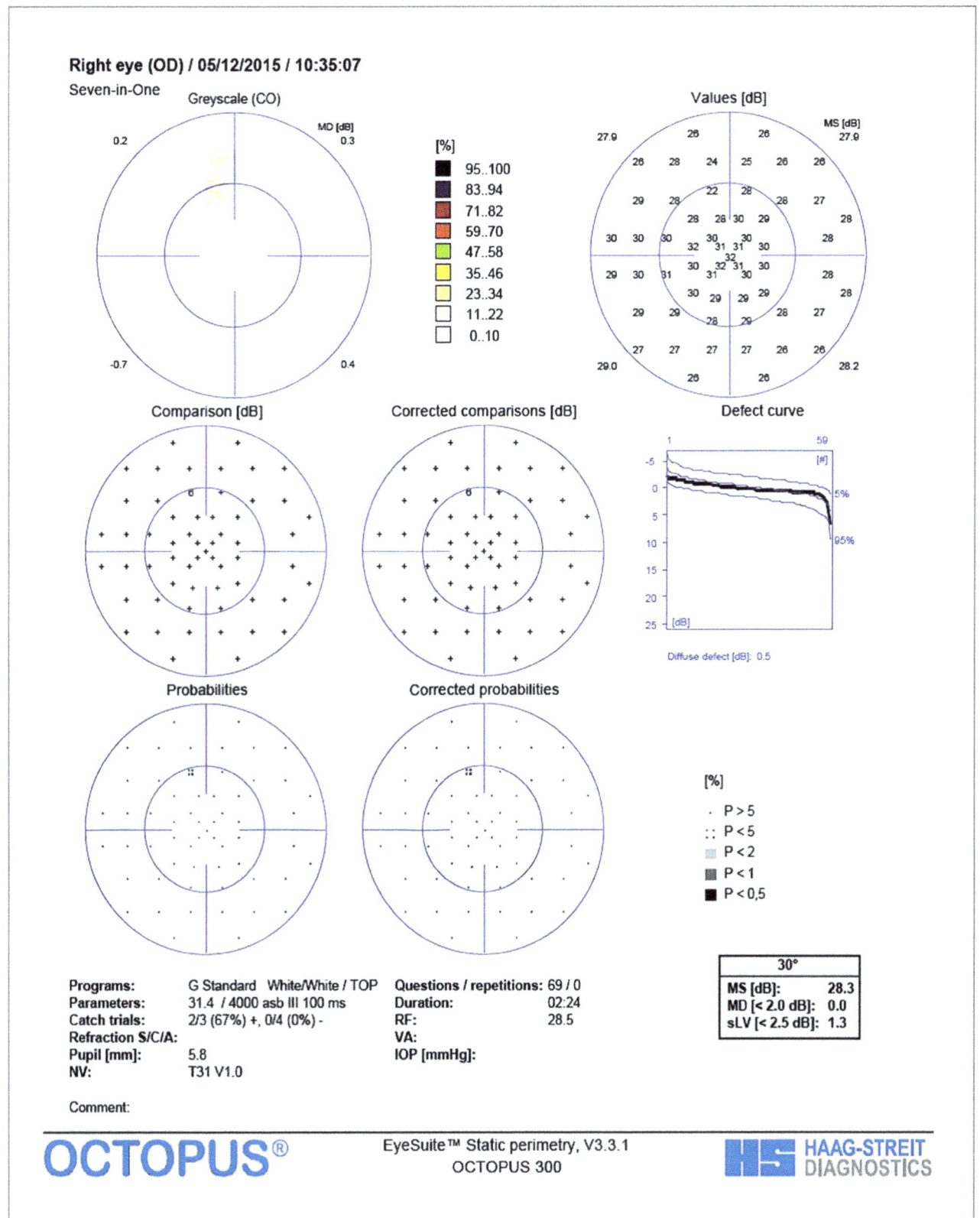

Fig. 4C

Figs. 4A to C: (A) Normal visual field (Octopus). Left eye of a 74-year-old patient tested with G Standard Dynamic Program; (B) Abnormal visual field (Octopus) right eye of a 52-year-old patient with inferior arcuate defect. Note the Babie curve depressed below the normal range; (C) Normal Octopus visual field, tendency-oriented perimetry.

CORRELATION OF FIELDS BETWEEN THE TWO PERIMETERS

Repeat visual field assessment is invaluable for confirming presence of visual field deficit, aiding localization of pathological lesion, and for recording improvement, stabilization, or deterioration of the underlying condition. Therefore, it is important that the same perimeter be used in the serial evaluation of a patient overtime. Even though the parameters of visual field loss show a good correlation between the two kinds of perimeters, the values from each may not be used interchangeably in the serial monitoring of patients.

With patients shifting between practices with different machines, it is important to have a general idea of intraperimeter comparisons. When interpreting progression by interpreting fields done on the two different perimeters, it is essential to keep in mind the effect of differing bracketing strategies, background illuminations on threshold values which impacts MD and PSD/(LV indices).[1-12]

NETWORKING AND COMPATIBILITY

The Humphrey machine can be connected to the office network and other Zeiss machines through FORUM eye care management systems **(Fig. 5)**. This establishes centralized data storage management and retrieval thereby increasing efficiency. It can be connected to the electronic health records to store data also.

The EyeSuite software with Octopus has the capability of connecting the machine to the other Haag strait machines such that the patient data can be accessed anywhere in the busy OPD **(Fig. 6)**. The software is compatible with standardized interfaces such as GDT and Digital Imaging and Communications in Medicine (DICOM) and can be transferred to EMRs thus reducing time and eliminating transcription errors.

MERITS AND DEMERITS

The Humphrey perimeter is used more extensively, and more ophthalmologists have been trained to read HFA visual fields, and therefore, find it easier to interpret. Also, as patients shift between practices, serial follow-up is easier if the next doctor has the same machine, even though a fresh baseline will need to be established to monitor progression. The Octopus perimeter is easier to use since the time taken for the field is less, and it does not require a dark room for perimetry. Fixation losses are not a concern during visual fields with the Octopus machines as stimulus projection is stopped when there is fixation loss and the perimetrist encourages the patient to refixate before testing is restarted. The direct projection system of the 300 series machines

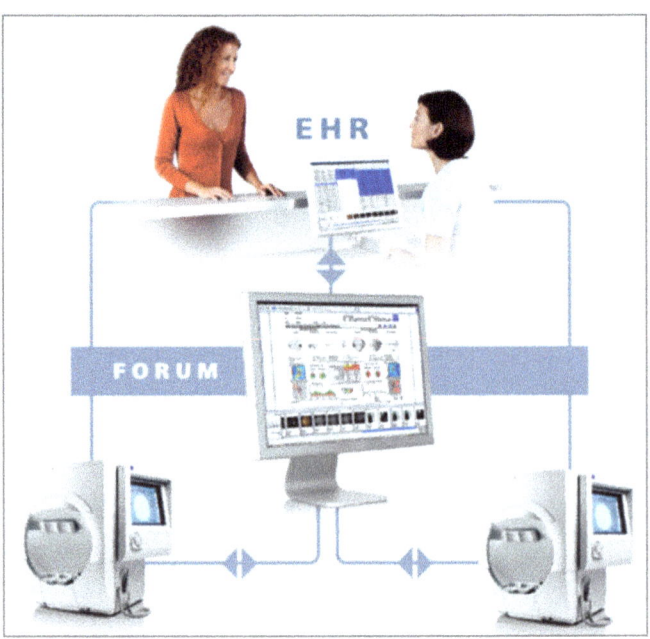

Fig. 5: Humphrey visual field connected to FORUM and electronic health record (HER). It can also connect to networked devices without Digital Imaging and Communications in Medicine (DICOM). *Source:* https://www.zeiss.com/content/dam/Meditec

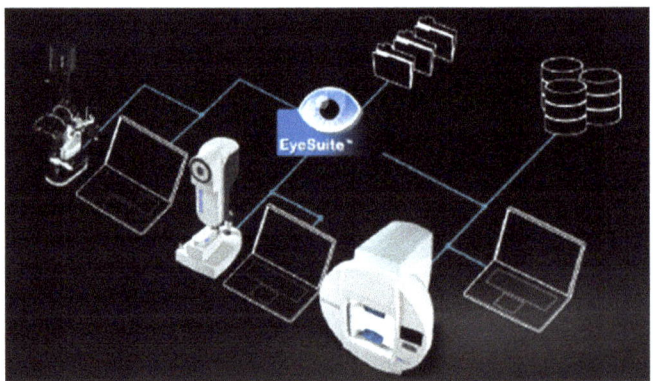

Fig. 6: Integration of EyeSuite with the Octopus 900. *Source:* http://www.haag-streit.com/products/perimetry/octopusr-900

implies that no near correction has to be added during perimetry. It is a compact machine and therefore requires less table space. Features unique to the Octopus include Polar diagram, cluster analysis and EyeSuite Trend analysis (all these features are discussed in detail in the preceding chapters on Octopus perimetry.

OCULUS PERIMETERS

The Oculus Easyfield is the smallest full-fledged perimeter on the market. It is designed for use as a visual field screener and as a threshold perimeter for immediate reexamination of any abnormal findings. Ideal for all common examinations of the central visual field up to 30°. It has an adjustable double chin rest and uses translucent eye shields for maximum patient comfort.

The Centerfield® 2 Perimeter has proven itself to be an invaluable instrument in the occupational health area. The unit performs static perimetry up to 70° eccentricity. It also meets the requirements of the German Ophthalmological Society's (DOG) Road Traffic Commission for conducting visual field testing in accordance with the regulations for the issuance of driver's licenses.

The Twinfield 2 Oculus device measures the full field of vision using both automatic, static perimetry, and automatic or manual kinetic examinations.

CONCLUSION

The best perimeter for your practice is the one you have. As long as it is used judiciously, and appropriate caution is exercised when interpreting the visual field report, the performance of each of the perimeters is comparable to the other. It is important that the same perimeter be used in the serial evaluation of a patient over time, especially to utilize the progression software of the device.

REFERENCES

1. Allingham RR. Shields' textbook of glaucoma. 5th edition. Philadelphia: Lippincott Williams and Wilkins; 2004.
2. Anderson DR, Patella VM. Automated static perimetry. 2nd edition. United States: Mosby. 1999.
3. Haag-Streit USA. (2015). Octopus Manual. [online] Available from: www.haag-streit-usa.com [Last accessed July, 2023].
4. Zeiss Group. (2015). Humphrey's Field Analyzer Manual. [online] Available from: www.zeiss.com [Last accessed July, 2023].
5. Ichhpujani P, Bhartiya S. Manual of Glaucoma, 1st edition. Delhi, India: Jaypee Brothers Medical Publishers; 2015.
6. Sharaawy TM, Sherwood MB, Crowston JG. Glaucoma, 2nd edition. Netherlands: Elsevier; 2014.
7. Nelson P, Aspinall P, Papasouliotis O, Worton B, O'Brien C. Quality of life in glaucoma and its relationship with visual function. J Glaucoma. 2003;12:139-50.
8. Weijland A, Fankhauser F, Bebie H, Flammer J. Automated perimetry: Visual field digest, 5th edition. Switzerland: Haag-Streit AG, Schlieren; 2004.
9. Lefrançoisa A, Valtot F, Barrault O. New diagnosis approaches: Our experience with Octopus Field Analysis (OFA V2.2), the new software for analysis of visual field (in French). J Fr Ophtalmol. 2009;32:3-14.
10. Naghizadeh F, Holló G. Detection of early glaucomatous progression with Octopus cluster trend analysis. J Glaucoma. 2014;23:269-75.
11. Holló G, Naghizadeh F. Evaluation of Octopus polar trend analysis for detection of glaucomatous progression. Eur J Ophthalmol. 2014;24:862-8.
12. Thomas R, George R. Interpreting automated perimetry. Indian J Ophthalmol. 2001;49:125-40.

SECTION 2

Visual Field Interpretation

3. **Single Visual Field Analysis**
   Alejandra Hernandez-Oteyza, Oscar Albis-Donado

4. **Octopus Perimetry: Analyzing the Single Field Report**
   Ann Mary Mathews, Mohana Sinnasamy, Murali Ariga

5. **Pearls and Pitfalls in Perimetry**
   Parul Ichhpujani, Neiwete Lomi, Savleen Kaur, Surinder Singh Pandav, Sushmita Kaushik

6. **Visual Field Progression**
   Yamunadevi Lakshmanan, Najiya Sundus K Meethal, Ronnie George, Shantha B, Vijaya L

7. **Visual Field Progression Analysis with Octopus Perimetry**
   Mohana Sinnasamy, Murali Ariga, Jayasudha Roopesh, Niranjana Balasubramaniam

8. **Visual Fields—An Overview**
   Ankur Sinha, Gitanjali Sharma

CHAPTER 3

Single Visual Field Analysis

Alejandra Hernandez-Oteyza, Oscar Albis-Donado

■ INTRODUCTION

Modern glaucoma diagnosis and follow-up require a tool that allows a quantitative assessment of visual field loss. This can be accomplished by automated static perimetry, a test that maps the retina's light sensitivity threshold at certain given locations of the visual field.[1-3]

The retinal nerve fiber layer (RNFL) is composed of the axons of retinal ganglion cells (RGC). Visual field testing allows the identification of characteristic patterns of photosensitivity loss of the retina that might reflect defects of the projections of the RNFL at the optic disc, or at other sites of the visual pathway.[1]

Humphrey's field analyzer (HFA) (Carl Zeiss Meditec Dublin, CA) is one of the most common devices used to perform automated static perimetry. It is most frequently used for the diagnosis and follow-up of glaucoma, but it can also be used in the assessment of different retinal and neurological disorders.

Humphrey's field analyzer projects stimuli on a white surface with a known illumination (31.5 asb). The size of the stimuli is usually Goldman size III, but in certain cases size V is used. The duration of the stimulus is fixed to 200 ms. The most commonly performed test uses a white stimulus over a white background, but HFA can also perform tests using a blue stimulus over a yellow background or a red stimulus over a white background.[2,4]

Humphrey's field analyzer allows for single field and for progression analysis. In this chapter, we will focus on the single field analysis, which uses the STATPAC software, capable of comparing the patient's results with a normative database composed of patients of the same age group.[5-7]

To analyze a single field analysis printout, we must first identify its portions and define a systematic order for the analysis. An example of the HFA single-field analysis printout can be seen in **Figure 1**.

■ IDENTIFYING INFORMATION

On the upper part of single field printout, we can find the patient's name, ID number, and birthdate, and the eye that is being tested. Correct spelling of the patient's name is crucial to allow future test comparison and progression analysis. When using different machines, a central database that uses FORUM and/or HFA-net can integrate tests from the same patient. It is also very important to enter the patient's birthdate correctly, as the machine will automatically calculate his or her age so that the STATPAC software can compare the results to the proper age group data **(Fig. 2)**.[8]

Going down in the printout, we then have information about the test being performed, whether it is a 24-2, 30-2, or 10-2 test **(Fig. 3)**. Recent upgrades also allow for 24-2C test, which combines the information of the 24-2 and 10-2 tests on the same printout **(Fig. 4)**.

We can identify three columns (formally four, in older versions) with general information about the visual field test. On the first column, we find the reliability indices, which will be further explained later on in this chapter. On the second column, we have additional information about the test, such as the stimulus size and color, the screen's color and brightness and the strategy. As mentioned earlier, stimulus size is usually Goldmann III but on cases with severe damage, a size V may be useful. Fundus' brightness for HFA is always set to 31.5 asb, so the stimulus brightness must also be higher, as compared to Octopus perimeters, for example. HFA has many test strategies available; the more common strategies are Swedish interactive threshold algorithm (SITA)-Standard, SITA-Fast, and more recently SITA-Faster. This column also contains additional patient's eye information, such as pupil size, visual acuity, and refraction used during the test (which should consider adequate age-corrected addition for the screen distance). If the patient's cylinder is <2D, spherical equivalent may be used. If the

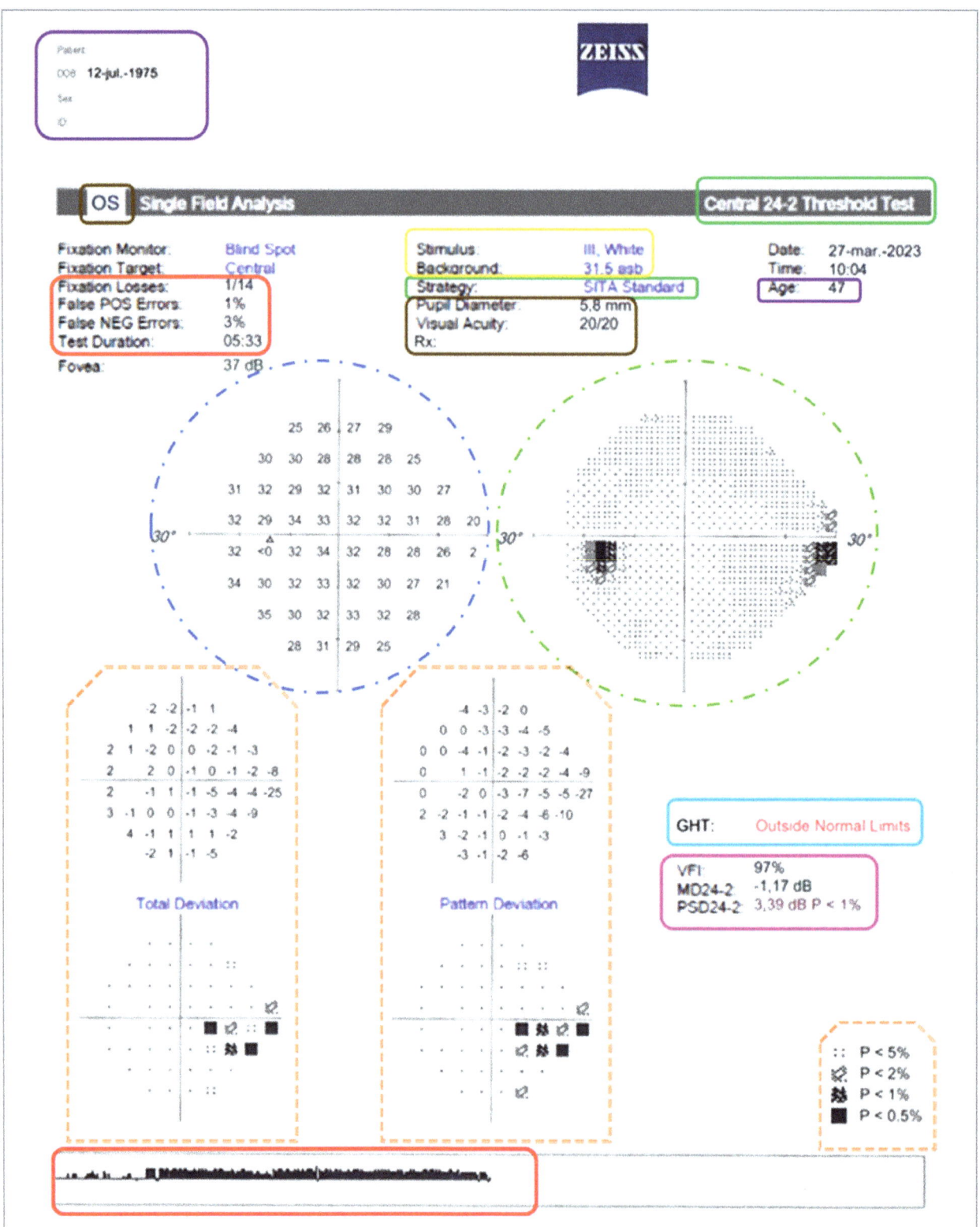

Fig. 1: 24-2 single field analysis printout. Purple: Patient's ID information (name, date of birth, sex, ID number, and age); Green: Test pattern and strategy chosen for the test; Yellow: Size of stimuli and background illumination of screen; Brown: eye tested, pupil size, visual acuity, refraction used; Red: Reliability indexes (fixation losses, false positive (FP) errors, false negative (FN) errors, test duration, and gaze tracker); Dotted blue: Raw numeric graph; Dotted green: Grayscale graph, Dotted orange: Total deviation and pattern deviation numerical and probability graphs; and probability scale); Light blue: Glaucoma hemifield test (GHT); Pink: Global indices [visual field index (VFI), mean deviation (MD), and pattern standard deviation (PSD)].

CHAPTER 3: Single Visual Field Analysis

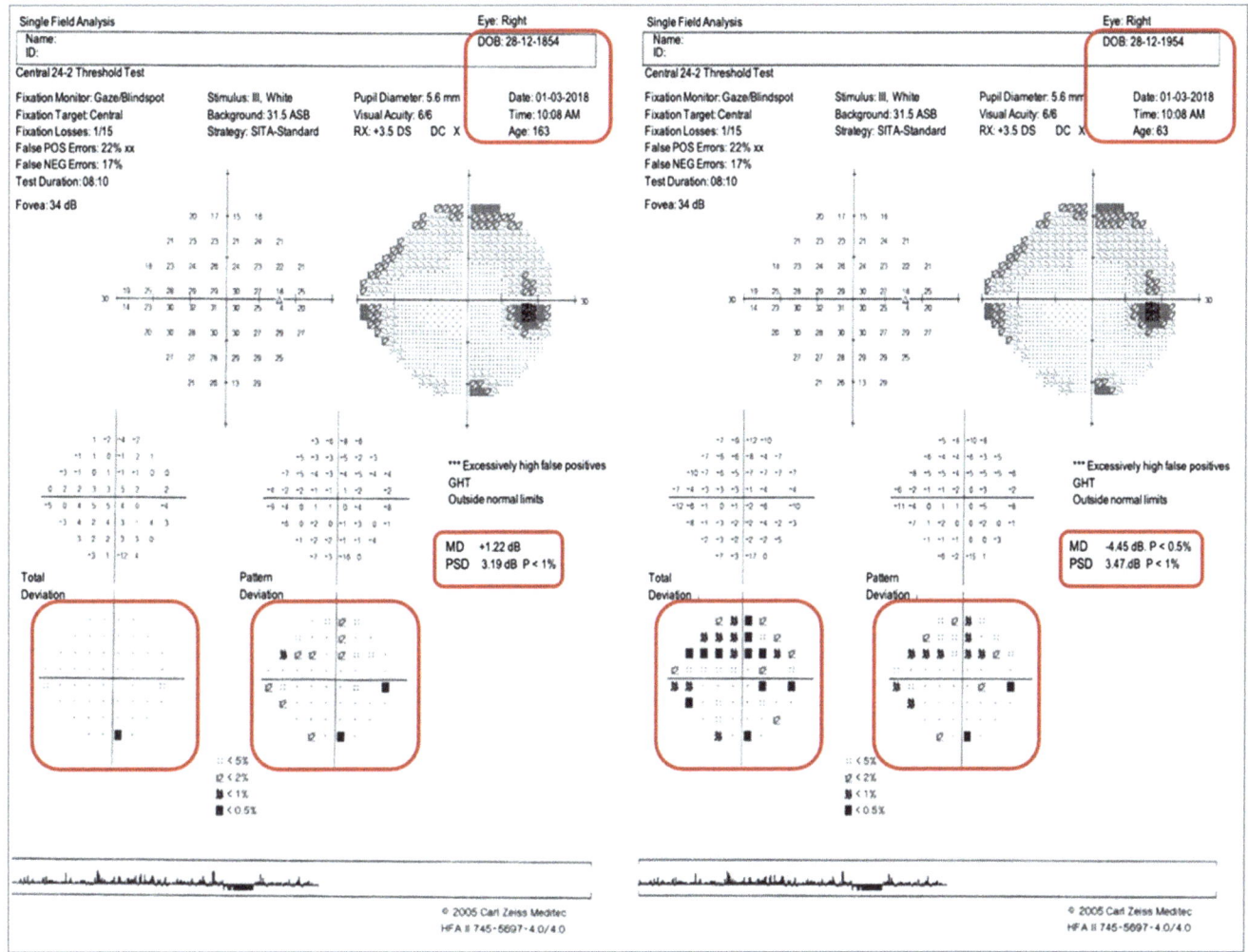

Fig. 2: On the left visual field the birthdate is mistyped, so the patient seems to be 163 years old. His retinal sensitivities are compared to the oldest age group of the normative database, so the mean deviation seems to be above the normal threshold for that age (+1.32 dB). On the right, when the birthdate is corrected, the retinal sensitivities are compared to the correct age group, so the mean deviation is now -4.45 dB, a better correspondence to the observed general depression and relative superior arcuate scotoma and nasal step.

patient uses contact lens, it is preferable to perform the test using the contact lens and using the proper near correction on the lens frame when necessary.[9]

Finally, the fourth and last column of the upper layout has the date and time of the test and the patient's age, to double-check that the birthdate is correct (*see* **Fig. 1**).

■ RELIABILITY INDICES

To assess the test's reliability, we have to analyze three parameters shown in the upper left corner of the printout (fixation losses, FPs, and FNs), as well as the duration of the test and the gaze tracking plot (found at the bottom of the page).[3]

1. *Fixation loses* are assessed by the Heijl–Krakau method, by identifying the location of the blind spot and then presenting 5% of the stimuli to such location. If the patient responds to these stimuli, it means he moved his gaze. We must consider that around 190 Goldmann size III stimuli fit in a normal blind spot. When fixation loses are >20%, a "XX" symbol appears next to the ratio of fixation loses/stimuli presented to the blind spot, to indicate a low reliability (*see* **Fig. 1**). Other sources of error that increase fixation losses are head tilting or improper position of the chin. Modern test strategies such as SITA-Faster turn off the fixation loses to decrease the test time.[3]

The gaze tracker is an additional aid to assess proper gaze direction. It uses an infrared light to detect the central reflex of the cornea with every stimulus and compares it to the pupil centroid position, and that way it is able to monitor blinking and eye movements. Downward peaks on the gaze tracker occur when the location of the gaze could not be determined, more commonly when

32 SECTION 2: Visual Field Interpretation

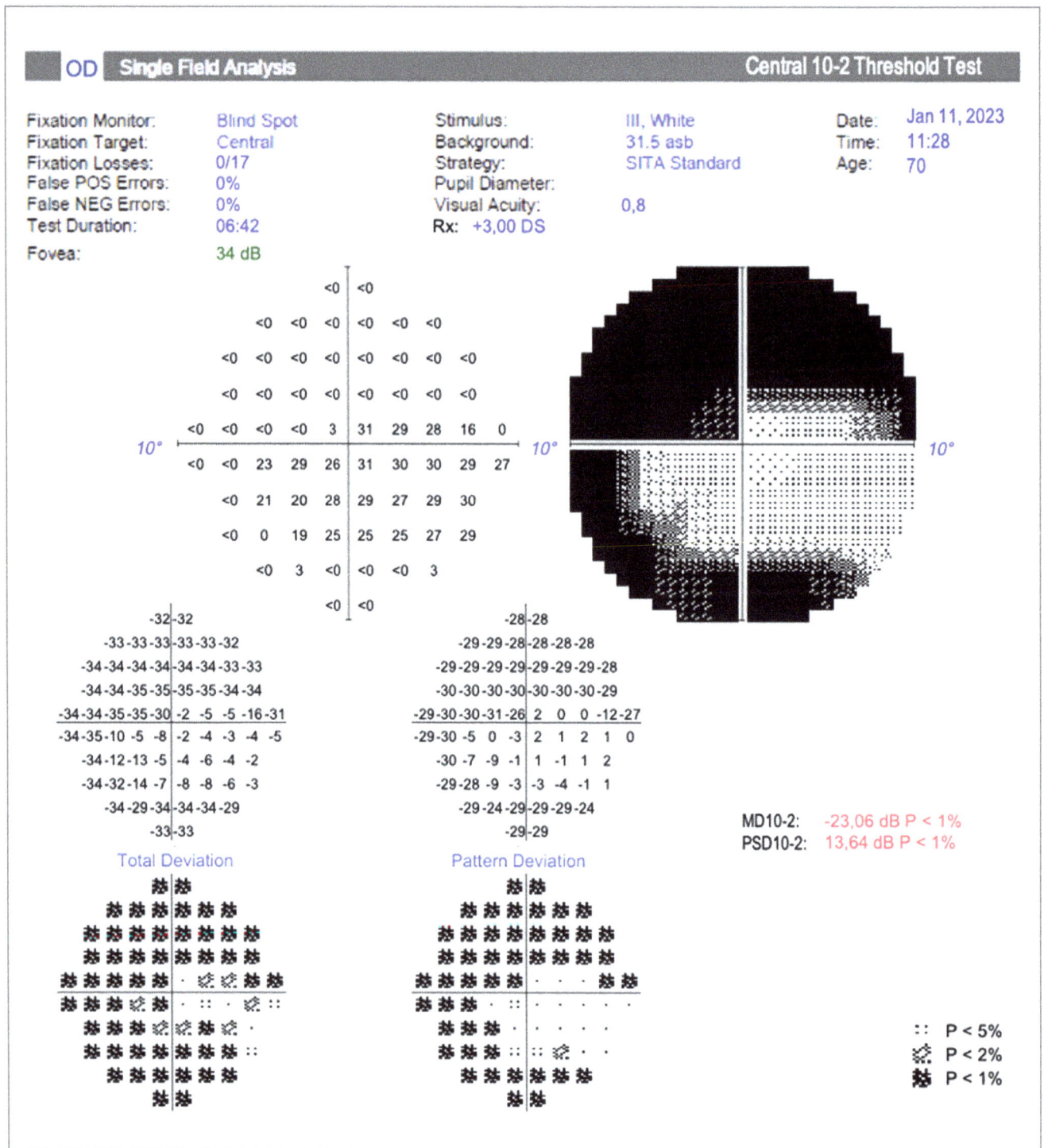

Fig. 3: 10-2 Single field analysis printout. Note the differences with the 24-2 printout, such as the blind spot cannot be seen (as it is found outside the central 10°), there is no glaucoma hemifield test (GHT), and no visual field index (VFI).

blinking; upward peaks are proportional in amplitude to the degrees of the deviation of the gaze (*see* **Fig. 1**).[8,10]

2. *False positive errors* rate measures how often the patient presses the response button without a visual stimulus being presented. Sometimes, an audible stimulus but not a visual one is presented, and if the patient responds, a FP is recorded. These patients are known as "happy triggers". In the SITA strategies, the algorithm detects the patient's normal response speed to stimuli, and FPs are registered when the patient responds too soon or too late to the

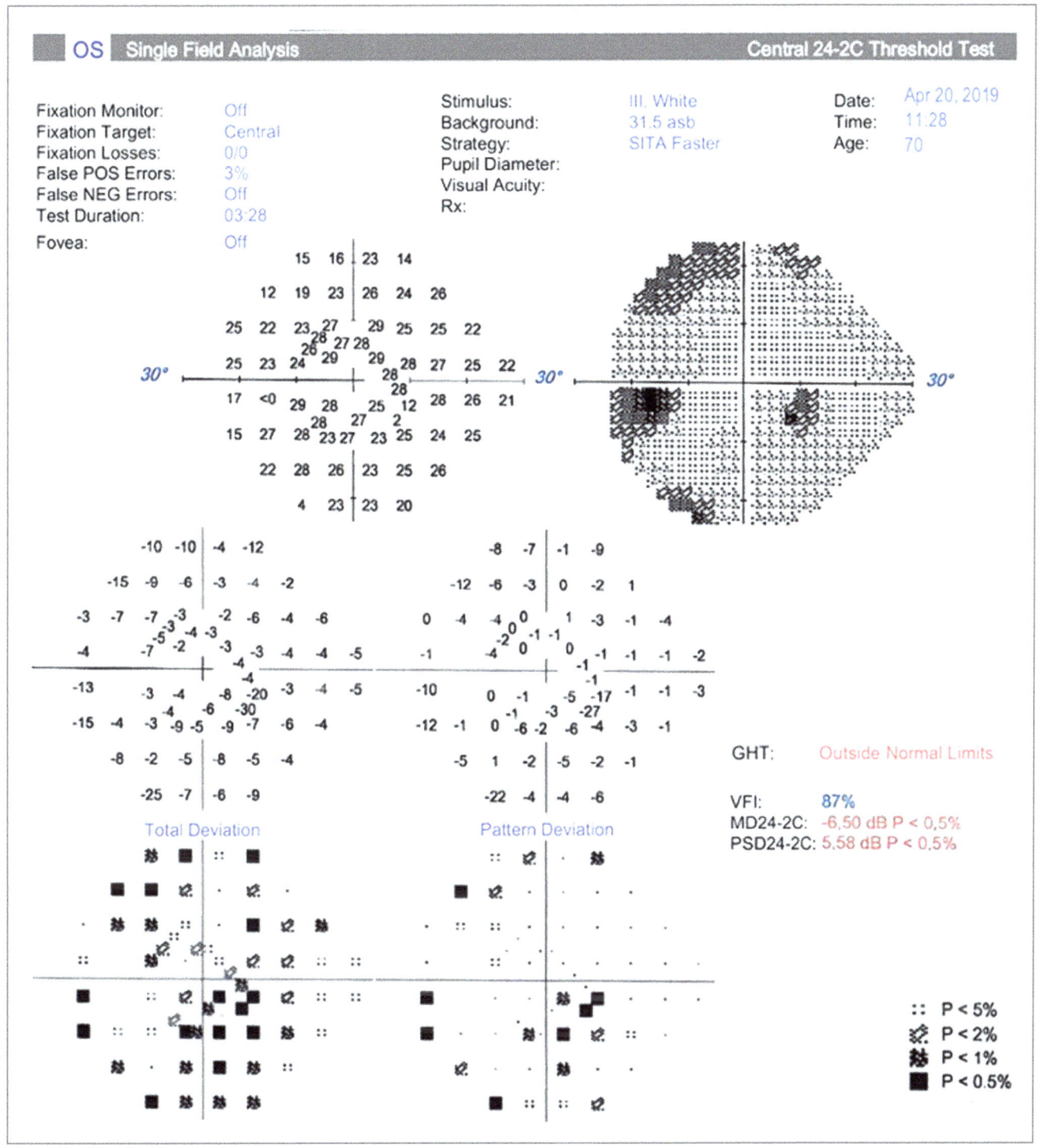

Fig. 4: 24-2C single field analysis printout.

stimulus being presented, compared to the response speed to previous stimuli during the course of the test. When the FP errors rate is high, it might be associated with abnormally high values in the raw numerical graph, a "white scotoma" in the grayscale graph, a legend that reads "excessively high FPs", a hemifield glaucoma test (HGT) that indicates "abnormally high sensitivity" and a very positive mean deviation (MD) **(Fig. 5)**.[2,3]

False positive errors are of major importance in determining the reliability of a visual field test. If the rate of FP errors exceeds 15%, this indicates low reliability and may result in exclusion of the test for future Guided

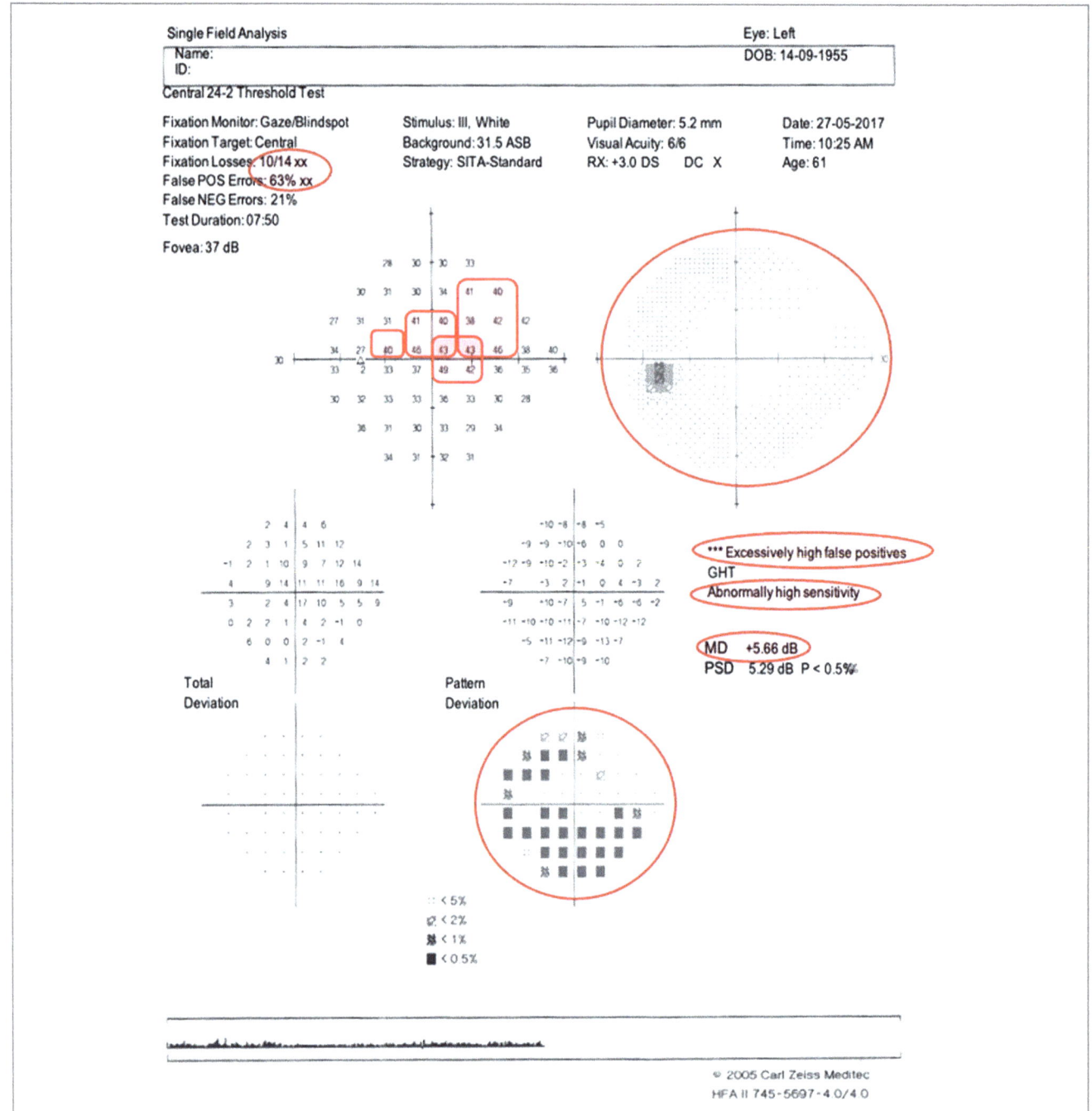

Fig. 5: A printout with a very high rate of false positives, at 63%. The numerical graph displays values higher than 40 dB, and the grayscale plot has a white scotoma. The legend reads "excessively high false positives," and the GHT indicates "Abnormally high sensitivity". Additionally, there is a positive mean deviation (MD) and the pattern deviation map appears to be worse than the total deviation map.

Progression Analysis (GPA). Additionally, if the rate of FP errors exceeds 33%, an "XX" symbol will appear next to the percentage of FP. Even a small number of FP errors (e.g., 5-10%) can invalidate a visual field test, particularly for research purposes.

3. *False negative errors:* The rate of FN is determined when a patient fails to respond to a stimulus that is 9 dB brighter at a spot where they had previously responded. This can be due to distraction or a compromised visual field due to advanced disease. A visual field with a high FN rate can appear worse than it actually is, or it may display a "cloverleaf pattern," which typically indicates fatigue during the test and is accompanied by a longer test duration. Similar to FPs, a FN rate exceeding 33% is displayed

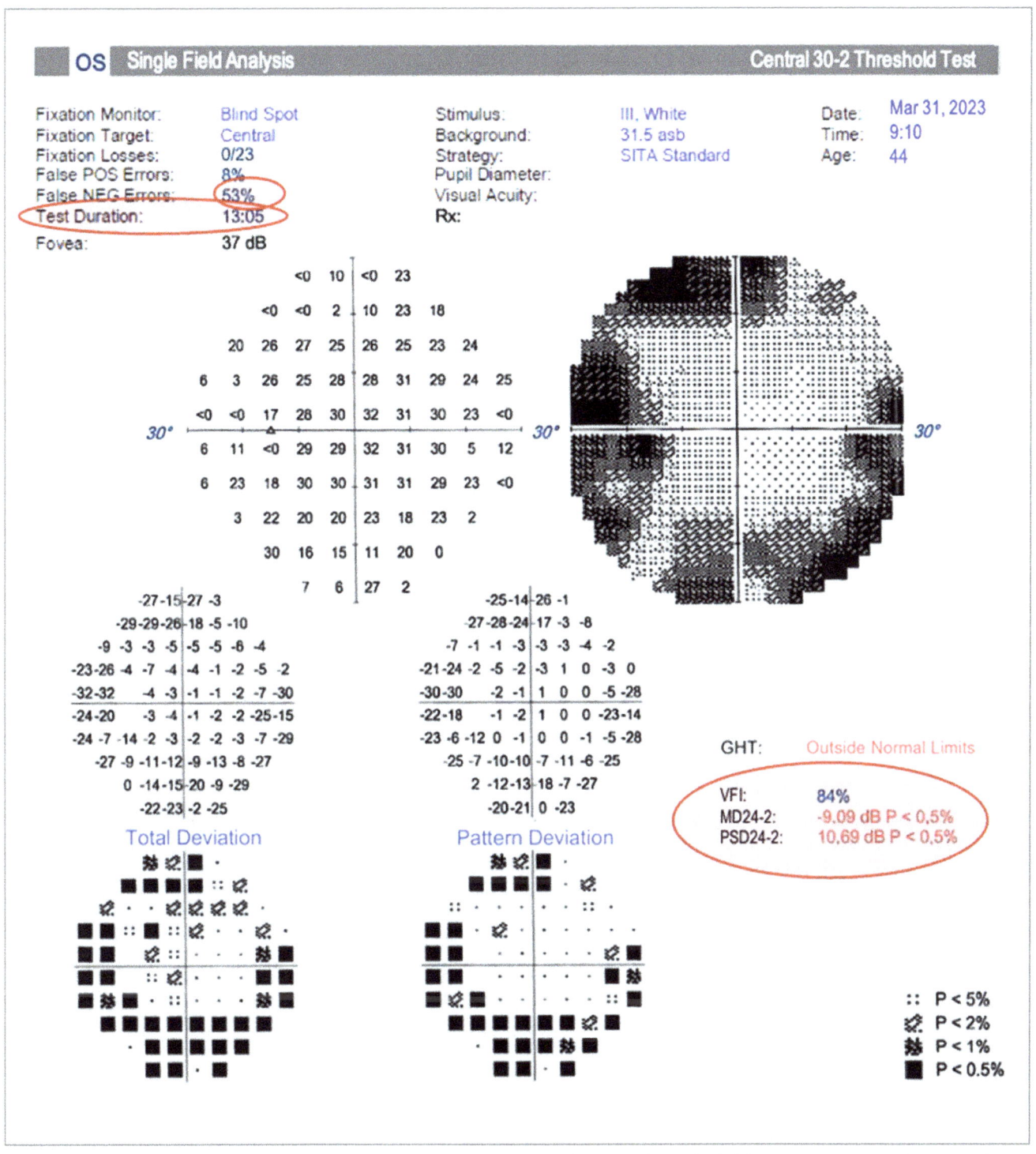

Fig. 6: Visual field printout of a 30-2 Single field analysis showing a clover-leaf pattern due to high false negatives (53%). We can see how the duration of the test is prolonged and the mean deviation (MD) is very depressed.

with an "XX" symbol next to the percentage of FN, and a FN rate exceeding 15–20% may indicate low reliability. If FN errors are too high due to poor cooperation or to a severely depressed fields, the printout reads "N/A" **(Fig. 6)**.

The HFA displays a "low patient reliability" legend when some of the reliability indices are altered. Low reliability indices can alter the result of the visual field **(Fig. 7)**.

The test duration depends on the strategy used. Normal test durations for a the classic 30-2 full-threshold test are

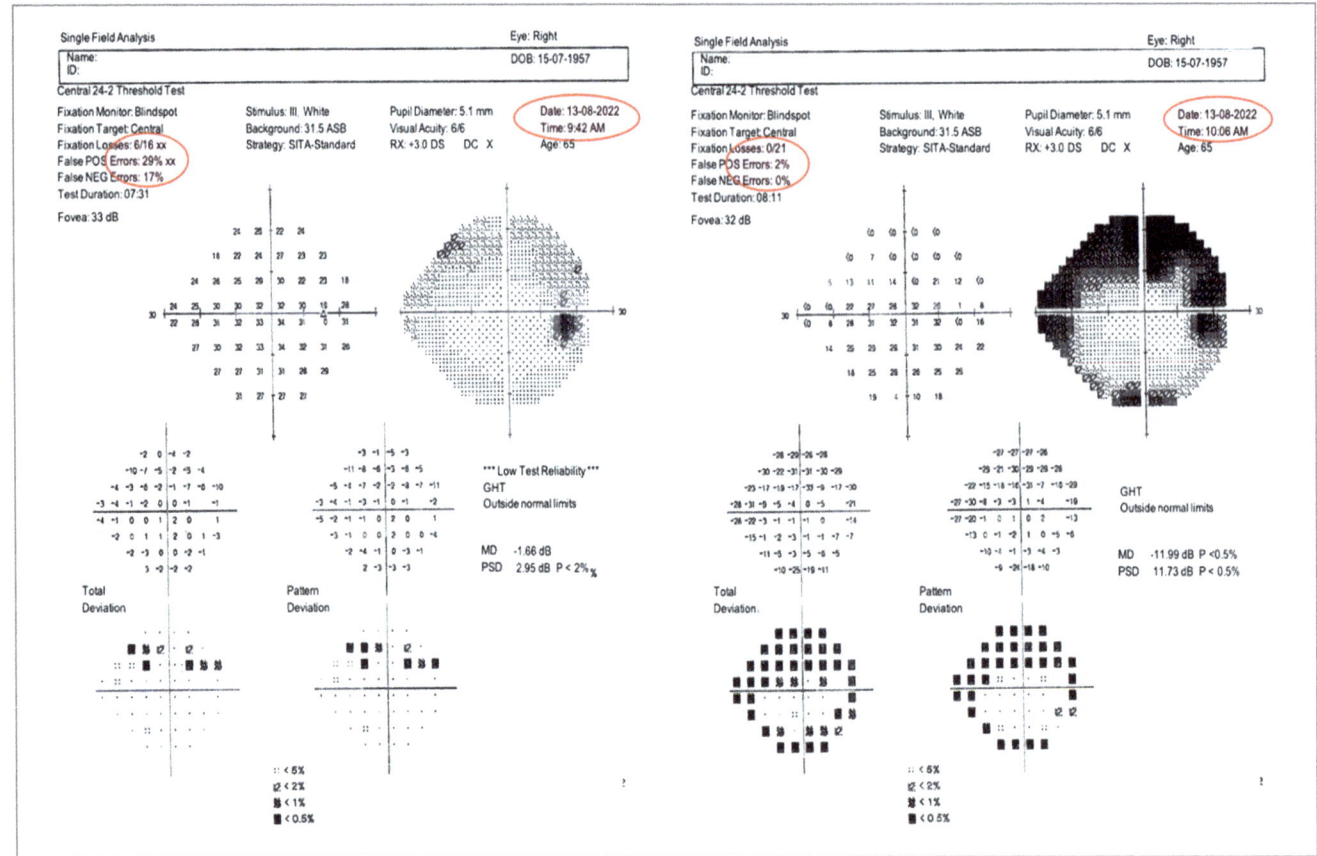

Fig. 7: Visual field test of a patient performed twice on the same day. On the left side, we can see an unreliable test due to a high rate of fixation losses, false positive errors, and false negative errors. On the right side, we can see the results of a more reliable test, which demonstrates a significant difference from the unreliable test, and better correlation to the actual glaucoma damage.

about 20 minutes, but for a 24-2 SITA-Standard, 24-2 SITA-Fast and 24-2 SITA-Faster tests, normal testing times are 7, 5, and 3 minutes, respectively (*see* **Fig. 1**).[11]

Below the reliability indices above mentioned, we find the fovea's sensitivity that normally ranges from 34 to 36 dB (*see* **Fig. 1**).

■ RAW NUMERIC GRAPH

This graph shows the raw number in dB of the retina sensitivity threshold measured at each location. It is important to keep in mind that sensitivity is measured in dB, which is a logarithmic scale that converts the ratio of background illumination to stimulus illumination, and it is necessary to interpret changes in sensitivity accurately. A sensitivity of 0 dB or <0 dB means that the patient was unable to detect a 10,000 asb stimulus at that location, which is the brightest stimulus available in HFA. When sensitivity is 10 dB, the brightness is decreased by a factor of 10, so a 10 dB sensitivity occurs when the retina can see a 1,000 asb stimulus. Similarly, a 20 dB sensitivity indicates that the retina was able to detect a 100 asb stimulus, and so on **Table 1**.[2,3]

TABLE 1: Equivalences of apostilbs to decibels in the Humphrey field analyzer.

Apostilbs	Decibels
10,000	0
1,000	10
100	20
10	30
1	40

The raw numeric graph can be very useful to assess damage and progression in visual fields, especially when assessing point-by-point progression.

In full threshold strategies when a value falls 5 dB above or below the expected value that spot is retested, thus displaying values in brackets. This is why full threshold strategies take a much longer time to perform (**Fig. 8**).

■ GRAYSCALE GRAPH

The grayscale graph is an extrapolation of the raw numeric graph, by assigning a grid of more or less intense gray tones to each number, depending on their sensitivity. Spots with higher sensitivity appear lighter and the less sensitive areas appear darker **(Fig. 9)**.[4]

This graph gives a fast overview of the pattern of visual field loss and is very useful when explaining the results to the patient. In the grayscale graph, we can also easily identify the previously mentioned "clover-leaf pattern".

■ DEVIATION MAPS

To understand these diagrams, it is essential to distinguish between generalized and localized defects. Although generalized depression might be the presenting sign of glaucoma, it is more commonly seen as an artifact produced by media opacities, most commonly cataracts, rather than a lesion of the retina or the optic pathways. We must remember that the goal of perimetry is to determine the sensitivity of the retina at each location. Cataracts absorb part of the intensity of the stimulus emitted by the perimeter, so the retina receives a less intense stimulus than the one sent by the device and the patient's response reflects a uniformly diminished hill of vision. In this scenario, the sensitivity of the retina might be correct, but the perimeter interprets it as if it were injured. However, generalized depression may also cover up a localized defect, and when present in eyes with clear media and good visual acuity it might be a sing of diffuse glaucoma damage.

On the contrary, a generalized elevation is the consequence of a patient who presses the button without a light stimulus, indicating a bad collaboration or a "trigger happy" response.

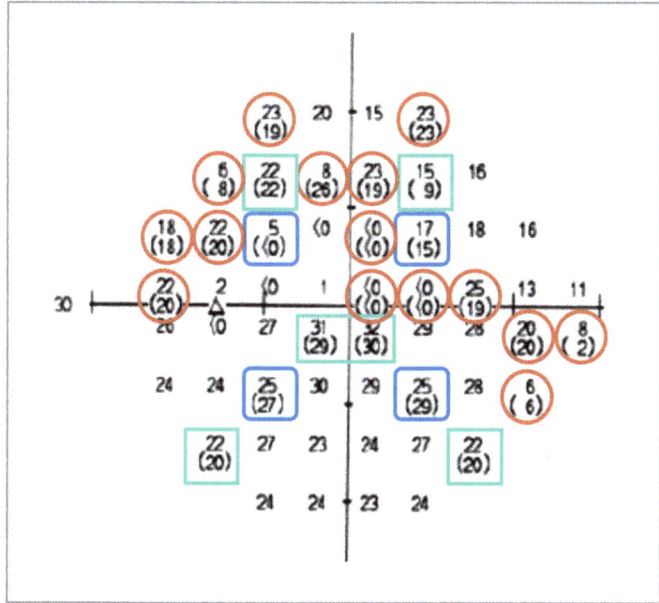

Fig. 8: The green and blue (cardinal spots) boxes are used to calculate short-term fluctuations and are always tested twice in full-threshold strategies. They are also the locations responsible for the clover-leaf pattern because they are examined first. Red circles indicate the locations that had to be retested. The value in brackets is from the second time the locations was tested.

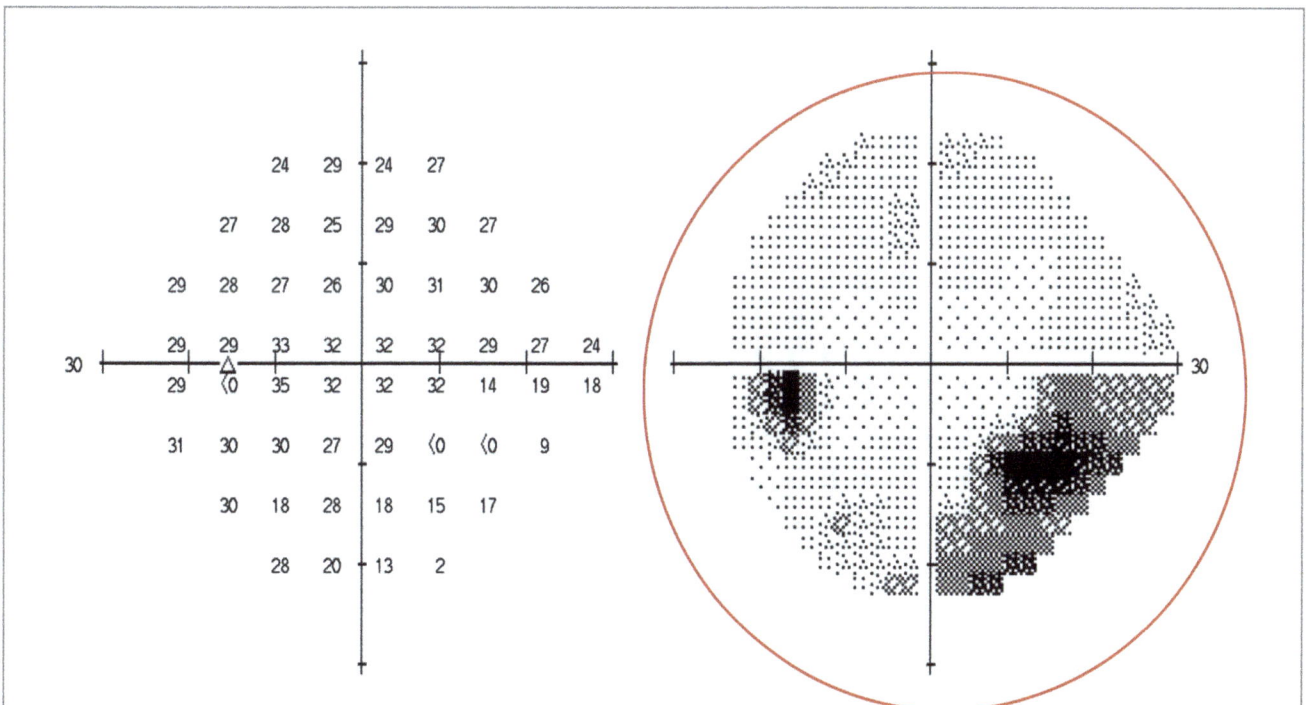

Fig. 9: In the greyscale graph (circled in red) we can see that spots with sensitivity of 0 dB appear black, spots with diminished sensitivity appear gray, and spots with higher sensitivity light gray. The blind spot can be identified as a black area in the lower-temporal quadrant.

Total Deviation Map

This plot represents a point-to-point comparison (difference) between the sensitivity of the patient and that of healthy patients of the same age. Therefore, it shows how much the patient deviates from what's normal for his age group at each location. If the sensitivity at a given location is the same as expected, the map displays a "0", but points with lower-than-normal sensitivities are expressed with a negative decibel value and spots with a higher sensitivity have a positive value (*see* **Fig. 8**).

Pattern Deviation Map

This plot also represents a point-to-point comparison between the sensitivity of the patient and that of healthy patients of the same age, but after adjusting the hill of vision, to dismiss the effect of generalized depression. It uses the seventh best sensitivity of the total deviation map as representative of generalized depression, and subtracts that value from all locations, highlighting subtle localized defects by increasingly darker probability symbols **(Fig. 10)**.[12]

The following example may better illustrate how to calculate the pattern deviation. After dismissing the most peripheral points and those adjacent to the blind spot, the seventh best value of the total deviation plot is found. Then, the sensitivity of this point is reset to 0 (which means zero deviation from normal) and the rest of the plot is adjusted accordingly **(Fig. 11)**.

Both the total deviation map and the pattern deviation map are expressed in numbers in the upper graph and in a probability map in the graph beneath them. In the later, statistical significance of the deviation at each point is plotted. The intensity of the gray indicates the probability

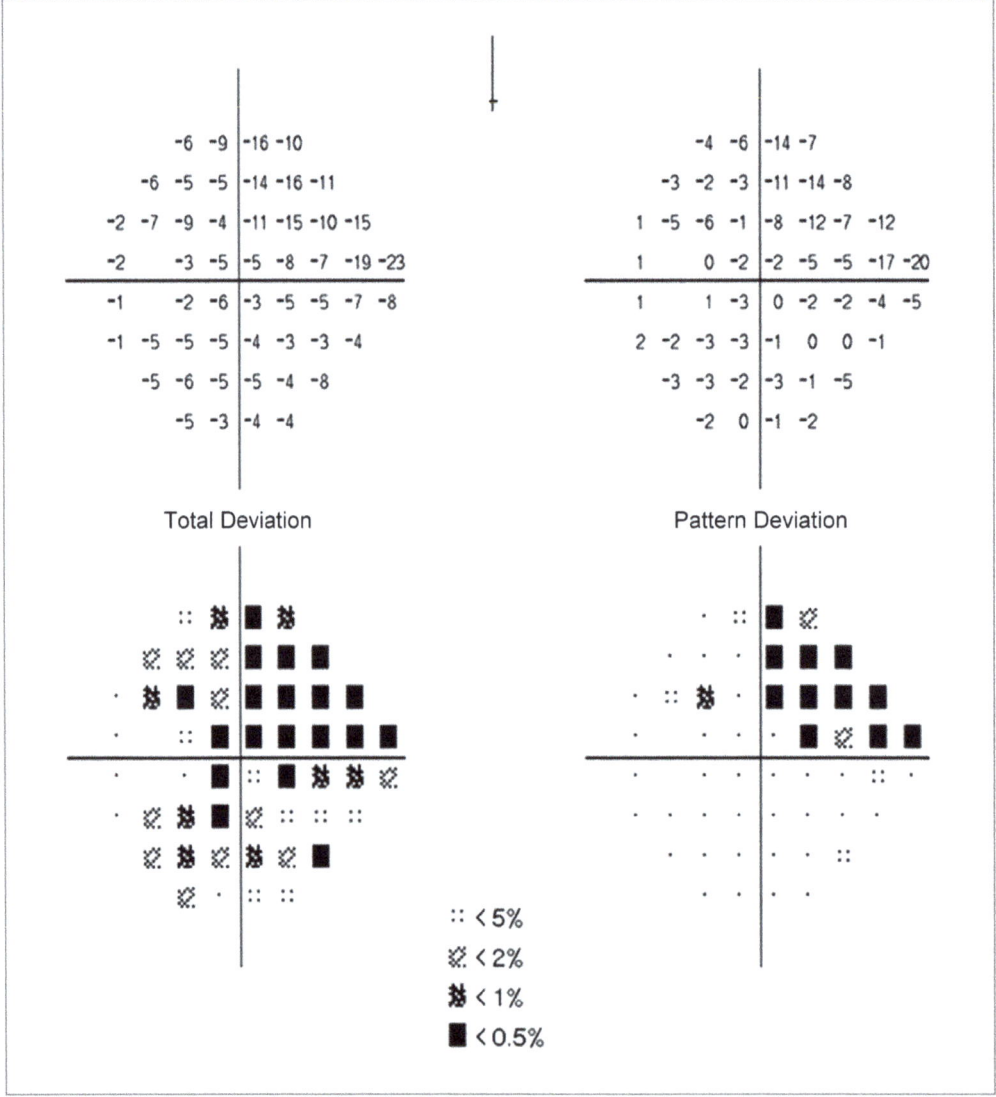

Fig. 10: Total deviation map and pattern deviation map. In this example, the seventh best value of the total deviation map is –3 dB, so the pattern deviation map shows all values as 3 dB better, effectively removing the generalized depression and highlighting the localized defect.

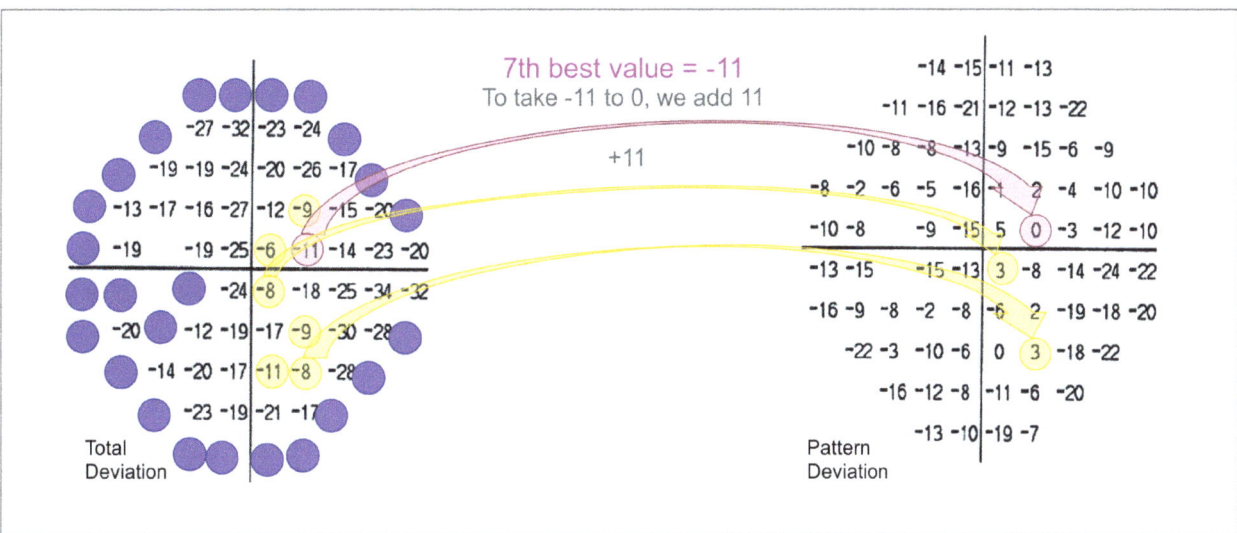

Fig. 11: Conversion from total deviation map to pattern deviation map. Purple circles are the values dismissed (peripherical and adjacent to the blind spot), yellow circles are the first to sixth best values, pink circle on the total deviation map is the seventh best value and is adjusted to 0 in the pattern deviation map. Yellow arrows represent how a –8 in the total deviation map is converted to three in the pattern deviation map.

that the deviation found in each point occurs in <5, 2, 1, and 0.5% of the normal population. The significance of each symbol is printed in the lower right corner of the printout, or between the two probability maps (depending on the software version of the HFA (*see* **Figs. 1 and 10**).

When glaucomatous damage is too severe, the pattern deviation map is not shown, instead, the printout shows a legend that reads "Pattern Deviation is not shown for severely depressed fields. Refer to total deviation." **(Figs. 12A and B)**.

The probability maps of the total deviation and pattern deviation maps must be compared between them to gain extra information. If they are similar, there is almost no generalized depression and the injury to the retina, the optic nerve or the visual pathway is real. If the total deviation map is worse than the pattern deviation plot, there is a generalized depression that may or may not be accompanied by a real lesion to the retina, optic nerve, or visual pathway. If, on the other hand, the total deviation map is affected but the pattern deviation map is clean (normal), this indicates a generalized depression without a localized defect. This can be due to cataracts, a small pupil, or a wrong refraction. If the pattern deviation map is worse than the total deviation map, we should double check the reliability indices, for we are probably dealing with a "happy trigger" patient **(Figs. 13A to C)**.

■ GLOBAL INDICES

They represent a global assessment of the visual field.

Visual Field Index

The visual field index (VFI) is a measurement that quantifies the percentage of residual visual field and healthy ganglion cells in a patient compared to normal subjects of the same age. This is done on a scale ranging from 0% (perimetrically blind) to 100% (normal field), as shown in **Figures 12A and B**.

The VFI takes into account the severity and location of the defects, with more weight given to central losses due to the larger number of ganglion cells devoted to central vision. Unlike other measurements, it is not heavily influenced by cataracts and other media opacities, making it a reliable tool to measure progression rate by trend analysis.

The calculation of VFI differs depending on the MD value. In cases, where the MD is better than –20 dB, it is calculated from the pattern deviation map. However, in cases, where the MD is worse than –20 dB, it is calculated from the total deviation plot and its value decreases accordingly.

Mean Deviation

The MD is the average of the values on the total deviation numerical plot. Negative values indicate that the mean sensitivity of the subject is lower than that of individuals of his same age. Positive values are supranormal. It tends to be near 0 dB in normal fields, since it expresses that most locations have values close to those expected for the age group.

The MD normal values range from +2 to –2 dB. MD from –2 dB to –6 dB indicate mild damage. Moderate damage has a MD of –6 to –12, and severe damage worse than –12 dB. A value of –24 dB or worse is usually associated with significant disability.

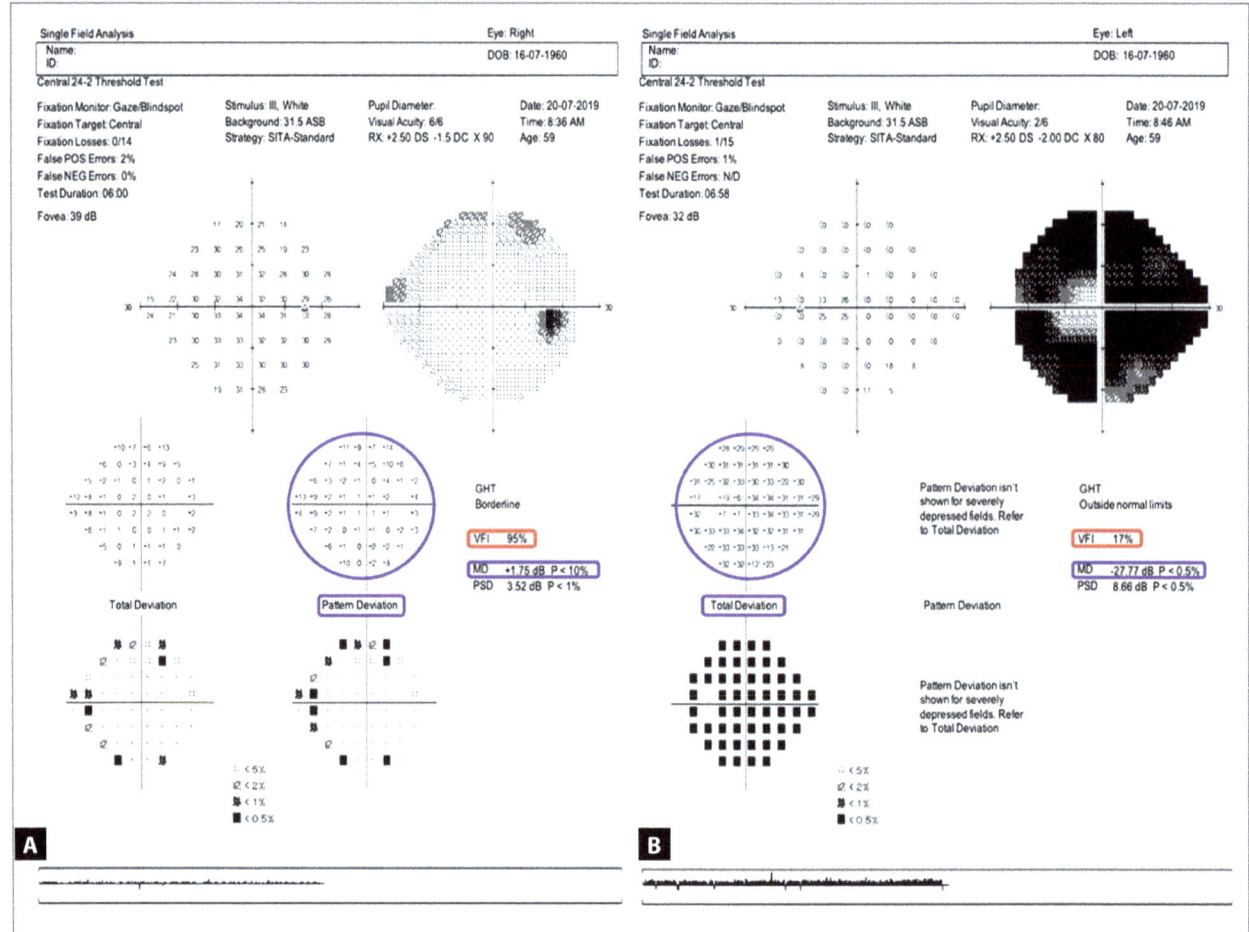

Figs. 12A and B: Visual field index (VFI). (A) Borderline visual field with a DM >−20 dB where the VFI of 95% was calculated from the pattern deviation plot. Note that despite 14 abnormal locations in the pattern deviation map, those locations are peripheral so the impact on VFI is not as strong; (B) Visual field with severe glaucomatous damage with a DM <−20 dB and a VFI of 17% that was calculated from the total deviation map.

It is commonly used for staging of visual field loss and also to measure the global rate of change overtime.

Pattern Standard Deviation

The PSD is the standard deviation of the MD, obtained from the total deviation numerical plot. It evaluates the changes in the shape of the hill of vision with respect to a pattern expected by age to estimate the amount of localized loss in a given visual field. A high PSD (>2.00) indicates there is a localized scotoma and it tends to increase if the scotoma worsens. It is not affected by generalized depression, but highly altered by localized defects, so it has a high sensitivity for early defects, but loses usefulness in advanced glaucomas, as the sensitivity loss becomes more homogenous.

Statistical Probability

If the values of any global index are outside the normal range, a p appears after the index with one of the following values: $p < 10\%$, $p < 5\%$, $p < 2\%$, $p < 1\%$ or $p < 0.5\%$. These p values indicate the statistical probability that the global index study is pathological with respect to a group of normal subjects of the same age.

■ GLAUCOMA HEMIFIELD TEST

The glaucoma hemifield test (GHT) evaluates asymmetry through the horizontal meridian. It compares the MD of five known zones in the superior hemifield with its five mirror zones in the inferior hemifield. All points evaluated are shared for both 24-2 and 30-2 patterns. The GHT gives one of six results:[13,14]

1. *Within normal limits:* There is no significant difference between the zones of the superior and the inferior hemifield. Sensitivity is approximately 99.5%.
2. *Outside normal limits:* The differences between the superior and inferior hemifield are greater than expected in 99% of the population. In other words, it is observed in <1% of normal subjects.

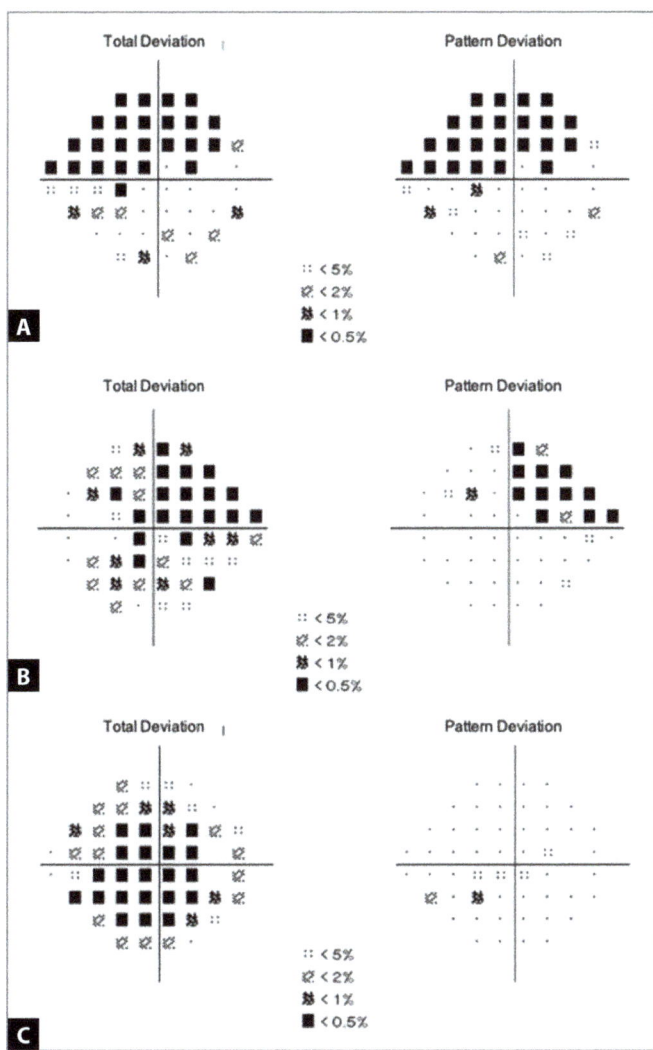

Figs. 13A to C: (A) The total deviation map is similar to the pattern deviation map; the defect is almost purely localized; (B) The total deviation map is worse than the pattern deviation map, and an additional localized defect is evident; and (C) The total deviation map is worse than the pattern deviation map, which means the defect is generalized depression.

3. *Borderline:* When differences in at least two zones are greater than expected in 97–99% of normal population. It is found in <3% but >1% of normal subjects.
4. *General reduction of sensitivity:* General sensitivity is below that expected in 99.5% of the normal population, but there are no differences between the superior and inferior hemifields of the visual field.
5. *Abnormally high sensitivity:* General sensitivity is higher than expected, that is >99.5%.
6. Borderline/general reduction of sensitivity

CONCLUSION

The Single-Field analysis is a critical tool in the diagnosis and monitoring of glaucoma and many neurological disorders of the visual pathways. Early detection of visual field defects is crucial for preventing irreversible damage to the optic nerve and preserving vision. Therefore, it is essential to have a solid understanding of the typical patterns of visual fields in glaucoma and those that are not glaucoma.

Analyzing a SFA requires a high degree of clinical expertise and attention to detail. It is important to pay close attention to the reliability indexes (fixation losses, FPs, and FNs), the GHT, and the global and local indices, including MD, and PSD. A small deviation from normal values could indicate early glaucomatous damage and warrant further investigation.

REFERENCES

1. Elze T, Pasquale LR, Shen LQ. Patterns of functional vision loss in glaucoma determined with archetypal analysis. J R Soc Interface. 2015;12(103).
2. Heijl A, Patella VM, Bengtsson B. The field analyzer primer: Effective Perimetry, 4th edition. Dublin, CA: Carl Zeiss Meditec Inc.; 2012.
3. Crabb DP. Visual Fields. Sherwood M, Hitchings R, Crowston J Shaarawy T. Glaucoma, 2nd edition. Philadelphia: Elsevier; 2014. pp. 109-22.
4. Mansoori T. Humphrey visual field printout: Illumination matters. Indian J Ophthalmol. 2019;67(8):1383-4.
5. Bengtsson B, Heijl A. Evaluation of a new perimetric threshold strategy, SITA, in patients with manifest and suspect glaucoma. Acta Ophthalmol Scand. 1998;76(3):268-72.
6. Akar Y, Yilmaz A, Yucel I. Assessment of an effective visual field testing strategy for a normal paediatric. Ophthalmologica. 2008;222(5):329-33.
7. Shirato S, Inoue R, Fukushima K, Suzuki Y. Clinical evaluation of SITA: a new family of perimetric testing strategies. Graefes Arch Clin Exp Ophthalmol. 1999;237(1):29-34.
8. Patel DE, Cumberland PM, Walters BC, Russell-Eggitt I, Cortina-Borja M, Rahi JS; OPTIC Study Group. Study of Optimal Perimetric Testing In Children (OPTIC): Normative Visual Field Values in Children. Ophthalmology. 2015;122(8):1711-7.
9. Miller BA, Gelber EC. Aphakic visual fields by automated perimetry. Ann Ophthalmol. 1990;22(11):419-22.
10. Gonzalez de la Rosa M, Pareja A. Influence of the "fatigue effect" On the mean deviation measurement in perimetry. Eur J Ophthalmol. 1997;7(1): 29-34.
11. Matsuda A, Hara T, Miyata K, Matsuo H, Murata H, Mayama C, Asaoka R. Do pattern deviation values accurately estimate glaucomatous visual field damage in eyes with glaucoma and cataract? Br J ophthalmol. 2015;99(9):1240-4.
12. Katz J, Quigley HA, Sommer A. Repeatability of the glaucoma hemifield test in automated perimetry. Invest Ophthalmol Vis Sci. 1995;36(8):1658-64.
13. Junoy Montolio FG, Wesselink C, Gordijn M, Jansonius NM. Factors that influence standard automated perimetry test results in glaucoma: test reliability, technician experience, time of day, and season. Invest Ophthalmol Vis Sci. 2012;53(11):7010-7.
14. Asman P, Heijl A. Glaucoma Hemifield Test. Automated visual field evaluation. Arch Ophthalmol. 1992;110(6):812-9.

CHAPTER 4

Octopus Perimetry: Analyzing the Single Field Report

Ann Mary Mathews, Mohana Sinnasamy, Murali Ariga

▪ INTRODUCTION

Single field reports give a cross-sectional assessment of the visual field at a particular point of time. This assessment is given in different formats with each format designed to give a feature of clinical relevance based on the raw data. Each representation is suited for a particular aspect of the visual field and aids in clinical decisions. This chapter aims to introduce the various representations of raw data with examples of normal and abnormal fields and an approach to interpret the single visual field reports of Octopus perimetry.

To study the progression of disease condition or to monitor the effect of management, progression analysis using software is ideally suited. It is used to study the visual fields recorded through different time periods to identify the progression of the condition and efficacy of management. This is discussed in detail in Chapter 7.

▪ PLOTS IN SINGLE VISUAL FIELD REPORTS OF OCTOPUS PERIMETER

In this test, the visual field of the central 30° is usually tested. This raw data is presented as a seven-in-one report in Octopus perimeter (**Fig. 1**). The approach to interpret this visual field is usually done in 10 steps. The seven-in-one report contains the following representations:
1. Details of the patient identification and examination parameters
2. Gray-scale presentation
3. Value table
4. Comparison table
5. Corrected comparison table
6. Comparison probability plot
7. Corrected comparison probability plot
8. Defect curve
9. Global indices
10. Cluster analysis and polar graph

Details of the Patient and Examination Parameters

The patient details (**Box 1**) are used to identify and compare the visual field of the patient to the normative database. Hence, the visual field representations in the report are influenced by the accuracy of the data entered. Inaccuracy in the date of birth may result in comparing the patient's visual field with age group that is different from the patient's age group. This can lead to false defects or false normal defects. Similarly, incorrect pupil size and uncorrected refractive errors can lead to diffuse reduction in the sensitivity. An example of patient and examination parameters from a visual field report is shown in **Figure 2**.

Reliability Indices

Next, the visual field report needs to be ensured whether it is reliable as it is vital before proceeding with using the result in clinical management. Many factors such as fatigue, difficulty in performing the test or intent to get a normal result or due to error in positioning the patient, or refraction are few reasons that can result in unreliable results.

Reliability indices in Octopus perimeter help to ascertain the reliability of a visual field report. The important among these indices are false-positive and false-negative answers. False positives and negatives >15% are marked in orange color and should be interpreted with caution; when false-positives and false-negatives are greater than 33% they are usually not acceptable and are marked in red.[1,2]

In case of interpreting the reliability factor and false-positive and -negative responses, it is important to understand that values >20% in false-negative responses can be seen in advanced glaucoma and retesting will not yield different results.

Also, the visual field examiner should be observing the patient throughout the testing duration and any deviation from normal should be documented in the report. Another factor that can affect the reliability of the report can be the

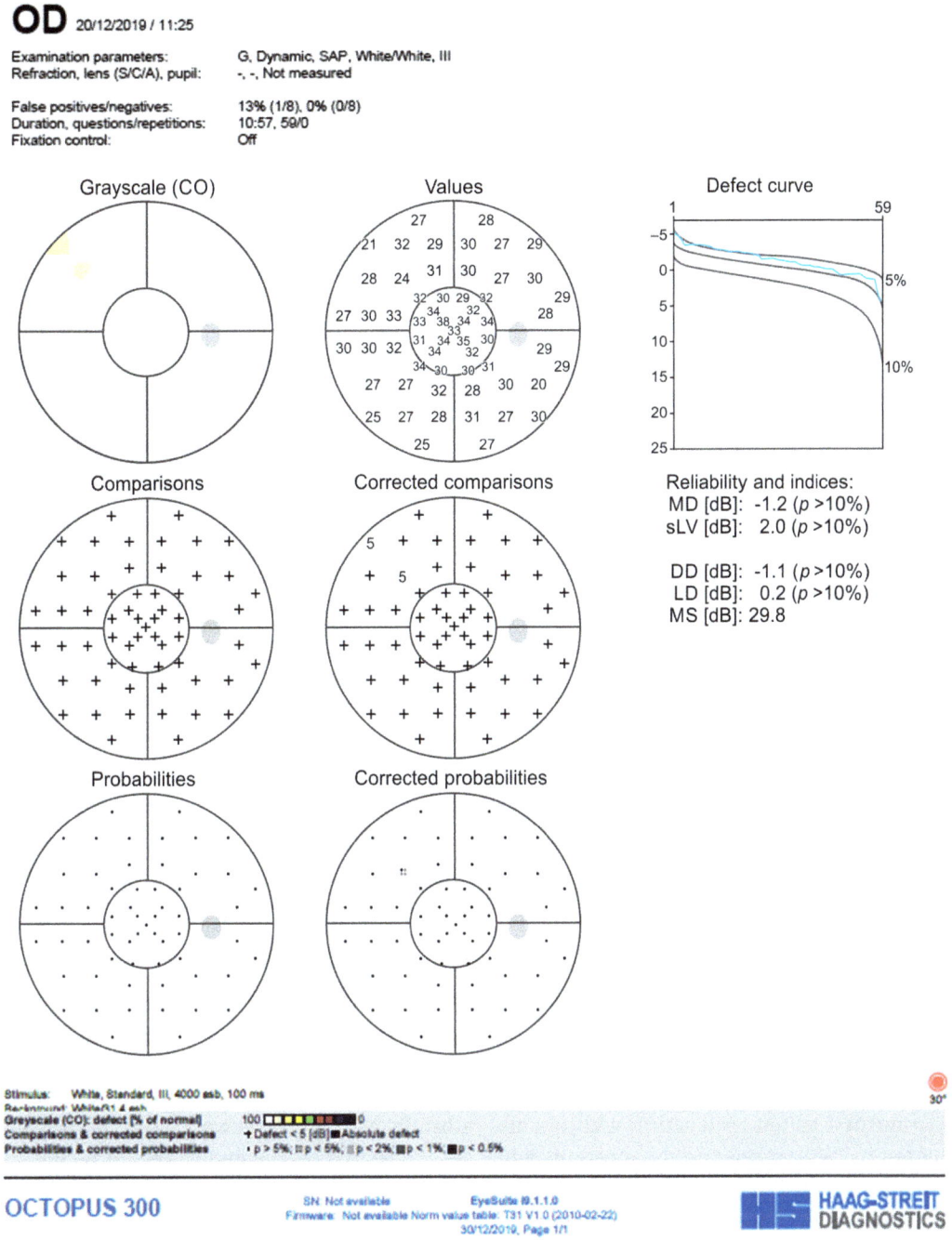

Fig. 1: Seven-in-one visual field report by Octopus perimeter.
(DD: diffuse defect; LD: local defect; MD: mean defect; MS: mean sensitivity; sLV: square root of loss of variance)
Courtesy: Haag-Streit Diagnostics.

long duration of testing as this suggests the patient's difficulty in performing the test and leads to fatigue in the patient.[3]

Grayscale

The grayscale representation of the visual field is color coded and offers a rough assessment of the central 30° field. The color used denotes the severity of the visual field defects. The darker the color, the greater is the reduction in sensitivity of the visual field. **Figure 3** shows grayscale representation of visual fields.

Value Table

Value table gives the threshold sensitivity of each test point in dB. It is right to the grayscale in the visual field report.

BOX 1: Parameters of patient and examination.
- Patient's name/hospital number
- Date of birth and age
- Eye tested
- Date and time of test
- Test pattern and strategy
- Stimulus type
- Maximum stimulus intensity and background luminance
- Refraction
- Pupil size

Surname, Name, 01/01/1933 (93 years) Right eye (OD)/01/25/2023/18:24:35	
Examination parameters:	G, Dynamic, SAP, White/White, III
Refraction, lens (S/C/A), pupil:	-, -, Not measured
False positives/negatives:	13% (1/8), 0% (0/8)
Duration, questions/repetitions:	10:57, 59/0
Fixation control	Off

Fig. 2: An example of patient and examination parameter displayed in visual field report.

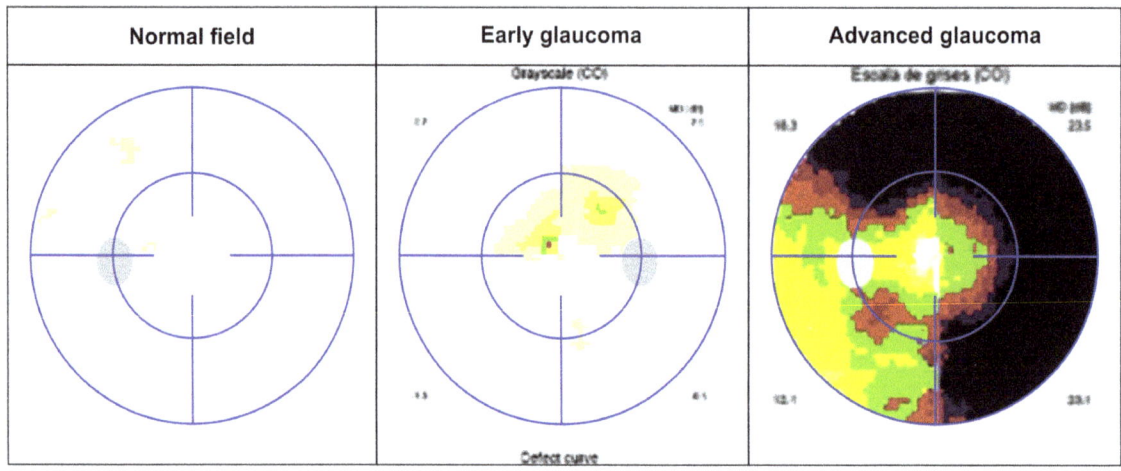

Fig. 3: Grayscale representation of visual fields seen in early and advanced glaucoma.

It is important to understand that the values are absolute and are not compared with the normal values. This is usually not used in clinical practice.

Comparison Table and Comparison Probability Plot

The comparison table gives the sensitivity compared to the age-corrected normal values. A location with normal sensitivity is denoted by "+" symbol and the locations with reduced sensitivity are denoted with the values. The black squares in this plot denote locations of zero sensitivity.

Comparison probability plot shows the statistical probability of the test location to have normal sensitivity. This plot is age corrected and is coded with dots and shades. The code is explained next to the plot in %, wherein $p < 5$ indicates reduced sensitivity while $p < 1$ indicates a strong probability that the test location has reduced sensitivity.

These plots are affected by both local and diffuse causes of visual field defects, and hence, it is prudent to understand that a defect in a particular location in these plots could be due to additive effects of both local and diffuse causes. For example, a test location showing a reduced sensitivity may be due to both cataract and glaucoma.

Corrected Comparison Table and Corrected Comparison Probability Plot

Subtle changes in field defects can be normal or reflect early glaucomatous changes. Fluctuations in the visual field can be seen in healthy eyes as well. In practice, differentiating normal and abnormal visual fields can be simplified by probability plots. To facilitate this, it is necessary to eliminate the effects of diffuse loss and study the defects caused only by the focal loss of sensitivity. The corrected comparison table and corrected comparison probability plot aid in eliminating the changes due to other causes, reflecting the defects due to local effect only. These are especially important plots in early-to-moderate conditions compared to advanced disease.

The corrected comparison table shows the values corrected for the effects of diffuse losses, reflecting the loss of sensitivities due to local defects only. Corrected comparison probability plot shows the probability that the field defects in the corrected comparison table are due to a disease condition and not due to normal fluctuations seen in healthy eyes. This is done by comparing the data with the field of health of a person of the same age. The darker the color in probability, the more severe the reduction in sensitivity.

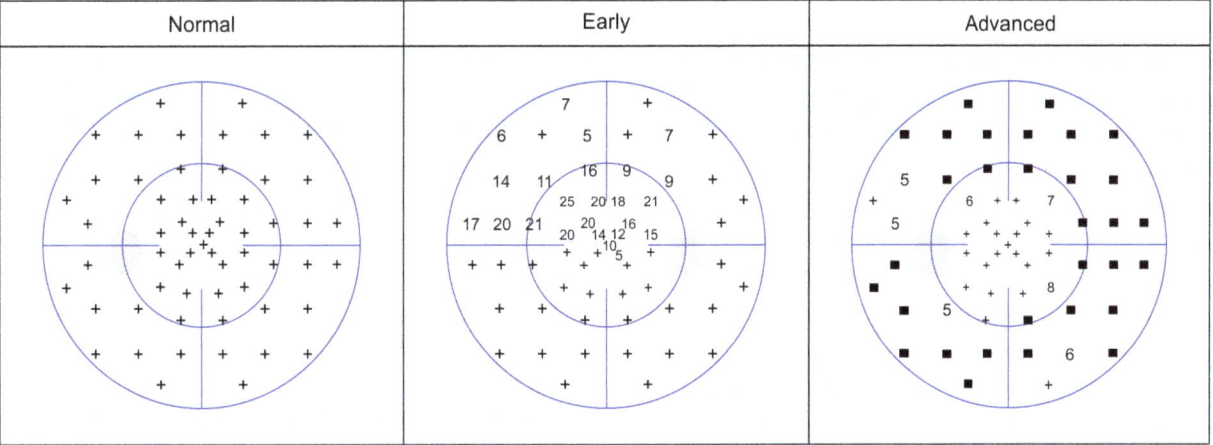

Fig. 4: Corrected comparison plot of visual field seen in early and advanced glaucoma.

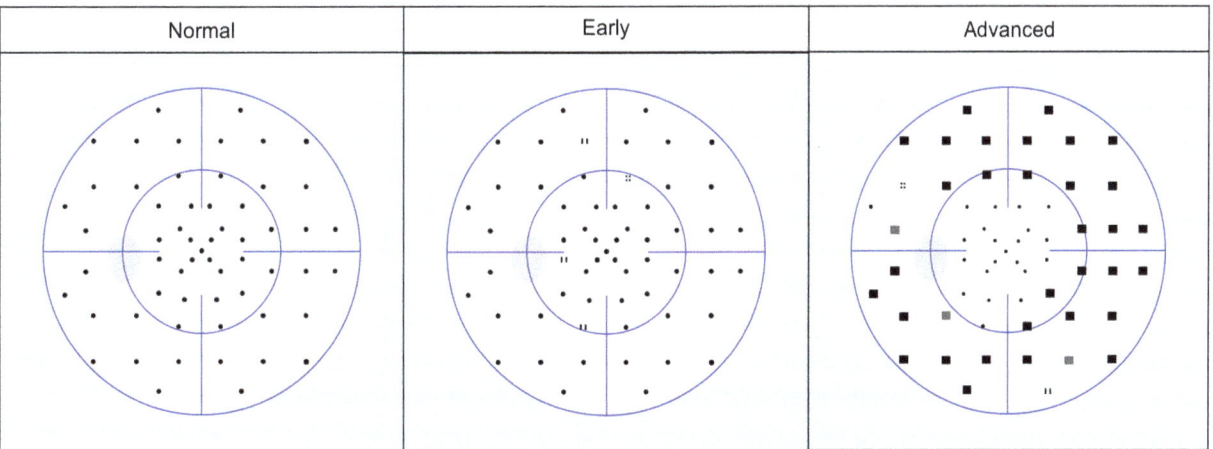

Fig. 5: Corrected comparison probability plot of visual field seen in early and advanced glaucoma.

Figure 4 shows corrected comparison plots and **Figure 5** shows corrected probability plots of visual fields seen in early and advanced glaucoma.

Defect Curve

Defect curve plots the sensitivity values of all the test locations with the highest sensitivity to the lowest from left to right. The plotted curve can be compared with the normal band given as the three blue lines in the plot with the upper and lower lines representing 90% confidence interval. This helps to differentiate between local and diffuse defects.[4]

When the test curve contains all its points within the normal values, it is a normal visual field. In case of diffuse defects, the test curve parallels the normal curve, but it is shifted below the normal curve. While in case of local defects, the curve remains within the normal band on the left side and falls steeply down on the right side as the points of lower sensitivities are plotted.

In clinical practice, it is not uncommon to see patients with both local and diffuse defects, such as having glaucoma and cataract in the same eye. In such cases, the curve is shifted below the normal band with steep descent in its right side, indicating the presence of both diffuse and local defects. **Figure 6** shows defect curves seen in local defect, in diffuse defect, and in combination of local and diffuse defects.

In clinical practice, when a defect curve shows a diffuse defect, it is important to look for a pathology causing it. If no pathology is identified, this indicates an unreliable test and should be repeated if appropriate.

Global Indices

Given in the right of the report are the global indices. They give quantitative assessment of the visual field which helps in grading the severity of field defects. These are as follows:
- *Mean defect (MD):* MD summarizes the overall sensitivity of the field and helps in assessing the progression of the

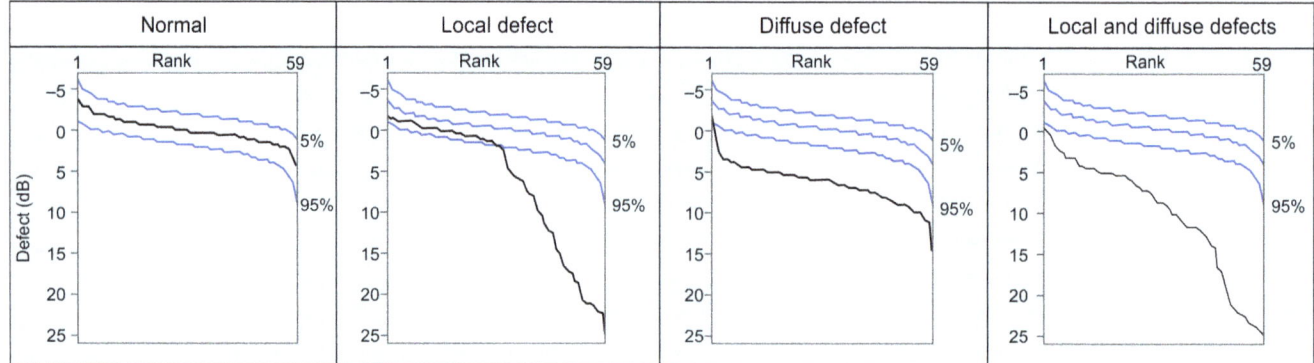

Fig. 6: Defect curves seen in local defect, diffuse defect, and in combination of both local and diffuse defects.

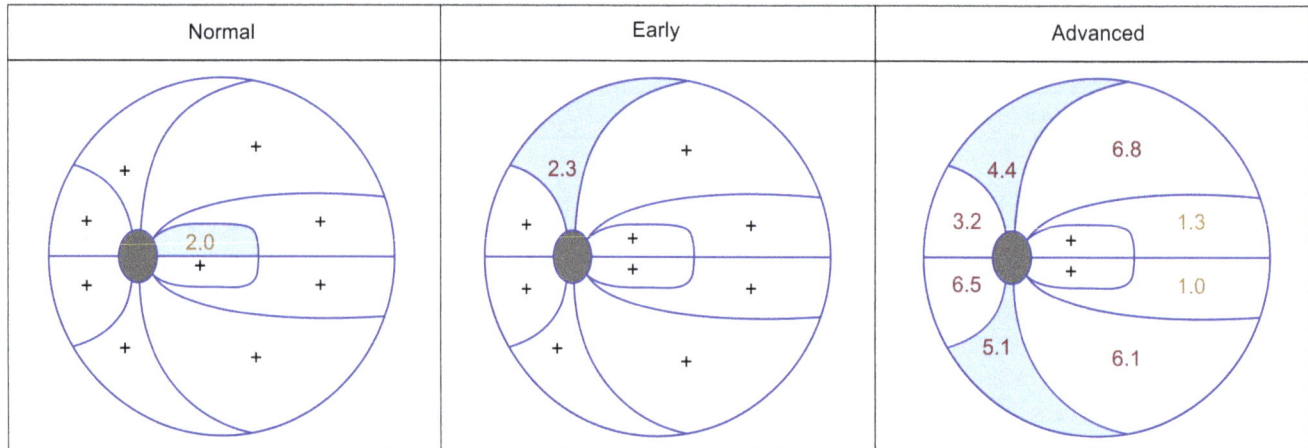

Fig. 7: Corrected cluster analysis of visual fields seen in early and advanced glaucoma.

disease.[5] It is influenced by both diffuse and local defects. The higher the MD, the greater the visual field defect.

- *Square root of loss of variance (sLV):* sLV provides the degree of variation in the sensitivities throughout the entire field. Unlike MD which gives an overall estimation of visual field defects, sLV helps in distinguishing the local and diffuse defects. If sLV is small, it indicates less variation among the sensitivities in the field. This may indicate both normal field and very advanced disease. In early-to-moderate severity, the variation is high, and thereby, sLV is high as well.

Cluster Analysis and Corrected Cluster Analysis

Cluster analysis gives the cluster mean defect of an individual cluster of the 10 clusters in the central 30° visual field and the corrected cluster analysis; the sensitivity values of clusters are corrected for diffuse loss of sensitivity such as cataract. It is highly sensitive to glaucoma and is designed specifically for it. This aids in identifying the exact location of reduced sensitivity structurally.[6,7]

During visual field testing, the test points in the central 30° visual field area are grouped into 10 clusters. All test points of a cluster follow the same retinal nerve fiber bundle. When there is a reduced sensitivity in a cluster in cluster analysis, it shows the structural location that is affected. This helps to identify the affected area structurally and correlate it clinically. For example, if cluster analysis shows reduced sensitivity of the cluster that represents a paracentral area, it warrants an urgent intervention to salvage the fixation area. **Figure 7** shows the corrected cluster analysis of visual fields seen in early and advanced glaucoma.

Polar Graph

The polar graph is a representation of sensitivities along the border of optic disc. In this representation, the sensitivities are represented as red bars plotted in the location of the corresponding disc edge. The length of the bar corresponds to the degree of reduction in sensitivity in that location. This plot aids in identifying the structural location of the affected neuroretinal rim and nerve fiber layer. These have been correlated with optical coherence tomography (OCT) results with good accuracy.[8] **Figure 8** shows the polar graph seen in early and advanced glaucoma.

CHAPTER 4: Octopus Perimetry: Analyzing the Single Field Report

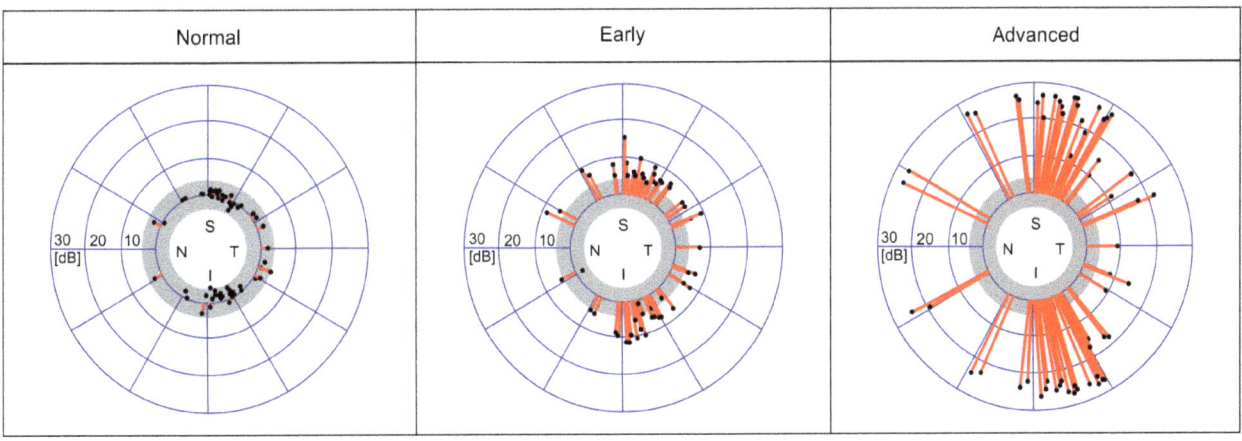

Fig. 8: Polar graph of visual fields seen in early and advanced glaucoma.

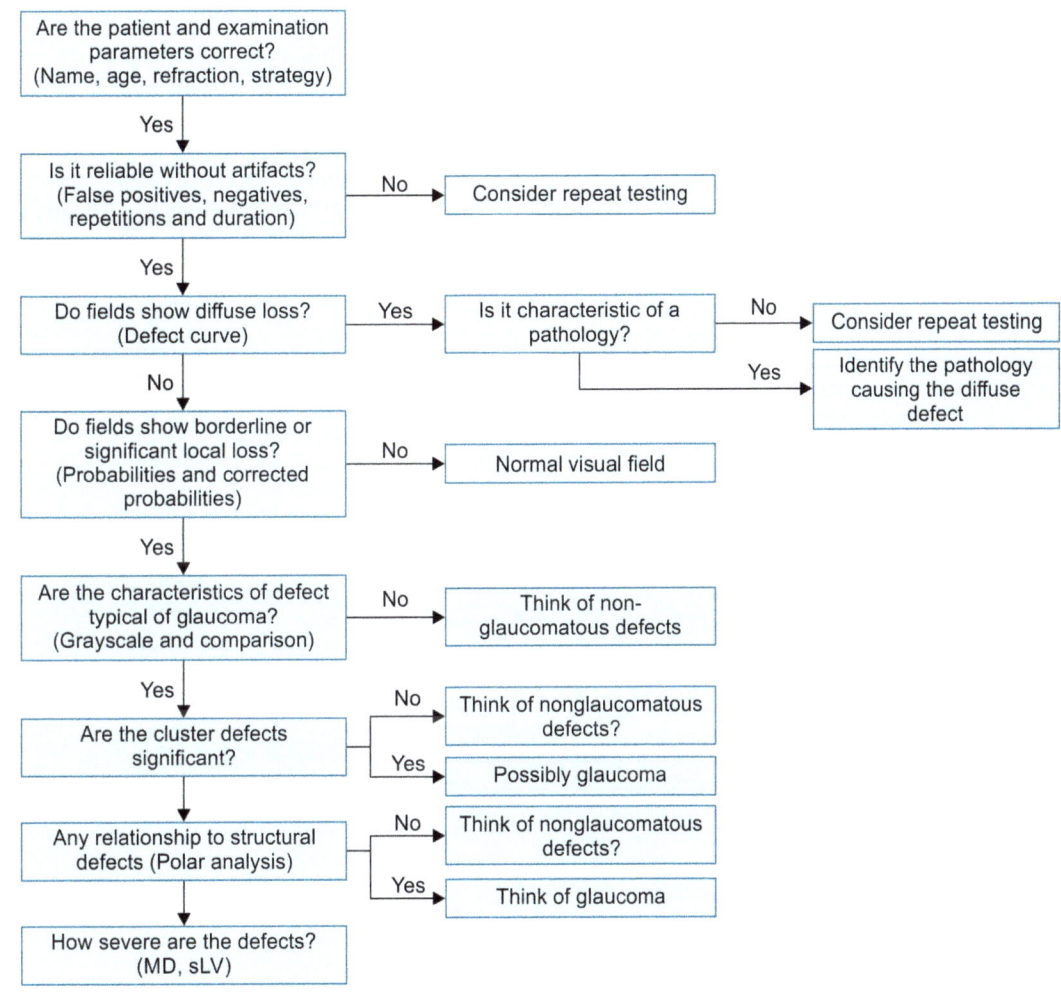

Flowchart 1: Step-by-step approach to interpret single Octopus visual field report.[9]

(MD: mean defect; sLV: square root of loss of variance)

APPROACH TO INTERPRET THE SINGLE VISUAL FIELD REPORT

The single visual field report in Octopus should be approached step-by-step, beginning from checking the patient identification and reliability. Diffuse loss if present is identified, and later the local defects are studied for severity and nature of the defect. Then the clusters affected are analyzed and are located anatomically with cluster analysis and polar graph. **Flowchart 1** shows a practical approach to interpret the visual field report from Octopus perimeter.

CONCLUSION

Single visual field report from Octopus perimeter consists of various representations, each highlighting a clinical aspect of visual field test. These plots designed to understand from the overall visual field sensitivity to studying each cluster of visual field in the central 30° facilitate identifying diffuse defects, local defects, depth, severity, and characteristic of field defects. These aid in diagnosing the condition causing the defect and its severity and in locating the retinal nerve fiber bundle spatially.

A structured approach in interpreting the single visual field report can offer the clinician a great wealth of information, thus helping in distinguishing between normal and abnormal visual field changes and identifying subtle changes early. It aids in early identification of glaucoma and initiation of management.

REFERENCES

1. Lee M, Zulauf M, Caprioli J. The influence of patient reliability on visual field outcome. Am J Ophthalmol. 1994;117:756-61.
2. Yohannan J, Wang J, Brown J, Chauhan BC, Boland MV, Friedman DS, et al. Evidence-based criteria for assessment of visual field reliability. Ophthalmology. 2017;124:1612-20.
3. Bengtsson B, Heijl A. False-negative responses in glaucoma perimetry: indicators of patient performance or test reliability? Invest Ophthalmol Vis Sci. 2000;41(8):2201-4. PMID: 10892863.
4. Bebie H, Flammer J, Bebie T. The cumulative defect curve: Separation of local and diffuse components of visual field damage. Graefe's Arch Clin Exp Ophthalmol. 1989;227:9-12.
5. Flammer J. The concept of visual field indices. Graefe's Arch Clin Exp Ophthalmol. 1986;224:389-92.
6. Naghizadeh F, Holló G. Detection of early glaucomatous progression with Octopus cluster trend analysis. J Glaucoma. 2014;23:269-75.
7. Gardiner SK, Mansberger SL, Demirel S. Detection of functional change using Cluster Trend Analysis in glaucoma. Invest Ophthalmol Vis Sci. 2017;58:BIO180-90.
8. Holló G, Naghizadeh F. Evaluation of Octopus Polar Trend Analysis for detection of glaucomatous progression. Eur J Ophthalmol. 2014;24:862-8.
9. Racette L, Fischer M, Bebie H, Holló G, Johnson C, Matsumoto C. Visual Field Digest: A guide to perimetry and the Octopus perimeter, 6th edition. Köniz, Switzerland: Haag-Streit AG; 2016.

CHAPTER 5

Pearls and Pitfalls in Perimetry

Parul Ichhpujani, Neiwete Lomi, Savleen Kaur, Surinder Singh Pandav, Sushmita Kaushik

■ INTRODUCTION

Visual field examination has been the gold standard to detect structural loss in glaucoma for decades now. The technique has undergone a paradigm shift from kinetic to static and now to automated perimetry. Automated perimeters make our work as glaucoma specialists much simpler but at the same time are not without their own limitations. Common pitfalls in perimetry at the time of testing as well as assessment can lead to misdiagnosis in many situations.

■ PRACTICAL PEARLS IN RECORDING FIELDS

- Always apprise the patient about the procedure before starting.
- Movements of the other eye can cause watering and discomfort; therefore, close the other eye well.
- The patient must be told that he/she can ask to pause the test in between if he/she is tired or his/her eyes are watering.
- The patient should have taken enough rest between right and left eye testing and ensure that he/she is attentive.
- If the patient has a poor attention span, one can select faster tests such as 24-2 SITA Fast. If a test result is abnormal or shows progression, always repeat the test.
- The patient should be reassured that during the field recording, >50% of the light spots will not be seen.
- Always record the visual fields on the same program which has been used earlier for better and meaningful comparisons.

Data Entry

Correct data entry is the most important step. The following entries must be carefully made:
- Date and time
- *Patient's name, hospital identification number, and date of birth:* For a correct sequential analysis of fields done over the follow-up visits, a patient's identification details must be entered exactly in the same fashion, as these details help to differentiate patients with the same name. A patient's perimetric outcomes are compared with a normative database of the same age group.
- *Best corrected visual acuity, pupil diameter, and spectacle prescription:* For sequential comparisons, one must look if any of these factors are changing:
  • A change in pupil diameter from 4 to 2 mm results in reduction of sensitivity by approximately 0.7 dB.
  • If the patient has been instilling pilocarpine or has senile miosis, dilate all miotic pupils to >2.5 mm for perimetry.
  • Refractive blur due to uncorrected refractive error will also cause diffuse increase in thresholds.
- *The eye being tested and the type of test:* Correctly enter the eye being tested and choose the appropriate type of test, namely 30-2, 24-2, 10-2, or macula test.
- Monitoring the fixation on the eye position monitor

Patient Placement

- The eye not being tested must be occluded with a nonprotruding patch, close to the nose to avoid obscuring the vision of the eye being tested.
- Discomfort resulting from poor posture will degrade the test performance; therefore, adjust the chair or the machine as per the patient's height. The buzzer must be in the patient's dominant hand.
- The eye being tested must be centered in the cross hairs of the eye position monitor. The chin holder may be adjusted by means of dials on the side of the machine.
- Lens must be placed as close to the patient's eye as possible. Eye lashes must not touch the lens. If the lens holder is positioned away from the patient, it may obscure the view of the test area. Always flip the lens holder out of the way for an emmetrope.

- Face mask-related artifacts have been commonly noted in the inferior field, followed by the central area. These artifacts could be mistaken for glaucoma progression damage. Therefore, if a patient is wearing a surgical face mask while performing perimetry, to reduce the breath-related and position-related artifacts, the mask must be secured with an adhesive tape on the superior border.

Instructions to the Patient

Clear instructions and counseling greatly increase the likelihood of obtaining useful data, particularly in those new to the test. The following key points must be emphasized:
- It is better to give a short demonstration to the patient, to apprise the patient as regards the target "flashes" and the concept of fixation.
- The patient must always look at the yellow light at the center. If the screen monitor shows that the patient is repeatedly looking away, then the test becomes meaningless due to fixation losses (FLs).
- While the patient is fixing on the central yellow light, the computer will flash light spots at random locations in their side field. The patient must press the button in their hand every time they see a flash of light.
- For a threshold test, at each location the machine tries to delineate the boundary between the visible and the invisible. One possibility is that there will always be some very faint lights that the patient does not see. The second possibility is that the lights very close to the boundary will be quite dim and the patient will be uncertain of their presence. The patient must respond if they perceive a dim flash.
- The patient should blink from time to time. Blinking just after they see a target is the best time as there is always a short interval between one target and the next.
- Typically, a threshold test takes about 10 minutes per eye.
- After completion of the test of one eye, the occlude is removed and time is given to the occluded eye to recover from its dark adaptation state.

Threshold Perimetry Analysis: Single-field Analysis

Check the patient's name, date of birth, and the refraction used.

Reliability Indices
- *Fixation losses:* From time to time, a target is flashed in the physiologic blind spot; if the patient is not looking at the yellow fixation light, he or she will see the flash and press the button. How many times the perimeter tested with flashes in the blind spot is depicted by the denominator, while the number of times the patient committed the mistake is depicted by the numerator. Frequent FLs compromise the sensitivity of the test to find early defects.

  Heijl–Krakau method of monitoring fixation: In patients with enlarged blind spots or with large visual field defects, low fixation loss indices must be interpreted with caution. Such patients, even if they make large eye movements, may not see the target probing for FL. The disadvantage of this method is that the results cannot be modified by fixation data.

  Newer, automated devices monitor actual eye position with video or infrared technology and either halt testing or exclude trials with improper eye position. The newer Humphrey field analyzers (HFA) use a video system to monitor the eye position and use the data to exclude trials in case of blinks.
- *False positives (FPs):* When the perimetry machine makes a soft click but does not show a target stimulus, an overly sensitive subject may press the buzzer. This will result in a high FP error and will lead to underestimation of the extent and severity of a defect. SITA strategy counts the number of anticipatory responses made too soon after a flash to be a considered as a response to the light.
- *False negatives (FNs):* Using brighter suprathreshold targets helps to enhance the comprehensiveness and accuracy of the visual field testing. The suprathreshold target is introduced in a region previously tested with targets of lesser brightness. If the patient fails to indicate its presence, this is noted as a FN error. A high FN rate implies attention or fatigue, and the printout will show scattered factitious elevations of threshold. For all these reliability indices, essentially an error rate of more than 20% suggests poor reliability. *Flagging* is indicated by an "*xx*" by the side of the abnormal value and the label of "*low patient reliability.*"
- *Time taken to do the test and the number of questions asked:* Some patients may confuse the perimetry machine's algorithms and not allow it to use its statistical shortcuts, leading to longer test duration. Patients with complex visual field defects, (e.g., a glaucoma patient with laser marks due to panretinal photocoagulation for diabetic retinopathy) have longer test duration.

  If the patient is poorly attentive, the technician must tailor the visual field to a faster strategy such as 24-2 SITA Fast.

  The SITA Faster (available on the HFA3) may have a higher number of unreliable tests compared with the SITA Standard test as the stimuli are presented more rapidly.

  Any unexplained progression in the visual field test must be repeatable. Always do visual field testing by using the same program, SITA Fast or SITA Standard.

Additionally, visual field done on two perimetry machines by different manufactures cannot be compared.

PRACTICAL PEARLS IN ASSESSMENT OF FIELDS

One should never comment on the presence or absence of glaucoma based on just the fields, until the patient has been examined **(Fig. 1)**. Old age, ailments, poor attention span, cataract surgery, and the presence of retinal or neurological disease may result in variation in fields and hence, a series of fields are needed to assess progression. If the first field is abnormal, one should repeat it, as 85% of patients will lose the defect on first field (*learning/practice effect*). Two visual fields with reproducible visual field defects are required before commenting on the pattern of the defect and pathology. When a diagnosis is questionable, then the course visual fields take over time along with a structural test such as optical coherence tomography (OCT) helps to arrive at the conclusion, whether it is a glaucomatous visual field defect or not.

Stimulus Size

Changing the stimulus size from Goldmann size III to size V increases the retinal sensitivity from 6 decibels (dB) to 10 dB. This phenomenon, known as "pathologic summation of Dubois-Poulsen," results in an exaggerated improvement in retinal sensitivity. A locus that is 0 dB with a size III stimulus may show an unexpected improvement to 20 dB when tested with a larger stimulus, for example, size V, which is why testing with a larger object may help identify those areas which have functional vision, especially in patients with advanced visual field defects.

PITFALLS IN AUTOMATED PERIMETRY

Like all other tests, perimetry also has several pitfalls. The visual fields should not be interpreted in isolation but must

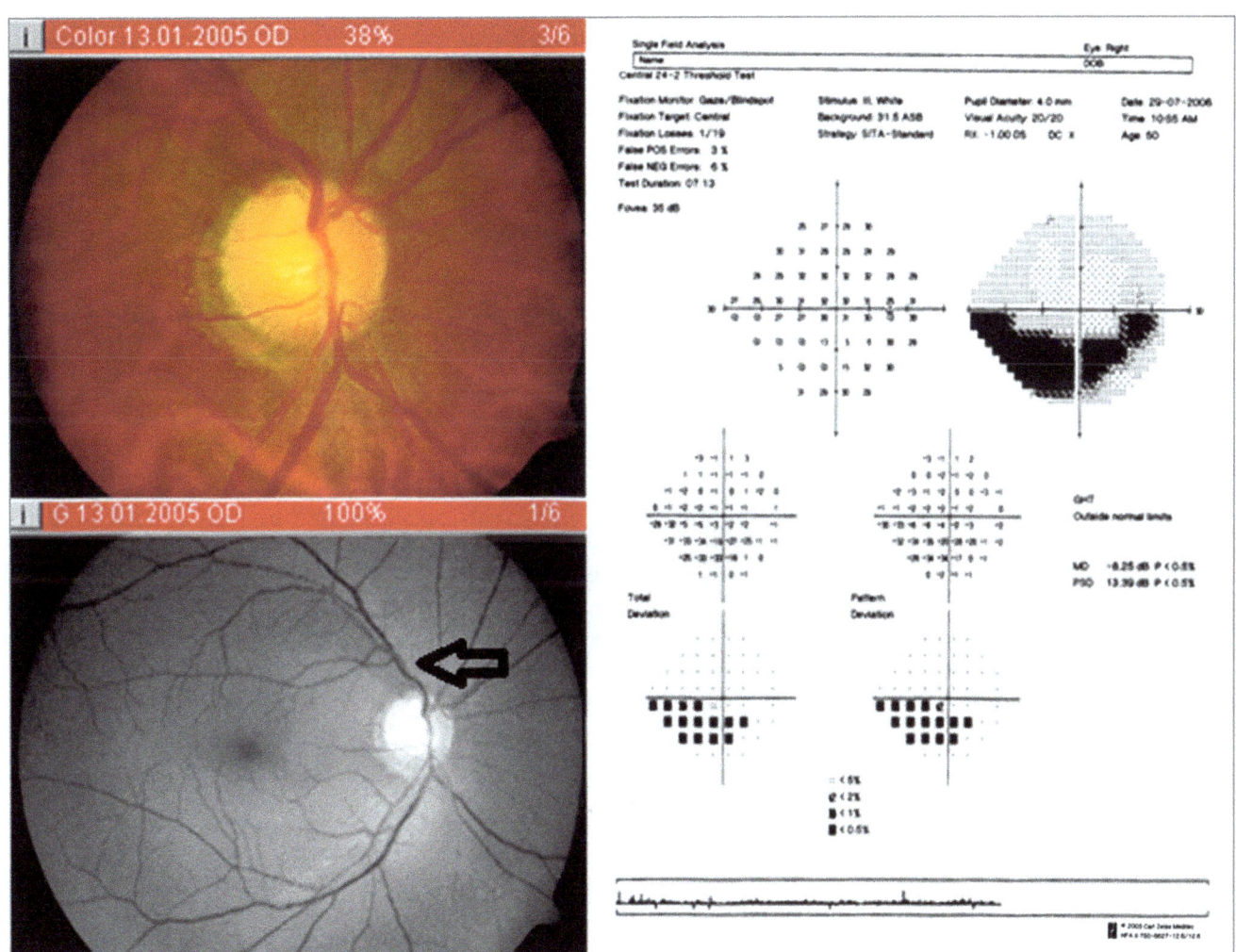

Fig. 1: A typical glaucomatous field defect. Clinical examination shows a superior notch in the right disc (right up) with corresponding retinal nerve fiber layer wedge defect (arrow) and inferior field loss (left).

always be clinically correlated. Nonglaucomatous optic disc and retinal pathologies also cause visual field defects leading to the misinterpretation of glaucoma diagnosis or progression. We illustrate a few clinical situations with fallacious field changes, which can lead to misdiagnosis.

Retinal Defects

Sometimes, retinal lesions can cause changes in the visual field similar to glaucoma (**Figs. 2 and 3**). A careful examination of retina and optic disc is necessary to rule out any such cause. Retinal pathologies generate deeper lesions in the visual field with absolute scotomas that have sharp borders and do not respect the horizontal meridian. This is in contrast to a glaucomatous visual field loss that has less clearly defined borders, but at the same time respects the horizontal meridian.

Neurological Causes

Neurological disorders are also very important when correlating visual field and optic disc changes because ganglion cell loss in neurological disorders also causes field defects. The visual field loss in neurological disorders respects vertical meridian unlike the glaucomatous visual field loss, which respects horizontal meridian (**Fig. 4**). Optic disc in such cases appears healthy or shows temporal pallor due to loss of papillomacular bundle and does not follow the ISNT (inferior ≥ superior ≥ nasal ≥ temporal) rule.

Sudden appearance of a vertical visual field defect in the field should raise the suspicion of a neurological abnormality.

When a nonglaucomatous cupping is noted, the Greenfield criteria give a guideline as to whether neuroimaging is warranted or not. Patients with age < 50 years, visual acuity < 20/40, optic nerve pallor more than cupping, and vertically aligned visual field defect require neuroimaging.

Preretinal Defects

With increasing age, the visual field gets depressed by virtue of reduction of light-difference sensitivity due to age-related loss of nerve fibers[1] and changes in the media. Deterioration of media clarity reduces illumination and therefore

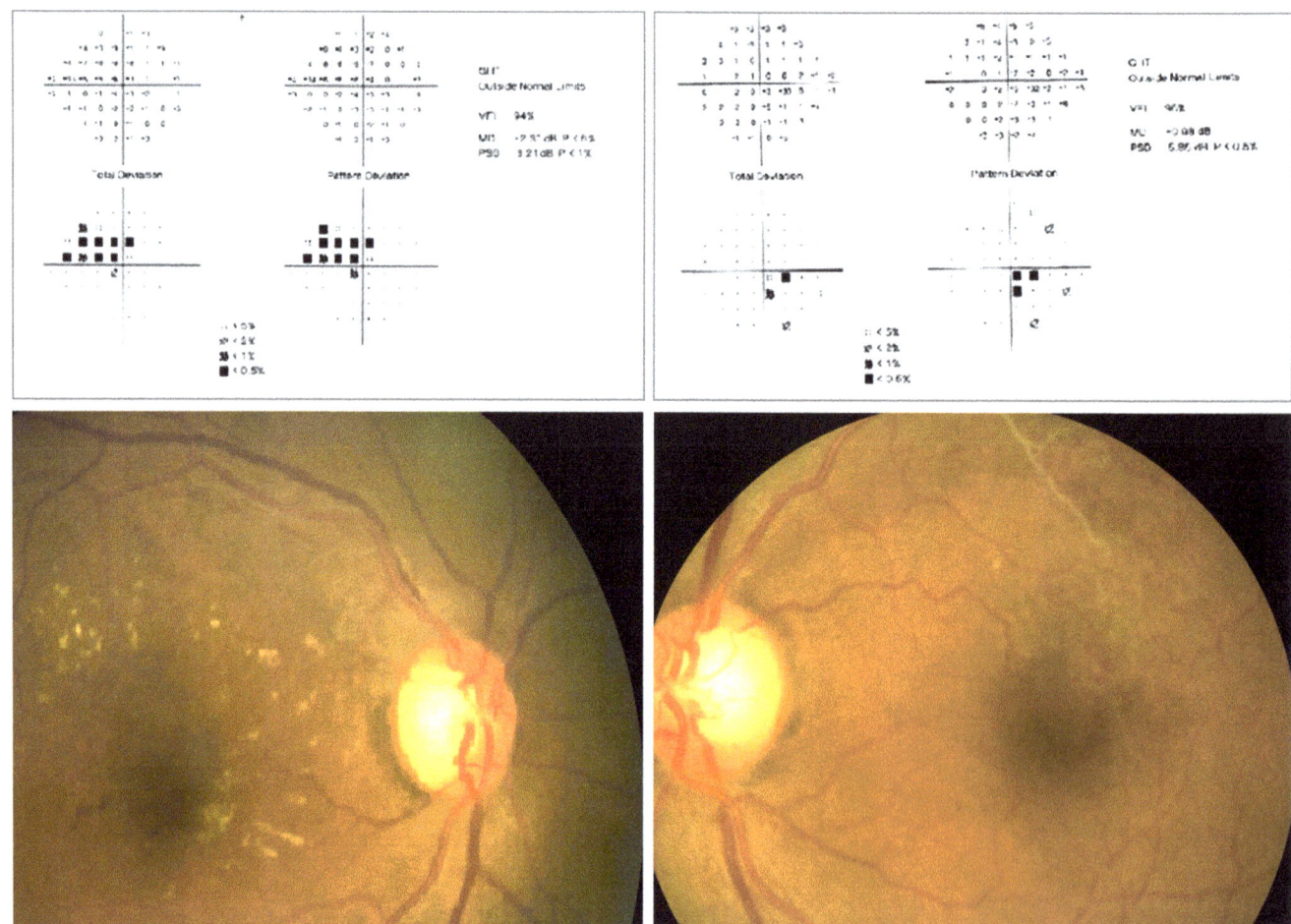

Fig. 2: Dilated examination revealed both eyes' cystoid macular edema.

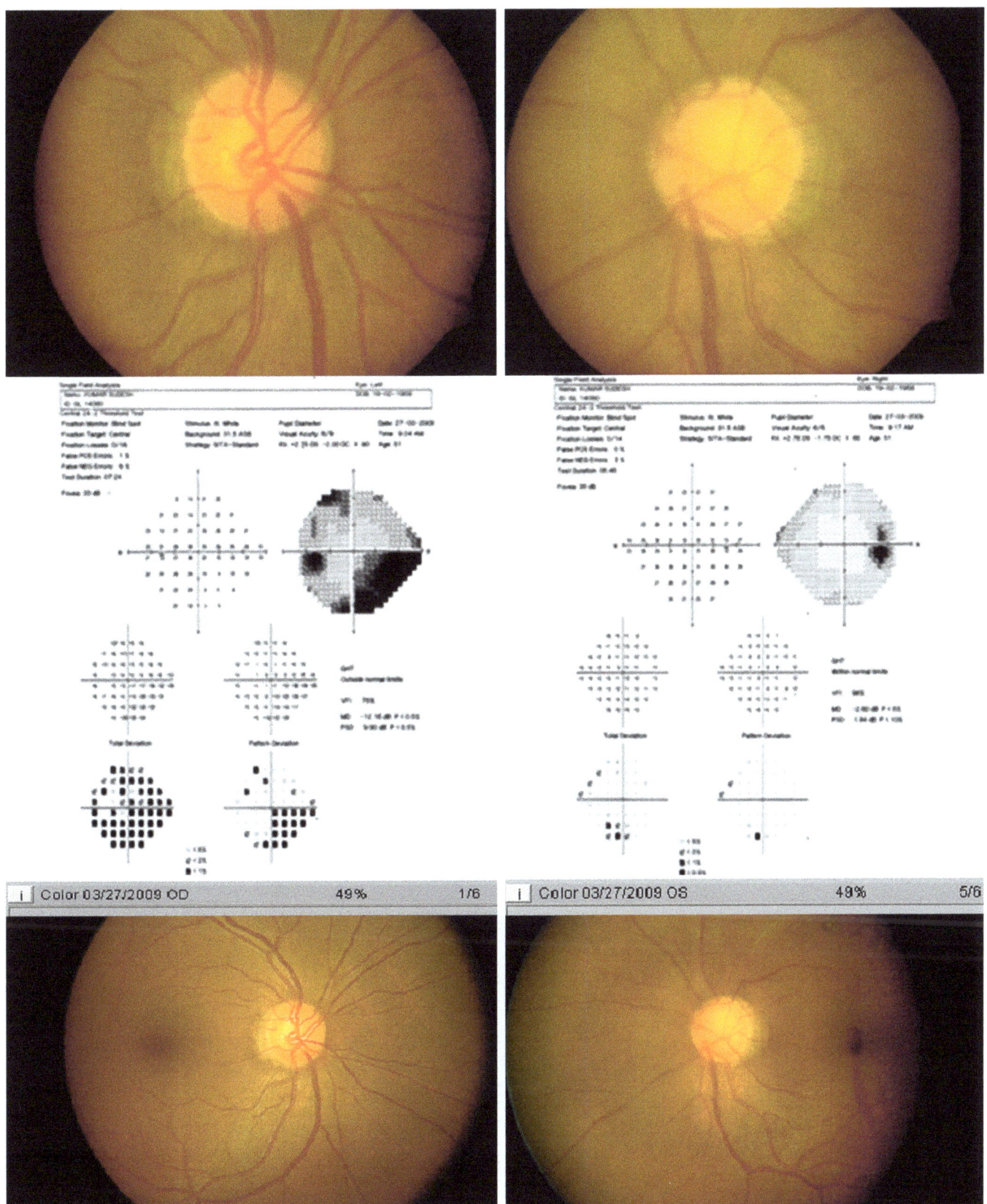

Fig. 3: A 60-year-old woman diagnosed with glaucoma and referred; IOP 16 mm Hg(RE), 12 mm Hg(LE); large Cup: Disc ratio LE> RE. VF showed RE normal and LE showed an inferonasal defect. Careful examination revealed a superotemporal branch retinal vein occlusion, which was lasered in the LE (below). (IOP: intraocular pressure; LE: left eye; RE: right eye; VF: visual field)

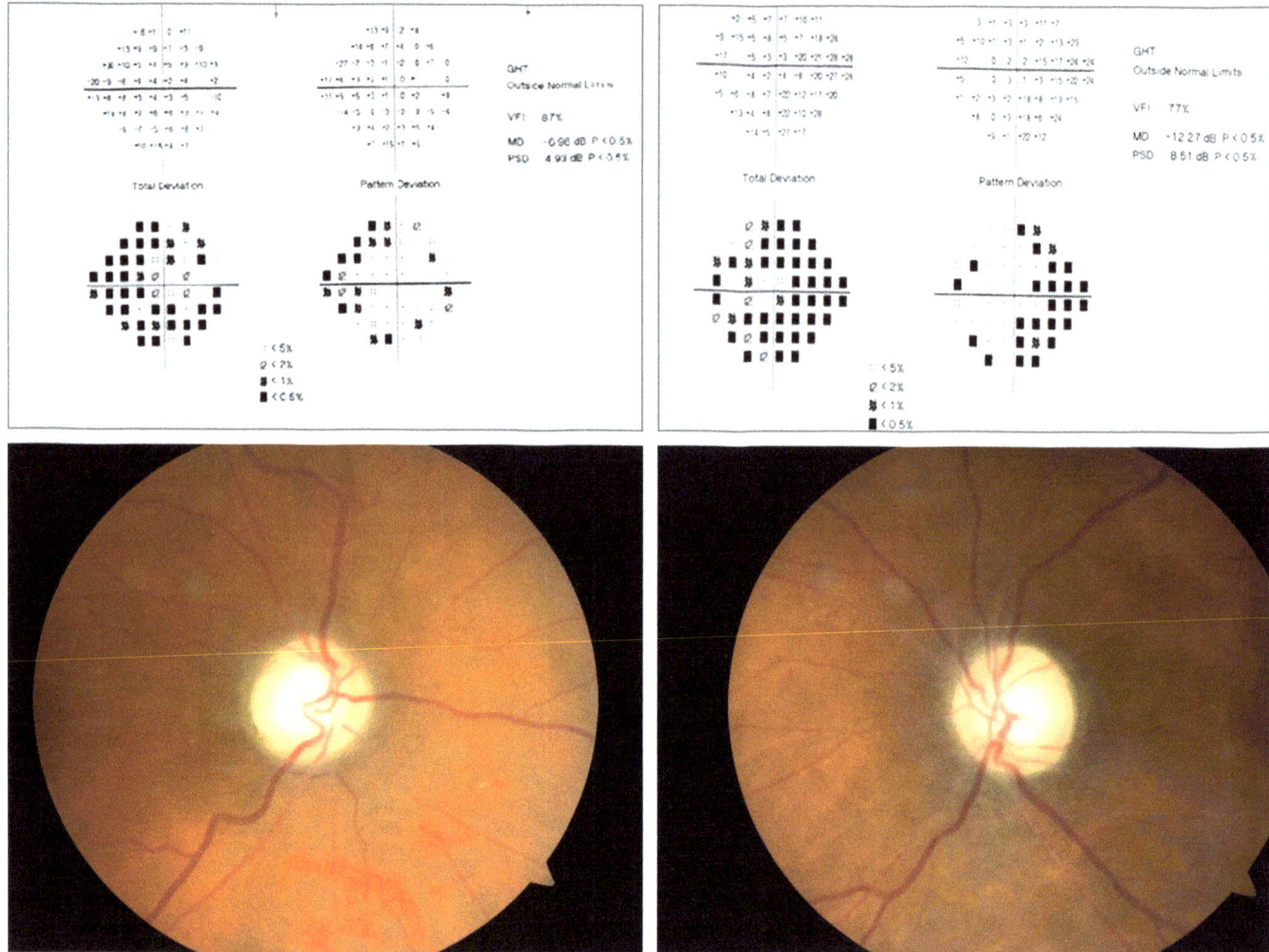

Fig. 4: Visual field defects in a 45-year-old female are significant but obey the vertical meridian. The discs are normal and hence rule out a glaucomatous field defect. Neuroimaging revealed a pituitary macroadenoma.

depresses the visual field and exaggerates the existing visual field defects.[2-4] For every decade of life, the size of the visual field decreases by 1–3°.

Cataracts or media opacities produce a diffuse depression on the total deviation plot causing the visual fields to be severely depressed, while the optic disc may be healthy **(Fig. 5)**. As per the reduced schematic eye, the nodal points of the cornea and lens are very close; therefore, they are considered as a single point, approximately 17 mm in front of the retina (close to the posterior lens surface). At this location, the visual information is inverted to the contralateral side. Therefore, the defects in the inferior hemifield appear as superior defects on the printout.

In a glaucoma suspect, localized defects due to media opacities could be attributed to progressive glaucomatous damage. A dilated examination must be done if a glaucoma patient has severely depressed visual fields.

After the cataract surgery, the previous value of mean deviation may decrease, while the pattern deviation may increase as more focal glaucoma defects will be revealed. Therefore, a new baseline should be set for progression analysis after cataract surgery.

False Depressions

Depression in the visual field can be due to some physiological phenomenon or some technical errors or inaccurate refractive correction that we should keep in mind while interpreting the perimetry printout.

Inexperienced Patient

A patient doing visual field test for the first time may have visual field defects that are known as *learning defects*. These mainly affect the midperipheral region and do not correlate clinically **(Fig. 6)**. These defects generally disappear on the sequential visual field testing or with the experience of perimetry. A lot of patients experience a visual field defect owing to the learning curve; therefore,

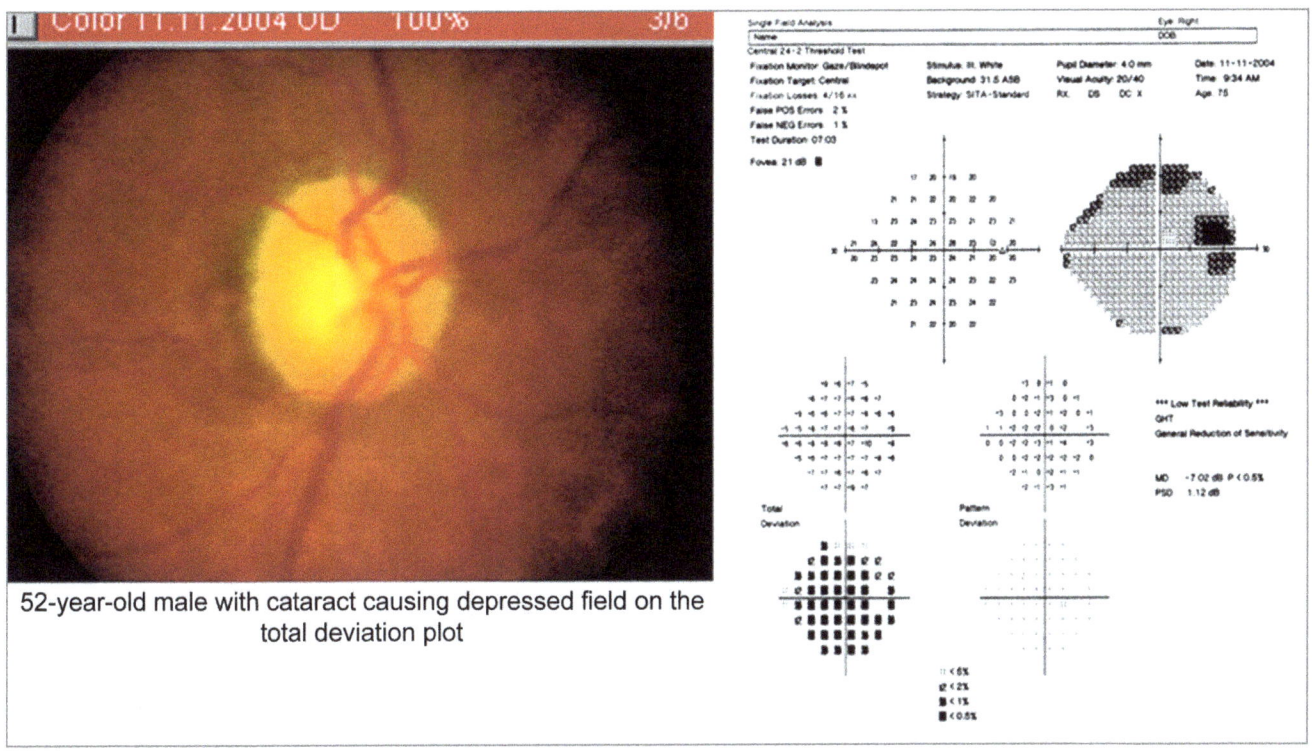

Fig. 5: Visual field changes due to cataract may be misleading. Cataracts produce defects evident as a diffuse depression on the total deviation plot causing the visual fields to be severely depressed, while the optic disc may be healthy.

a demonstration test must be done.[5,6] With experience of maintaining fixation and consistently responding to stimuli, patients respond even to more dim stimuli and also those stimuli that are presented further away from the central point of fixation.[7,8] If the first test is unreliable, one must repeat the second test at a later stage. The second test (if reliable) should be taken as the baseline. The most common artifact in the first test is an overall reduction in sensitivity of the visual field. Localized visual field defects must be carefully correlated clinically, as they can be because of optic disc edema and other optic nerve head pathology; these must not be ignored as artifacts. Localized visual field loss can be detected by probability plots, despite overriding reduction in sensitivity.

Fatigue

As the test progresses, a long test strategy causes fatigue that mainly affects the mid-peripheral region. Hence, the sensitivity of these points decreases as compared to the surrounding points hat appears as a scoot main the visual field. To avoid these, a fast strategy should be adopted. Also, we should follow the visual field of the same strategy on the subsequent follow-up.

Artificial tears may be instilled prior to the visual field test to reduce fatigue due to dry eyes.

Physiological/Pathological Ptosis

Glaucoma is a disorder of an elderly age group and due to aging, senile ptosis can occur. Other conditions such as congenital ptosis or a case of third nerve palsy may produce a superior artefact.[9-11] Ptosis results in a marked drop in sensitivity from normal values to 0 dB in the superior field of vision.[12] This pseudoscotoma is seen in about 1–2% of all central threshold perimetry examinations. This may appear in both eyes if bilateral or just one eye, or the second eye tested if fatigue related. The lid can be taped open with a micropore tape to prevent this **(Figs. 7 and 8)**.

Refractive Errors

The trial lens must be properly placed close to the testing eye in the trial frame. For patients with very high refractive errors, contact lenses must be used to avoid rim artifacts. The patient's habitual near-point correction is not suitable for perimetry as it is set for a different distance (i.e., 40 cm vs. 33 cm).

With the new HFA3 using the liquid lens technology, trial lenses are not needed and therefore, lens-induced errors are not there. To prevent these artifacts, the lens must be inserted in the trial frame correctly. Additionally, the correcting lens must be in proximity to the testing eye. Very high refractive errors have a higher risk of rim artifacts; in such cases, the

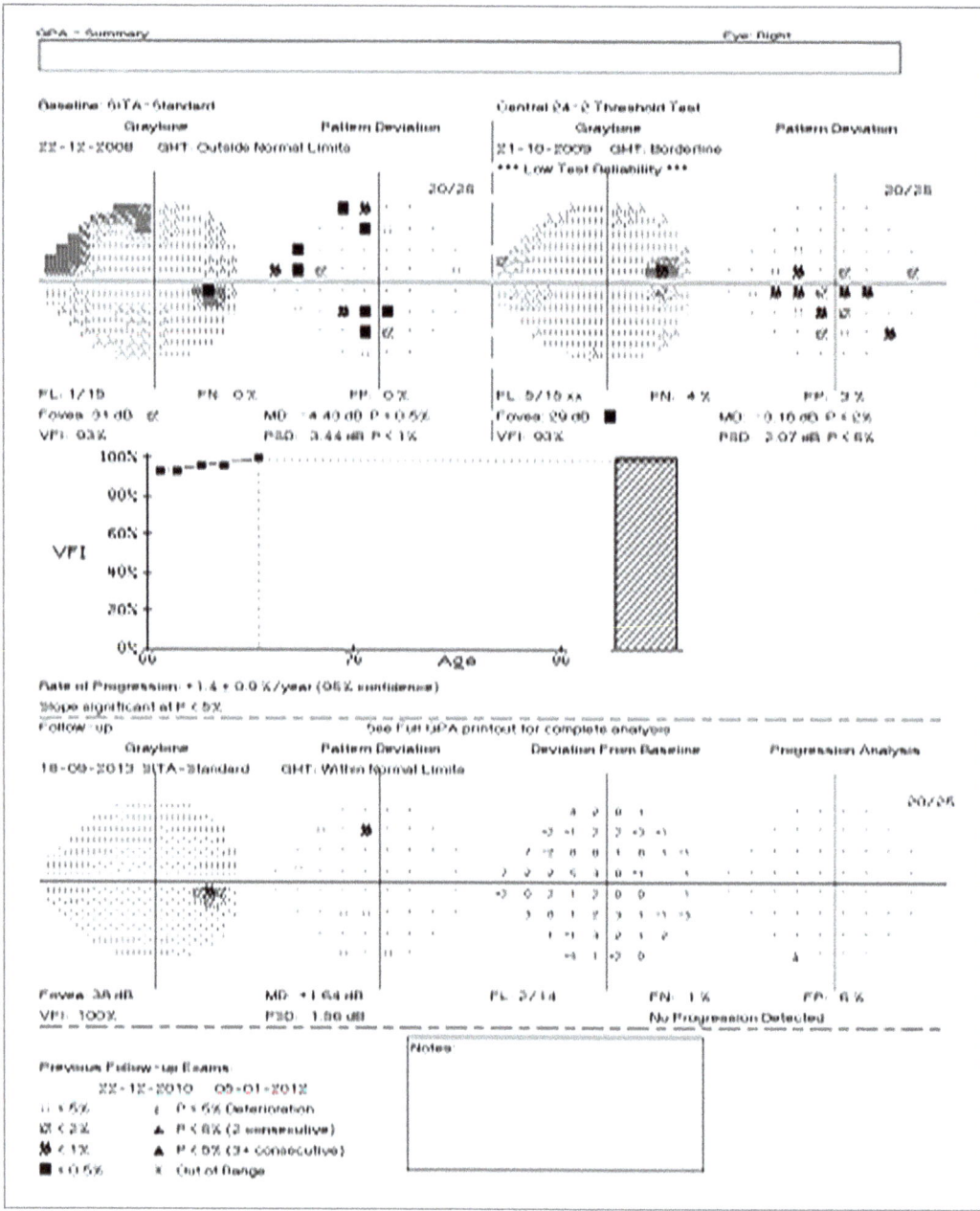

Fig. 6: Learning curve.

use of contact lenses is preferred. The patient's habitual near-point correction is not suitable for visual field testing. This is because it is measured for a different distance (i.e., 40 cm vs. 33 cm).

Additionally, care must be taken such that the lens does not touch the eyelashes as it may hinder blinking.

Use of Miotics

Even the use of miotic therapy can lead to a defective field loss involving the peripheral field; hence, there is a problem when assessing patients on miotics.[13-16] Miosis has the effect of reducing the sensitivity of the visual field and can amplify the magnitude and extent of preexisting visual field impairments. When the diameter of the pupil is <2 mm, it results in exaggerated visual field loss due to reduced intensity of the stimulus as well as the background.

Low Reliability Indices

Reliability indices are important factors to be considered for the interpretation of the visual field. However, these may sometimes be misleading if clinical parameters, both intraocular and extraocular, are not considered.

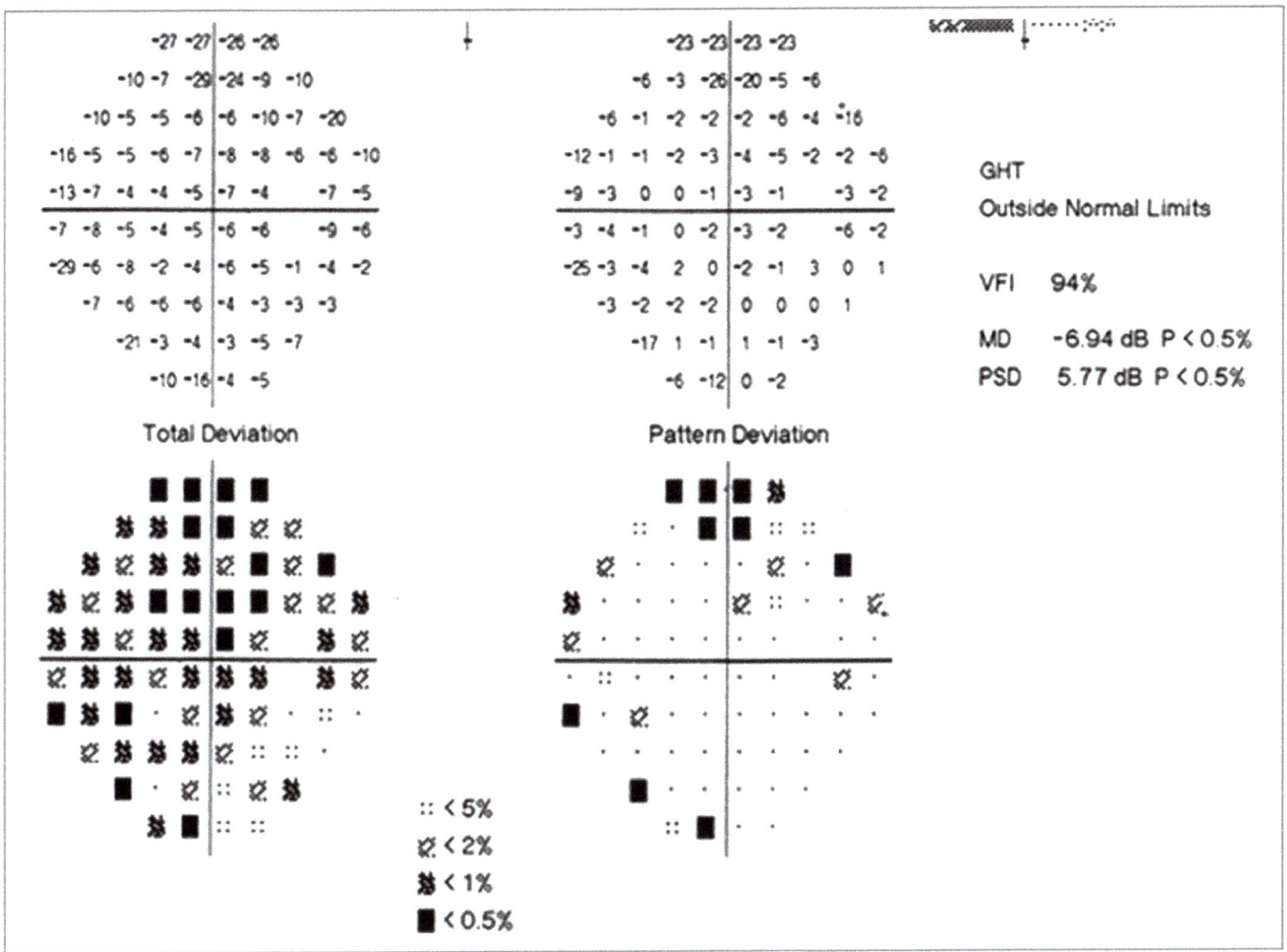

Fig. 7: Superior field defects in a patient with ptosis due to third cranial nerve palsy. (GHT: glaucoma hemifield test; MD: mean deviation; PSD: pattern standard deviation; VFI: visual field test)

Fixation instability: This can result from poor fixation, nystagmus, a ill-defined blind spot, or head movement during the test. Visual field result may be reliable in some of these instances if the patient has been closely observed during the catch trials.

During the test, a stimulus is administered at a level above the threshold that is detectable by the patient, based on a certain decibel value that has previously elicited a positive response. Consequently, the patient is expected to respond to this stimulus. However, if they fail to respond, it is considered a FN. In individuals with preexisting visual field defects, the occurrence of FN is often higher compared to individuals with normal visual fields. This implies that FNs are more likely to indicate true visual field defects rather than merely reflecting the patient's lack of reliability.[17] High FNs are also seen in early onset of visual loss because of varying responses in loci of relative scotomas. These high FN scores may also suggest fatigue.

During the visual field test, the projection device clicks without presenting a stimulus or moves. When the patient acknowledges the stimulus by responding to a click, it is categorized as a FP. A high FP score is often observed in patients who tend to be overly responsive, pressing the response button frequently even when they have not actually perceived any stimuli. As a result, these patients continue to respond to both real and nonexistent stimuli, leading to subsequent presentations of stimuli at progressively higher sensitivities. This process can extend beyond the upper limit of 51 dB if the patient persists in pressing the response button. Consequently, the mean deviation value increases significantly (shifting toward the positive), thus creating artificial abnormalities in the pattern deviation. This deviation from the standard therefore produces abnormally elevated sensitivity, rendering the visual field results unreliable.

SECTION 2: Visual Field Interpretation

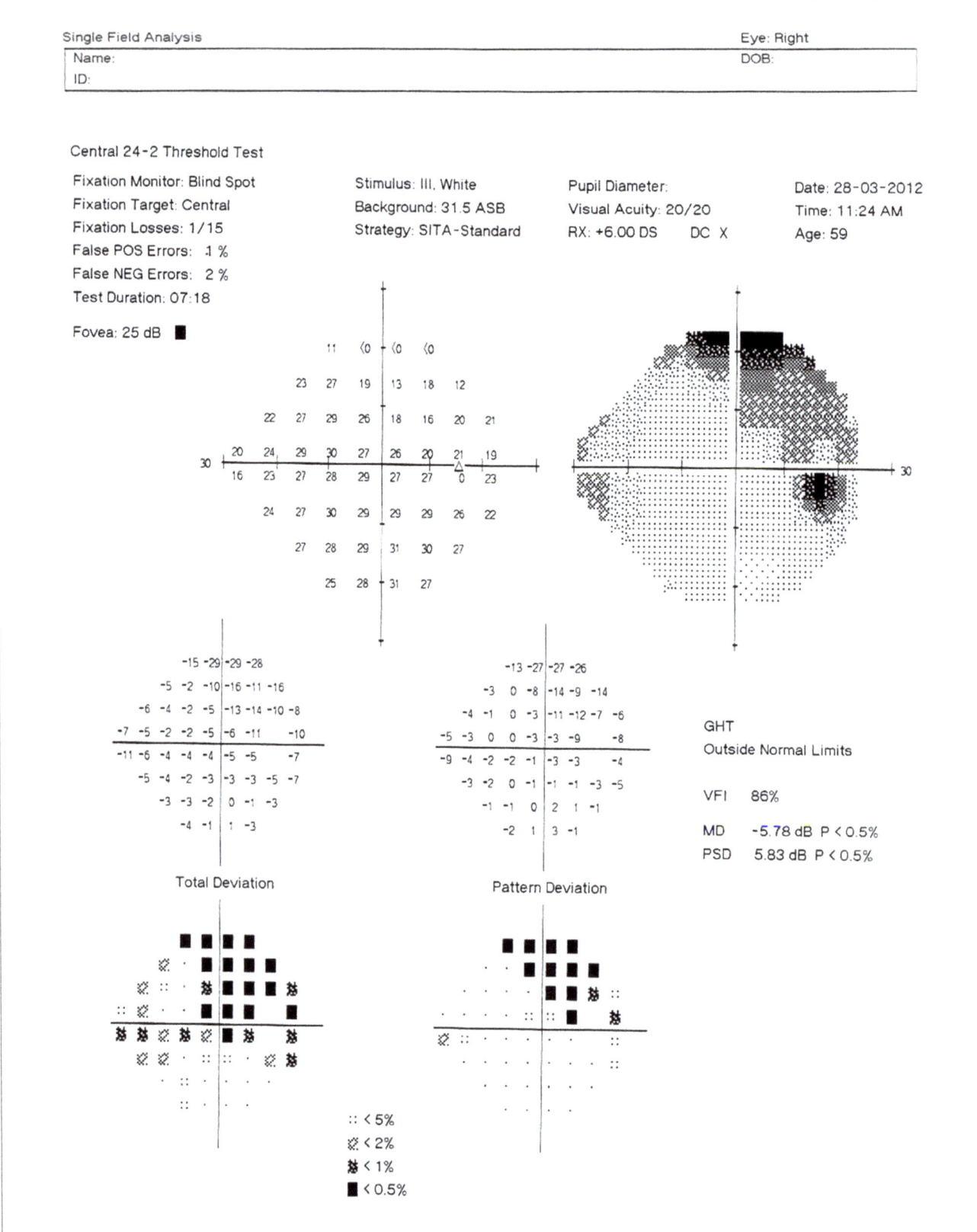

Fig. 8A

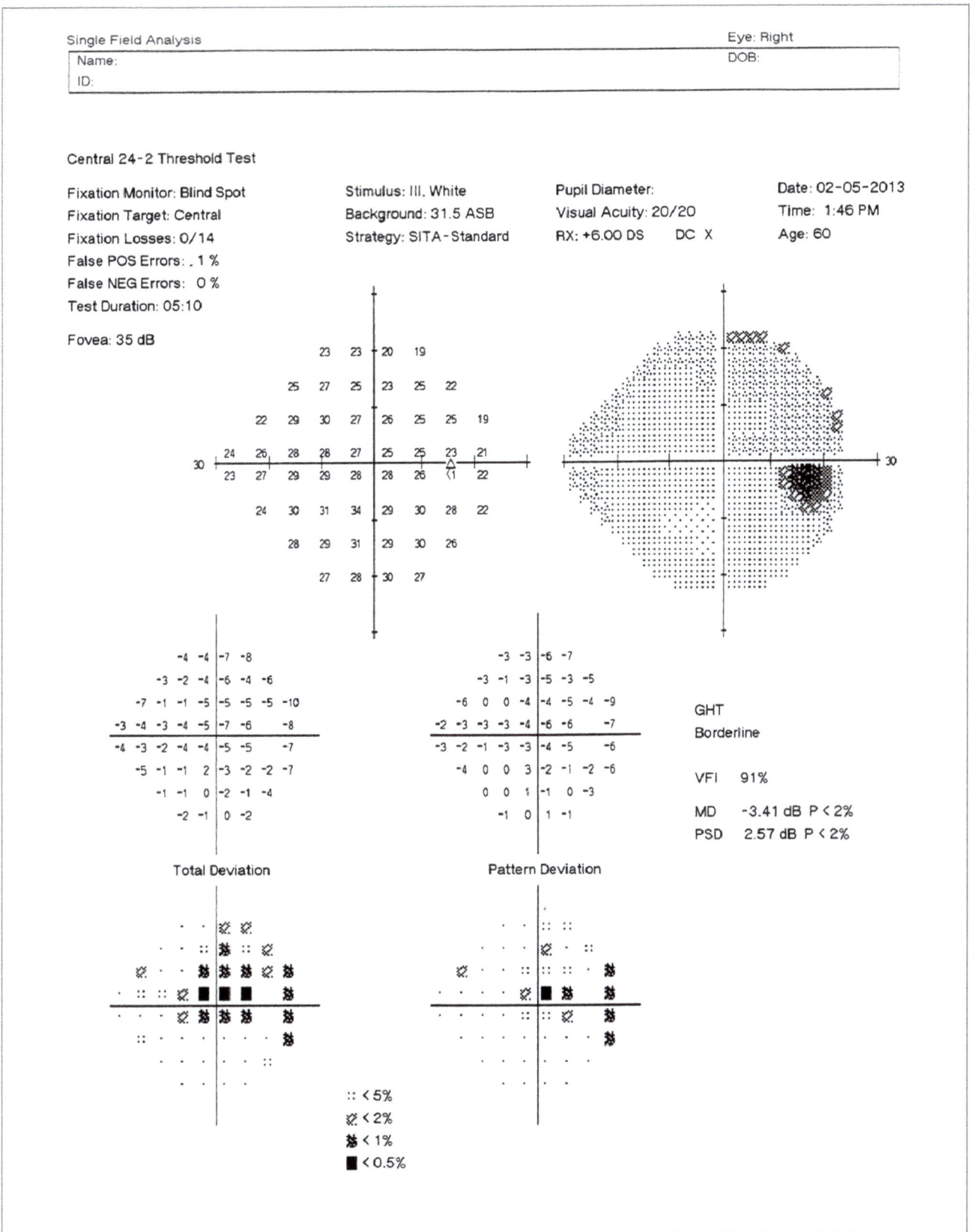

Fig. 8B

Figs. 8A and B: Superior visual field defect in a patient with ptosis and visual fields of the same patient in the same sitting, after taping the upper lid. (GHT: glaucoma hemifield test; MD: mean deviation; NEG: negative; POS: positive; PSD: pattern standard deviation; VFI: visual field index)

Lens Rim Defects

Poorly positioned lenses often interfere with visual perception.[18-20] Visual field defects related to a lens artifact are usually located between 25° and 30°. Wide aperture lenses must be positioned close to the eye. When there is a significant decrease in sensitivity at a specific tested point, dropping below 0 dB, while neighboring points closer to the fixation point do not exhibit a similar decline, it raises suspicion of a lens rim defect. This observation suggests that the decreased sensitivity is localized to that specific point and is not a general characteristic of the surrounding area.

Observer Interpretation

When analyzing the printout, it is important to avoid relying solely on the grayscale representation, as it may not accurately depict localized areas of visual field loss when there is a concurrent diffuse visual loss. Moreover, further progression of an existing visual field defect might go unnoticed. Consequently, relying solely on the grayscale interpretation may lead to an inaccurate assessment of the extent of visual loss. In some cases, this approach can result in a false diagnosis of progressive visual field loss. It is worth noting that variations in grayscale print quality can occur due to factors such as using a new printer ribbon or cartridge. Therefore, the probability plots must be taken into consideration, as these indicate the actual extent of visual loss.[6] One must get a 10-2 test done for a patient who has characteristic macular ganglion cell thinning on OCT or one or more abnormal points in the central 10° of a 24-2 test. The central points of a 24-2 test must be evaluated carefully, as a single depressed point (rather than the customary cluster of points) may be significant.

■ CONCLUSION

Following points must be remembered for a good perimetric outcome:

- The perimetrist must communicate with the patient.
- The patient must be comfortably positioned for good lumbar support. The forehead rest alarm must be activated.
- If there is no dedicated perimetry room, light-dimming curtains must be installed around the perimeter and earmuffs should be given to the patient.
- The operator's comments regarding the patient's performance and the accompanying circumstances can provide valuable insights during interpretation of the results. These comments may shed light on any factors that could have influenced the test outcomes and help in understanding the context of the findings.
- In order to ensure accuracy and reliability, it is important for the technician to periodically review the field analyzer manual, which typically includes a list of potential operator errors. Familiarity with these potential errors allows the technician to identify and rectify any mistakes that may have occurred during the testing process. Regular review of the manual thus helps in maintaining the quality of the testing procedure and ensures that the results are as accurate as possible.
- For an absolute presbyope or cycloplegic patient, add +3.00 sphere to the distance correction. For an intermediate presbyope, the rule of thumb is to add +0.50 sphere to their habitual add.
- Look for distinctive patterns such as the "clover leaf" or "inverse clover leaf" on the grayscale as these suggest that the test data is not reliable.
- To ensure accurate measurements, it is recommended to enable the foveal threshold measurement option. This feature allows for precise assessment of the central visual field, which is particularly important in evaluating conditions, such as macular degeneration.
- In case the patient has central vision defects, utilizing the diamond fixation target may be beneficial. These targets help patients with impaired central vision to maintain fixation during the test, resulting in more reliable visual field assessments. The impact of central vision defects on the overall test results can thus be minimized, allowing for a more accurate evaluation of the peripheral visual field.
- "Baseline fields" should be established as soon as possible and be updated as needed.
- Consider the influence of coexisting conditions on the perimetric outcome. Never interpret the visual fields in isolation.

■ REFERENCES

1. Balazsi AG, Rootman J, Drance SM, Schulzer M, Douglas GR. The effect of age on the nerve fiber population of the human optic nerve. Am J Ophthalmol. 1984;97:760-6.
2. Spaeth GL. The management of cataract in patients with glaucoma: A comparative study. Trans Ophthalmol Soc U K (1962). 1980;100:195-205.
3. Guthauser U, Flammer J, Niesel P. Relationship between cataract density and visual field damage. Doc Ophthalmol Proc Ser. 1987;49:39.
4. Guthauser V, Flammer J. Quantifying visual field damage caused by cataract. Am J Ophthalmol. 1988;106:480-4.
5. Anderson DR. Automated Static Perimetry. St Louis: CV Mosby; 1992.
6. Rowe FJ. Visual field analysis with Humphrey automated perimetry. Parts I and II. Eye News. 1998;4(6):6-10;5(1):15-9.

7. Werner EB, Adelson A, Krupin T. Effect of patient experience on the results of automated perimetry in clinically stable glaucoma patients. Ophthalmology. 1988;95:764-7.
8. Autzen T, Work K. The effect of learning and age on short-term fluctuation and mean sensitivity of automated static perimetry. Acta Ophthalmol (Copenh). 1990;68:327-30.
9. Meyer DR, Stern JH, Jarvis JM, Lininger LL. Evaluating the visual field effects of blepharoptosis using automated static perimetry. Ophthalmology. 1993;100:651-8.
10. Klingele J, Kaiser HJ, Hatt M. Automated perimetry in ptosis and blepharochalasis. Klin Monbl Augenheilkd. 1995;206:401-4.
11. Federici TJ, Meyer DR, Lininger LL. Correlation of the vision-related functional impairment associated with blepharoptosis and the impact of blepharoptosis surgery. Ophthalmology. 1999;106:1705-12.
12. Cahill KV, Burns JA, Weber PA. The effects of blepharoptosis on the field of vision. Ophthalmic Plast Reconstr Surg. 1987;3:121-5.
13. Mikelberg FS, Drances M, Schutzer M, Wijsman K. The effect of miosis on visual field indices. Doc Ophthalmol Proc Ser. 1987;49:645.
14. Lindenmuth KA, Skuta GL, Rabbani R, Musch DC. Effects of pupillary constriction on automated perimetry in normal eyes. Ophthalmology. 1989;96:1298-301.
15. Webster A, Luff A, Canning C, Elkington A. The effect of pilocarpine on the glaucomatous visual field. Br J Ophthalmol. 1993;77:721-5.
16. Edgar D, Crabb D, Rudnicka A, Lawrenson J, Guttridge N, O'Brien C. Effects of dipivefrin and pilocarpine on pupil diameter, automated perimetry and LogMAR acuity. Graefes Arch Clin Exp Ophthalmol. 1999;237:117-24.
17. Katz J, Sommer A, Witt K. Reliability of visual field results over repeated testing. Ophthalmology. 1991;98(1):70-5.
18. Zalta AH. Lens rim artefact in automated threshold perimetry. Ophthalmology. 1989;96:1302-11.
19. Henson DB, Earlam RA. Correcting lens system for perimetry. Ophthalmic Physiol Opt. 1995;15:59-62.
20. Donahue SP. Lens holder artifact simulating glaucomatous defect in automated perimetry. Arch Ophthalmol. 1998;116:1681-3.

CHAPTER 6

Visual Field Progression

Yamunadevi Lakshmanan, Najiya Sundus K Meethal, Ronnie George, Shantha B, Vijaya L

INTRODUCTION

Visual field (VF) progression can be defined as either deepening of existing scotoma and enlargement of the scotoma or development of a new scotoma in the VFs.[1,2] The factors that are likely to cause a change in VF are disease progression, variability or fluctuation, learning curve, or a combination of any of these factors. Evaluating the changes in the VF over a period of time is one of the standard techniques used to assess the disease progression in glaucoma.[3-6] The real challenge for clinicians is to differentiate the true disease progression from other biological and nonbiological variability.[1-22]

CHALLENGES IN ASSESSING THE VISUAL FIELD PROGRESSION

Visual field testing, being a psychophysical test, is subjected to a lot of variability such as short-term fluctuation, long-term fluctuation, the subject's cognitive function, the test strategy that determines the duration of the test, stimulus size, cataract or other media opacities, pupil diameter, alertness during the test, and other artifacts.[7-14] The VF of a normal subject fluctuates on repeated testing, and this fluctuation is greater in glaucomatous eyes. The peripheral threshold points show greater variation than the central points. Points depressed because of glaucomatous damage tend to fluctuate more than the normal threshold points.

Since there are multiple sources of variability in VF, an adequate number of tests are required to differentiate between test-retest variability and actual progression.[15]

A minimum of six VFs over a 2-year period is recommended to comment on the stability of VF.[20] Hence, it is an arduous task to differentiate the true change (progression) from any other variability (fluctuation and artifacts) that can either mask or mimic the glaucomatous change.

There are various methods used to analyze the progression of VF. Paul et al.[16] reported that there are 301 different methods that we can choose to analyze the progression of VF. The methods for assessing the progression of glaucomatous VF can be broadly classified into four types:[18]
1. Subjective analysis
2. Defect classification systems
3. Event analysis
4. Trend analysis

Subjective Analysis

It requires a competent examiner to subjectively assess a series of VFs in order to comment upon the stability of VF. This method is reported to have only moderate inter-rater and intra-rater agreement. The Humphrey field analyzer (HFA) provides an overview printout that can print a maximum of 16 VF visits of a patient with three visits on every single page in a chronological order. It provides all information that we get in a single field analysis printout that includes patient demographic data, tested eye, test program and strategy, glaucoma hemifield test (GHT), visual acuity, pupil diameter, reliability indices, foveal threshold, global indices, gray scale, and total and pattern deviation for each visit. It can combine results from the 24-2 and 30-2 programs, but not the 10-2.

Defect Classification Systems

Defect classification systems classify the VF into stages, and any change in the stage between visits determines the progression of VF. Examples of such classification systems are the Glaucoma Staging System (GSS I and II), Advanced Glaucoma Intervention Study (AGIS), and Collaborative Initial Glaucoma Treatment Study (CIGTS).[19] GSS stages the VF from 0 to 5 according to mean and pattern standard deviation of the VF, 0 being normal and 5 being advanced field loss. The AGIS and CIGTS use scores ranging from

0 (normal) to 20 (worse VF), and worsening of score from baseline confirms the progression. These staging systems are not routinely used to judge progression in the clinic.

Event Analysis

Event analysis is an empirical method that determines progression by comparing the point-by-point thresholds from the latest VF test (follow-up) with the first two VF tests (baseline). Humphrey's glaucoma progression analysis (GPA I) and guided progression analysis (GPA II) provide the event analysis. The event analysis highlights any statistically significant ($p < 0.5\%$) depression from the baseline that is larger than the expected clinical variability and provides symbols along with simple plain language message whenever changes show a significant and consistent loss. This analysis is based on the criteria used in the Early Manifest Glaucoma Trial (EMGT). When significant deterioration ($p < 0.5\%$) is noted from the baseline in the same three or more points for two or three consecutive follow-up visits, the progression analysis gives a message of "possible progression (PP)" or "likely progression (LP)." When neither of these changes occurs, no message will be shown. The difference between event analyses of GPA I and II is that the latter does not show progression analysis for severely depressed VF, i.e., with mean deviation (MD) < −20 decibels (dB).

Trend Analysis

Change in sequential VF over time is detected using the linear regression model and also provides the rate of progression (ROP) per year. Humphrey's GPA I and GPA II provide the MD and visual field index (VFI)-based trend analysis, respectively. Progressor is another software that provides a pointwise linear regression-based trend analysis. The basic tenets of event and trend based on GPA I and II are discussed further.

Glaucoma Progression Analysis

Even though the HFA can provide GPA I event analysis for a minimum of three VF visits, it is best to have at least five VF tests to analyze progression. The GPA I event printout report is interpreted in the following steps:
1. The first page of the GPA I report is labeled the Glaucoma Progression Analysis—Baseline. The first two selected tests form the baseline. The baseline report will have patient details that include the name, identification number, date of birth, and the tested eye. It also displays the grayscale plot, raw data, total deviation, pattern deviation, foveal threshold, reliability indices [fixation losses (FL), false positive (FP), false negative (FN), and gaze tracking parameters], global indices [(MD and pattern standard deviation (PSD)], visual acuity, and pupil diameter of the selected baseline reports.
2. Below the baseline report, the GPA I also provides the summary plot of the MD of all visits along with the MD slope and its significance level using the simple linear regression model **(Fig. 1)**.
3. The rest of the printout is labeled the "Glaucoma Progression Analysis—Follow-up," which contains all the follow-up visits selected for GPA I analyses with three follow-up visits printed on one single page. It also provides the test date, reliability indices, global indices, GHT, pupil diameter, visual acuity, and four plots. The four plots are gray scale, pattern deviation probability plot, deviation from baseline, and progression analysis. The gray scale and pattern deviation probability plot are the same as in the single field analysis printout.
4. Deviation from baseline compares the pattern deviation of each point from the follow-up test with the averaged baseline pattern deviation values and gives the difference in dB. A negative threshold indicates a worsening point, a positive threshold indicates an improvement (likely due to long-term fluctuation or a learning curve), and 0 indicates no change from baseline **(Fig. 2)**.
5. Deviation from baseline is again a plot with numbers. Not everyone is good at interpreting numbers and that too in a busy clinical day. Hence, this progression analysis plot makes the job easier. This plot gives the statistical significance of decibel change shown in deviation from the baseline plot for each point using five symbols as follows:
   - △ Deterioration from baseline at $p < 5\%$ occurred for the first time
   - ▲ Deterioration at the same point noted in two consecutive visits
   - ▲ Deterioration at the same point noted in three consecutive visits
   - X Out of range (the baseline threshold value is significantly less to analyze progression)
   - ● Stable

Apart from this, it also provides one of the following GPA I alert messages—PP, LP, and no progression.

Possible progression: If three or more points show deterioration in at least two consecutive tests[20]

Likely progression: If three or more points show deterioration in at least three consecutive tests

No progression detected: If the above criteria are not met, this message is displayed.

Analysis of the Glaucoma Progression Analysis Report:
1. Confirm that the chosen baseline represents the actual baseline status of the patient. Establishing the baseline test is very crucial as the rest of the follow-up tests will be

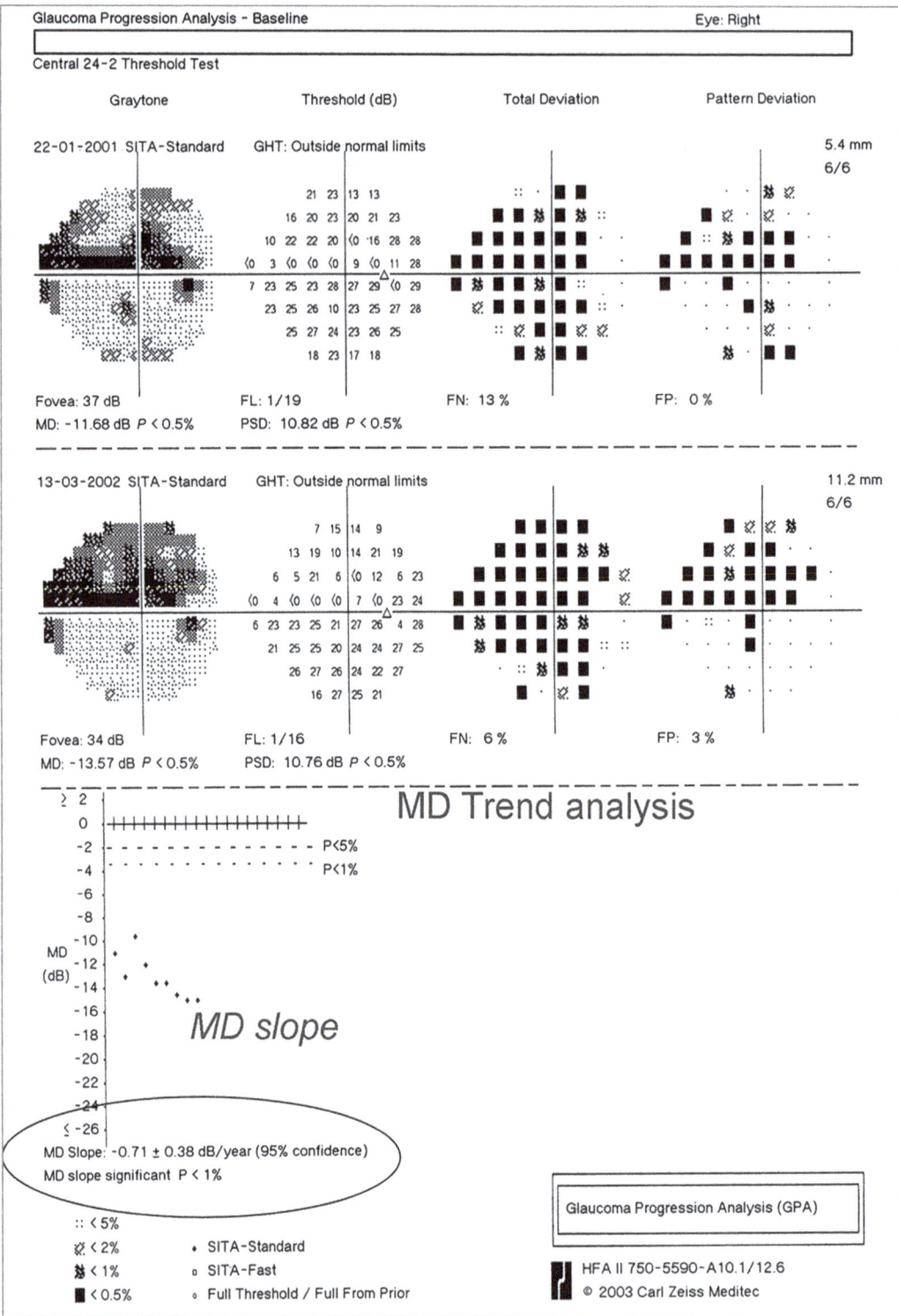

Fig. 1: Glaucoma progression analysis (GPA I). (GHT: glaucoma hemifield test; FL: fixation losses; FN: false negative; FP: false positive; MD: mean deviation; PSD: pattern standard deviation)
Courtesy: Carl Zeiss Meditec© (2003).

compared and analyzed with the baseline reports, which might underestimate or overestimate the progression. The examiner can choose and reestablish the baseline whenever indicated.

2. *Indications for reestablishing the baseline:*
   a. Look for marked learning curve patterns and artifacts in the baseline report that are likely to mask the progression. Look for reliability indices

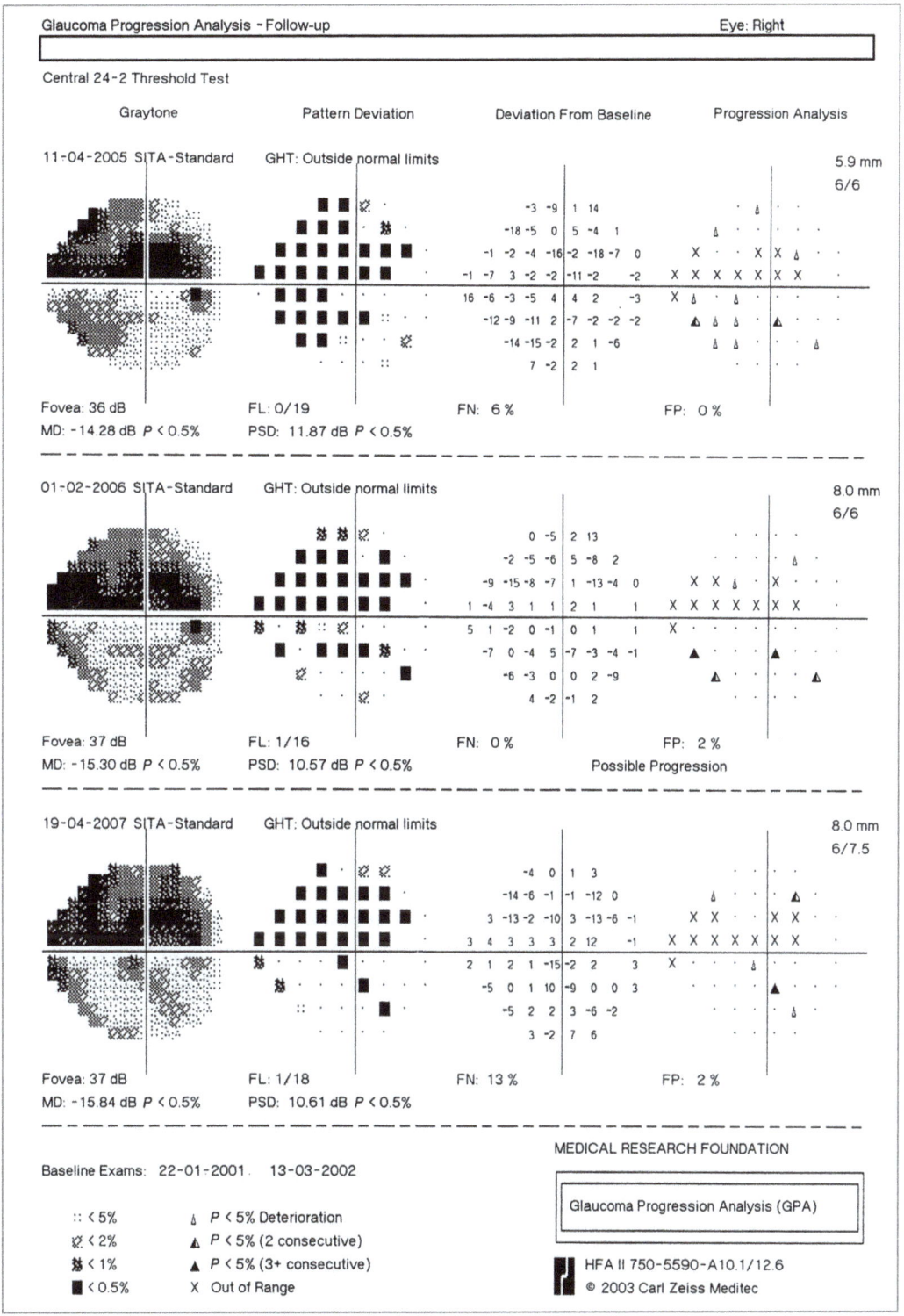

Fig. 2: Deviation from the baseline. (GHT: glaucoma hemifield test; FL: fixation losses; FN: false negative; FP: false positive; MD: mean deviation; PSD: pattern standard deviation)
Courtesy: Carl Zeiss Meditec© (2003).

(recently added feature offers the ability to real-time monitor the gaze tracking parameters for each tested location—**Fig. 3**), rim/edge artifact, and whether the VF correlate with the clinical findings. Use two reliable repeatable fields, preferably done within a short time interval, to establish the baseline.

b. Consider if a patient underwent cataract surgery or a yttrium-aluminum-garnet (YAG) capsulotomy since

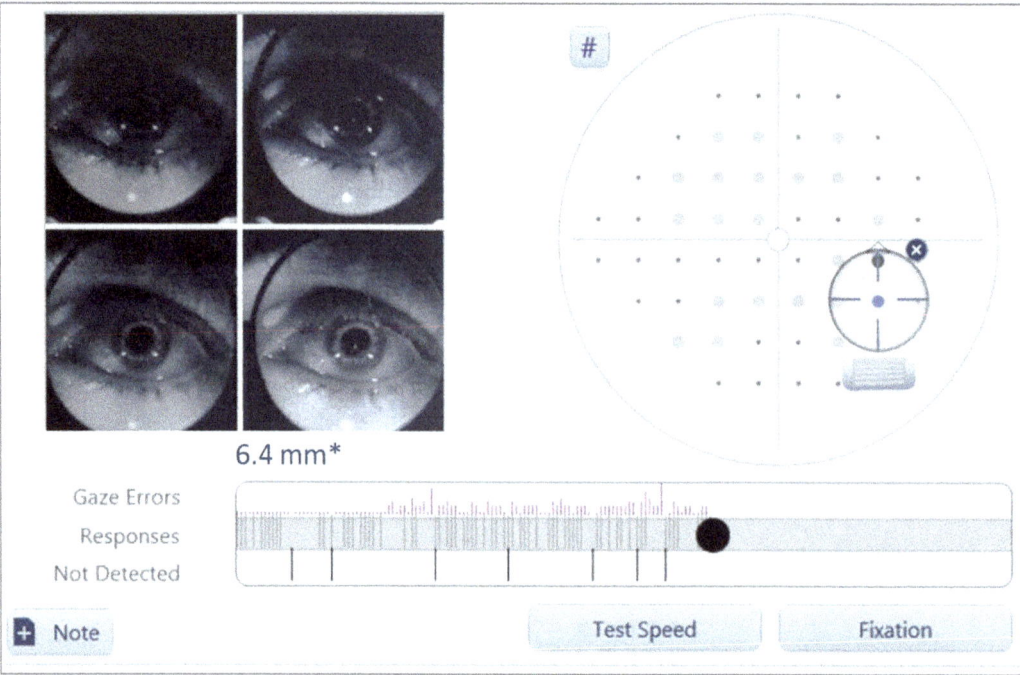

Fig. 3: Real-time monitoring of the fixation stability using gaze tracking method.

there could be an improvement in overall threshold points following either event. If we continue with the earlier baseline, the GPA I could show an improvement on follow-up visits that can actually mask any progression due to glaucoma. So, it is highly recommended to change the baseline in such a situation.

c. The baseline has to be reestablished when there is a significant change in the defect pattern or there is a significant intervention, such as glaucoma surgery. For instance, a patient presenting with an early superior arcuate scotoma, who over the years requires retinal laser photocoagulation for a retinal condition will require a new baseline established to incorporate any defects secondary to the laser. If an eye with progressing glaucoma undergoes a trabeculectomy or a major treatment change, the baseline should be changed again to detect any progression in the follow-up. If we continue to use the initial baseline fields, all follow-up visits will show progression, thus overestimating the progression. Unless we reestablish the baseline, we may not be able to measure the true progression.

3. If the GPA I shows progression with/without a stable clinical condition, look for confounders such as progressing cataract, posterior capsule opacification in pseudophakia, and other anterior/posterior segment changes before concluding that the patient has progressed.
4. It is noteworthy to look for the location of the points that show progression. Is it a single point or a cluster of points showing progression? Are they central points or peripheral/edge points showing progression? The central points are less likely to fluctuate as compared to peripheral points.
5. It is always advisable to maintain the same test strategy while analyzing and labeling the progression. Since different test strategies have different threshold algorithms and different normative databases, they may not be directly comparable.
6. Once the requirement of reestablishing the baseline and the confounding factors is ruled out, confirm progression only if points show progression at least in two –three successive follow-up visits.
7. It is recommended to repeat the test within a short interval to confirm/rule out progression.
8. Mean deviation, being a global index of VF, is unlikely to show progression unless there is a drastic change in follow-up VF. A significant slope in a field with an early defect is unlikely for this reason. Assessing the standard deviation of MD slope gives us an idea about the long-term fluctuation of the patient VF.
9. Mean deviation is affected by cataract and miotic pupils. Keep in mind the limitations of using the MD trend analysis before labeling a VF as progressed.

Guided Progression Analysis

The GPA II also provides us with event and VFI trend analyses. The event analysis of GPA II is the same as in GPA I, except that the former does not show progression analysis for MD values depressed >–20 dB. The VFI[20] is a measure of VF status expressed as a percentage of a normal age adjusted VF ranging from 0 to 100%. 0 indicates perimetrically blind and 100 indicates a normal field of vision. It is centrally weighted (depressed central points are given more weightage than similar depression in peripheral points) to correlate with ganglion cell density and visual function. It is also less affected by cataract and other media changes as compared to MD. A comparison between event- and trend-based analyses of VF progression is provided in **Table 1**. The VFI trend analysis of GPA II plots the VFI at all visits included for analysis taking into account the subject's age and gives a linear regression analysis of VFI over time. Based on the rate at which the VFI is changing over time, it provides us with the ROP in percentage (%)/year and classifies the probability that this slope is statistically significant. A slope that is significant at $p < 5\%$ would be considered to be statistically significant progression. The ROP, e.g., 2%, 3%, or 10%/year, would be important in deciding whether this rate is clinically likely to result in visually significant impairment in the patient's lifetime. To help make this decision, the VFI printout also projects the anticipated change in VFI over the next 2–5 years. This projection requires a minimum of five visits over a 2-year period of time. Keep in mind that this projection is based on the trend noted in the fields included for analysis and assumes that the same ROP will continue.

How to read and analyze the VFI trend analysis report?
1. We can either get a complete GPA II printout **(Fig. 4)** or a summary in a single page.
2. The GPA II summary provides both event and trend analyses. It has three sections, the baseline tests at the top, last/current VF test with event analysis at the bottom, and the VF history and trend in the middle **(Fig. 5)**.
3. The VF history has two plots, the VFI plot and the VFI bar. In the VFI plot, the VFI of all included visits will be plotted against the patient age and provides the linear regression analysis of VFI over the time. The VFI bar is a histogram that indicates the present VFI and the predicted VFI in the next 2–5 years if the result of regression analysis is displayed **(Fig. 6)**.
4. It also provides the ROP of the VFI and its significance level (displayed below the VF history).

Analyzing the GPA II printout:
1. Confirm that the chosen baseline represents the actual baseline status of the patient.
2. Look for reliability indices, rim/edge artifacts, and confounders (discussed earlier) to rule out the need for reestablishing the baseline, although the VFI is less likely to get affected by cataract.
3. Look at the slope of the VFI plotted over time to determine the progression of VF. Improving VFI over age (positive slope) represents a marked learning curve, changes in media clarity, or long-term fluctuation of the initial visits selected for analysis. Decreasing VFI over age (negative

TABLE 1: Comparison between event and VFI trend-based analyses of visual field (VF) progression.

	Event	Visual field index (VFI) trend
Analysis	Compares with baseline	Looks for trend over time
VF visits	At least five	Five to seven visits over 2 years
Early change	Sensitive	Not sensitive
Confounders	Affects the analysis	Less affected
Rate of progression	No information	Provides progression rate
Future prediction	Not possible	Possible

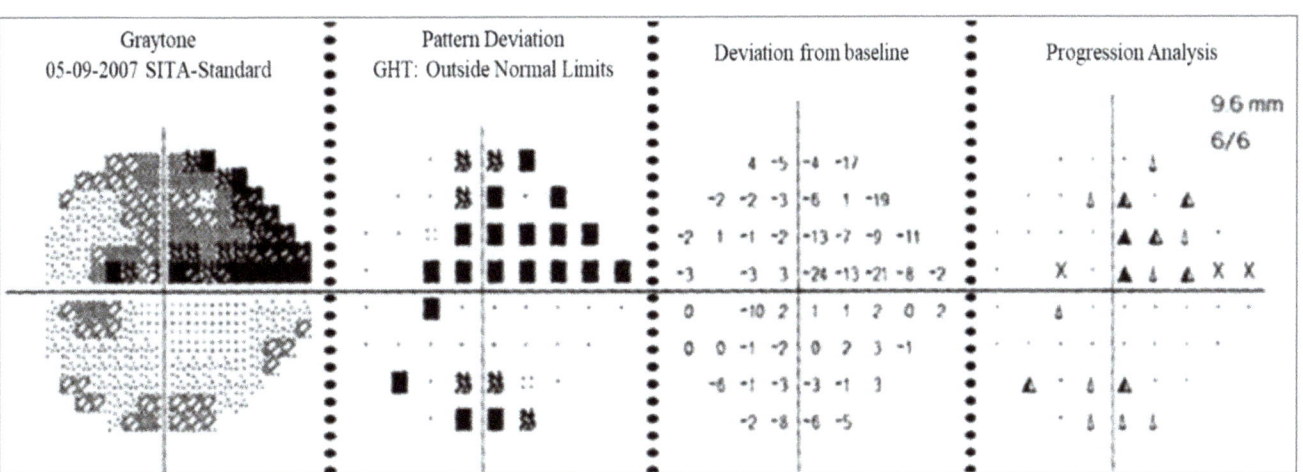

Fig. 4: Complete GPA II printout. (GHT: glaucoma hemifield test; GPA II: guided progression analysis)

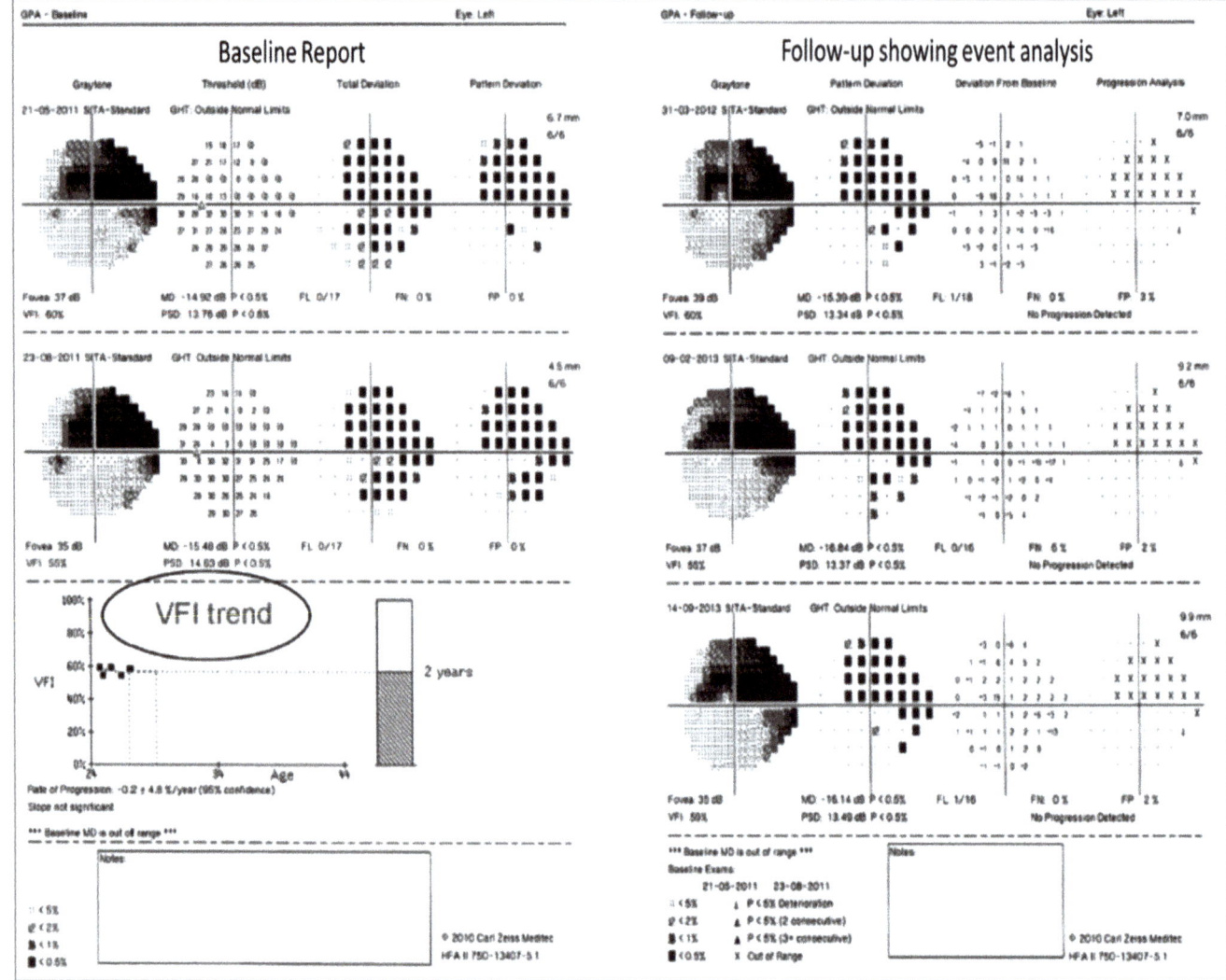

Fig. 5: GPA II summary showing event and trend analyses. (GPA II: guided progression analysis; VFI: visual field index)

slope) represents progression of VF. Not all VFI trends with negative slope represent progression. We need to confirm the progression only after looking into VFI ROP and its significance level.
4. It is desirable to maintain the same test strategy while analyzing and labeling the progression.
5. Once again, progression must be confirmed on repeat testing a short time later.
6. VFI, being a global index of VF, is unlikely to show early progression localized to a small region in the VF. The event analysis is however likely to detect this.
7. It is always best to integrate both event and trend analyses to confirm the progression.

The following examples illustrate some of the factors to be kept in mind while assessing progression with event and VFI trend analyses. We will discuss the case under four categories:

1. Confounding factors that mask/mimic VF change
2. Importance of subjective analysis rather than going by message given by the progression software
3. Significance of reestablishing the baseline
4. Practicality of having more number of VF visits/follow-ups

1. *Confounding factors that mask/mimic VF change*
   a. Gradual increase in cataract might mimic changes in a glaucomatous VF defect. Here is an example of a patient with the overview printout **(Fig. 7)** showing progressing VF from generalized reduction in sensitivity (first visit) to superior defects (fourth visit). Once the patient underwent cataract surgery, the VF became normal (last visit). Hence, it is important to rule out contribution of cataract for the change in VF and also to reestablish the baseline after cataract surgery **(Fig. 8)**.

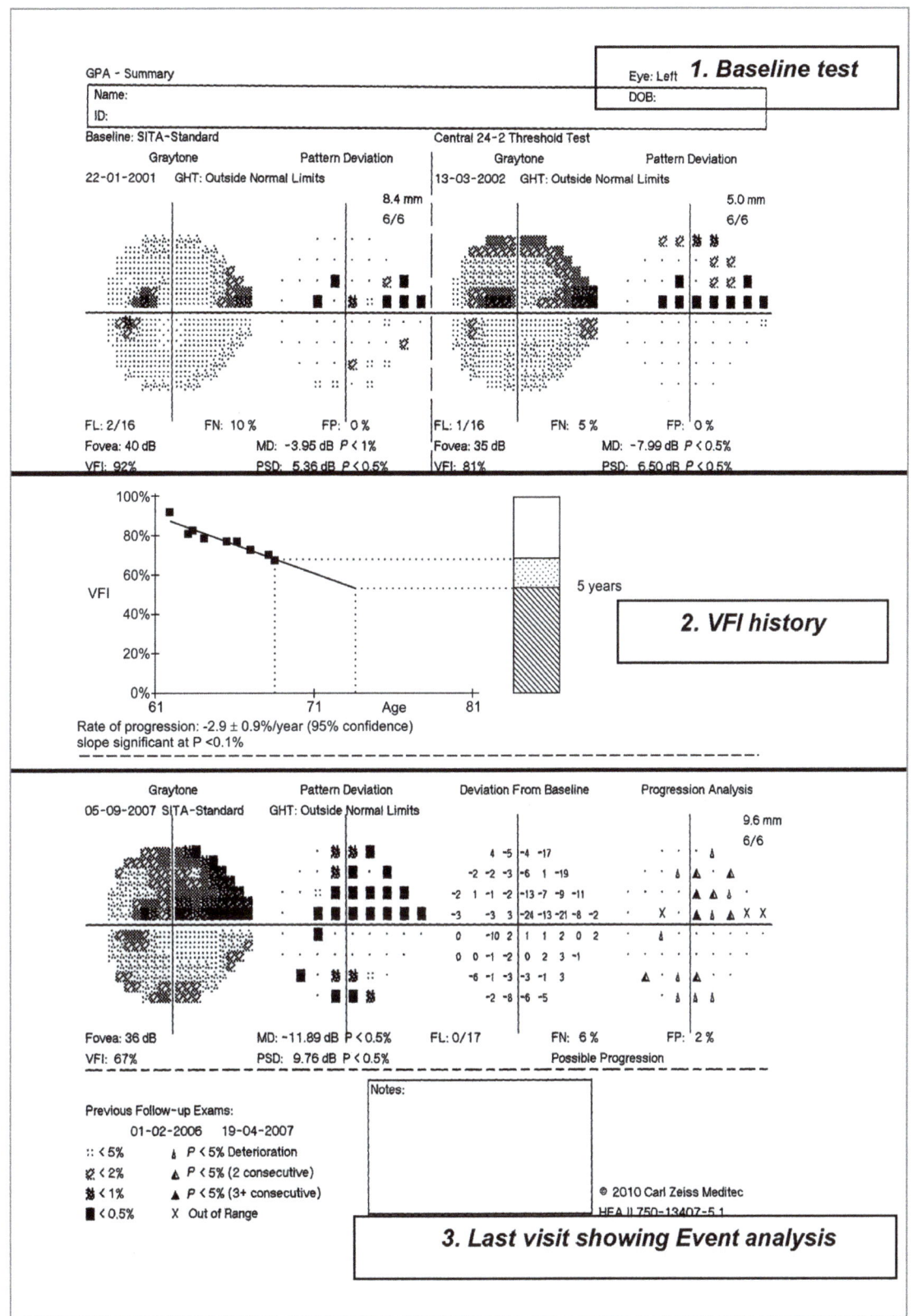

Fig. 6: VFI plot and bar. (GHT: glaucoma hemifield test; GPA II: guided progression analysis; FL: fixation losses; FN: false negative; FP: false positive; MD: mean deviation; PSD: pattern standard deviation; VFI: visual field index)
Courtesy: Carl Zeiss Meditec© (2010).

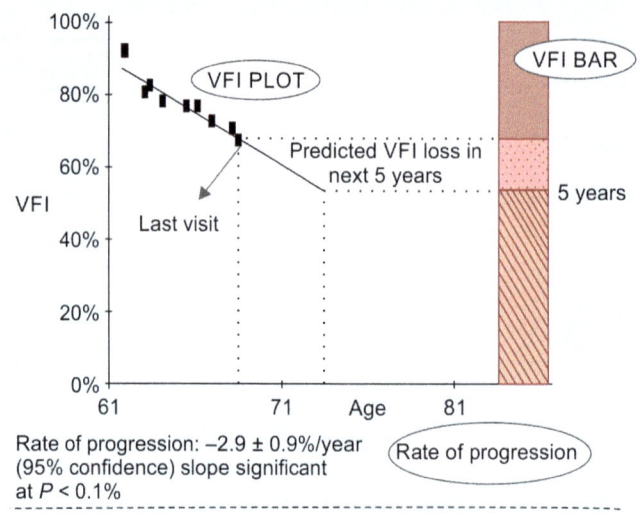

Fig. 7: Overview printout showing progression. (VFI: visual field index)

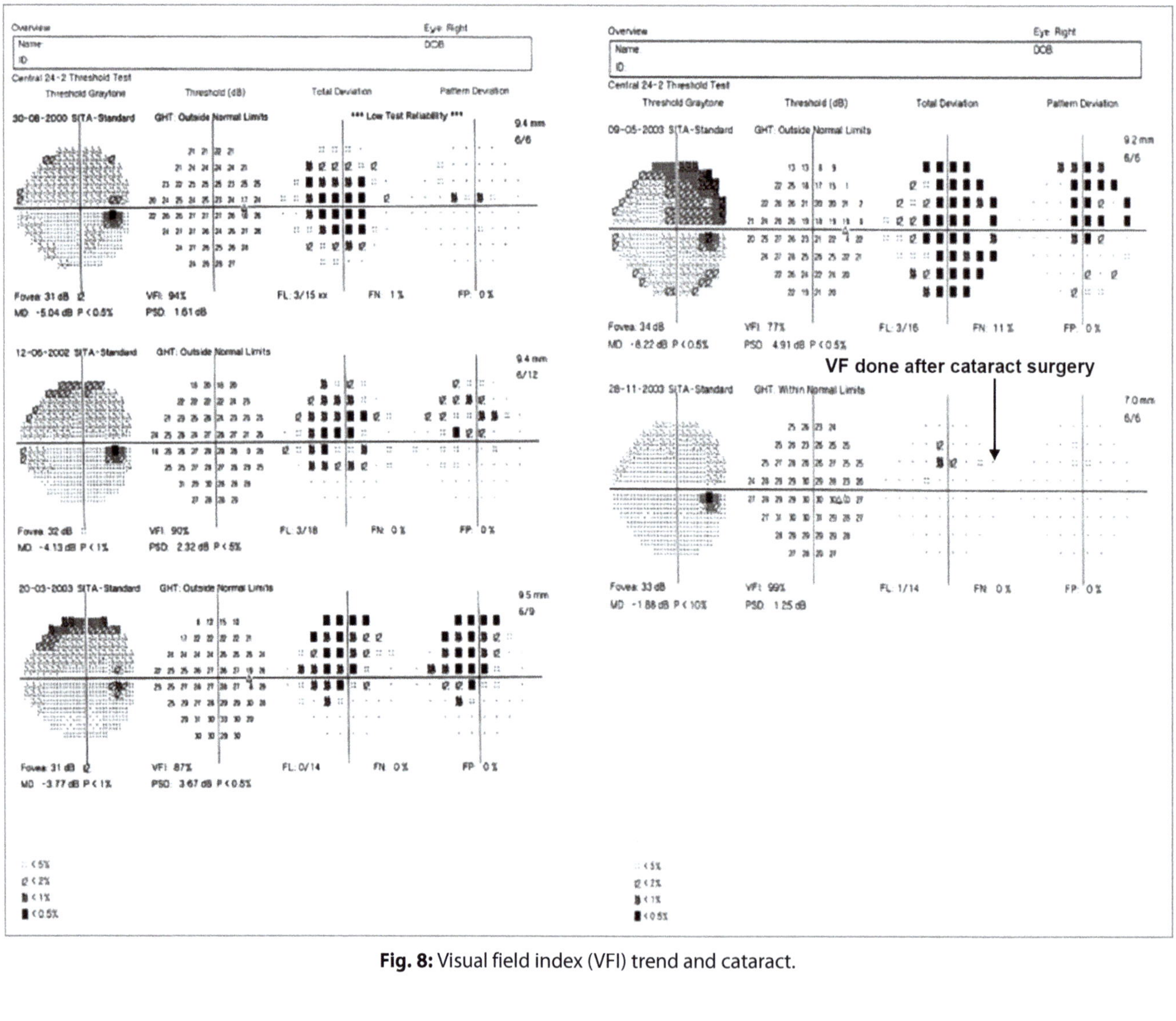

Fig. 8: Visual field index (VFI) trend and cataract.

b. A sudden change in VF should be repeated to confirm the change in defect pattern/progression. Here is an example **(Fig. 9A)** in which the VFI trend shows a sudden dip in the fourth visit (almost 11% decrease in VFI), although both the trend and event analyses are stable. The single field analysis (SFA) printout of that particular visit clearly shows a rim artifact that has contributed to the change in VFI **(Fig. 9B)**. The next two follow-up visits look almost stable. We can also note an increased standard deviation of the VFI ROP that is likely due to fluctuation.

c. It is well known that some patients might have learning effect for almost —two to three VF visits. Here is an example, in which the VFI trend of this subject **(Fig. 10)** shows a positive slope in which the VFI improved from 52% (first visit) to 65% (last visit). This fluctuation is also reflected in ROP that has been estimated to fall in between 16.2% and –4.4% per year.

2. *Importance of subjective analysis:* These GPA printouts that emphasize the subjective analysis of the location of progressing points rather than going by the overall message/ROP slope given by event/trend analysis:

a. It is worthwhile to subjectively analyze the location of progressing points before confirming the change in VF. In this example **(Fig. 11)**, although the VFI trend appears stable, the event analysis gives a message of possible progression. When we look at the progression analysis, the four points that showed progression were located in the outer ring. On follow-up with further VF visits, the edge points that showed progression in event analysis were now stable and the analysis was suggestive of stable VF on both event and trend analyses **(Fig. 12)**. As we know, peripheral points tend to fluctuate more than central points, we need to confirm the progression with further follow-up.

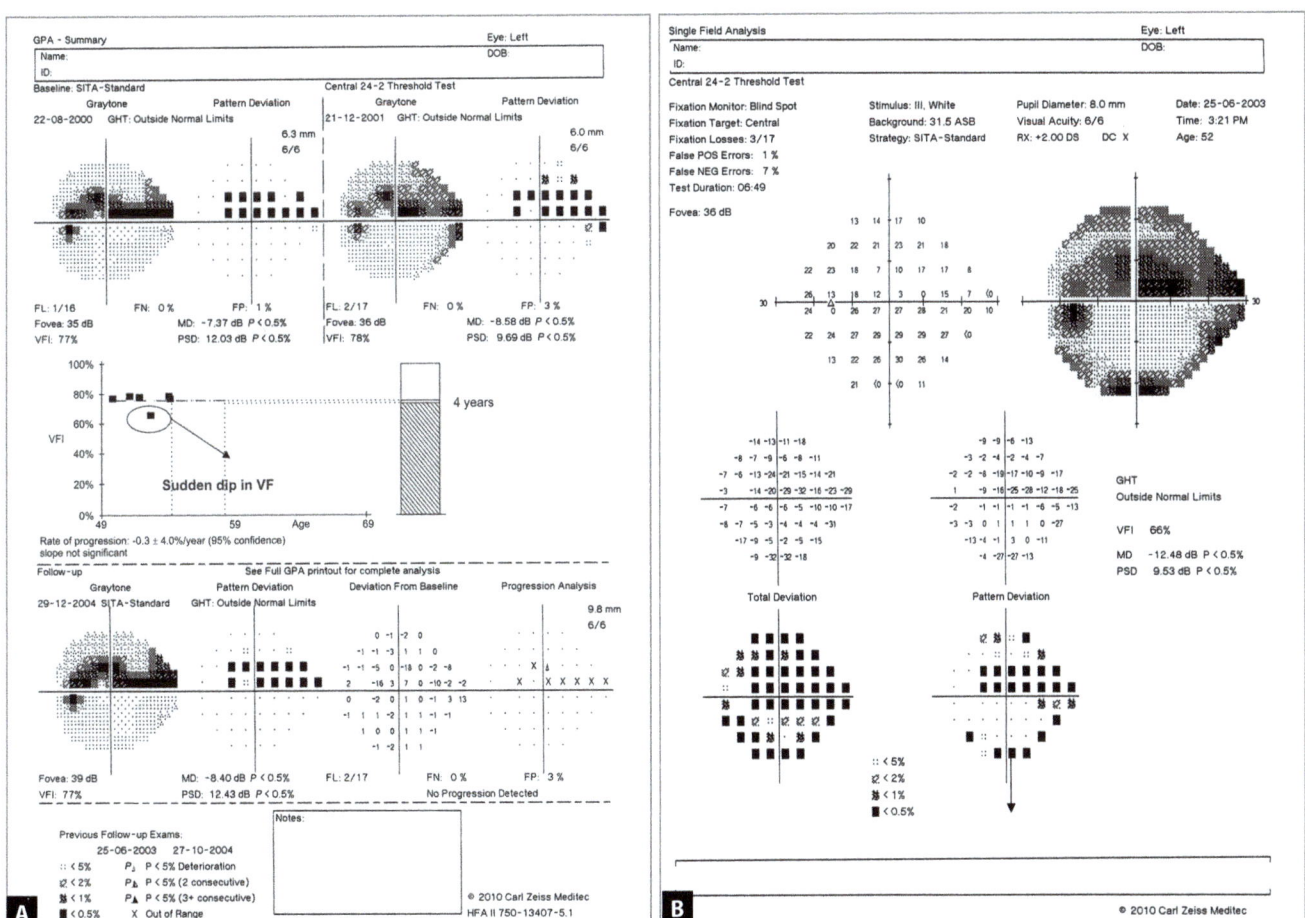

Figs. 9A and B: (A) VFI trend showing a sudden dip; (B) Rim artifact. (GHT: glaucoma hemifield test; GPA II: guided progression analysis; FL: fixation losses; FN: false negative; FP: false positive; MD: mean deviation; NEG: negative; POS: positive; PSD: pattern standard deviation; VFI: visual field index)
Courtesy: Carl Zeiss Meditec© (2010).

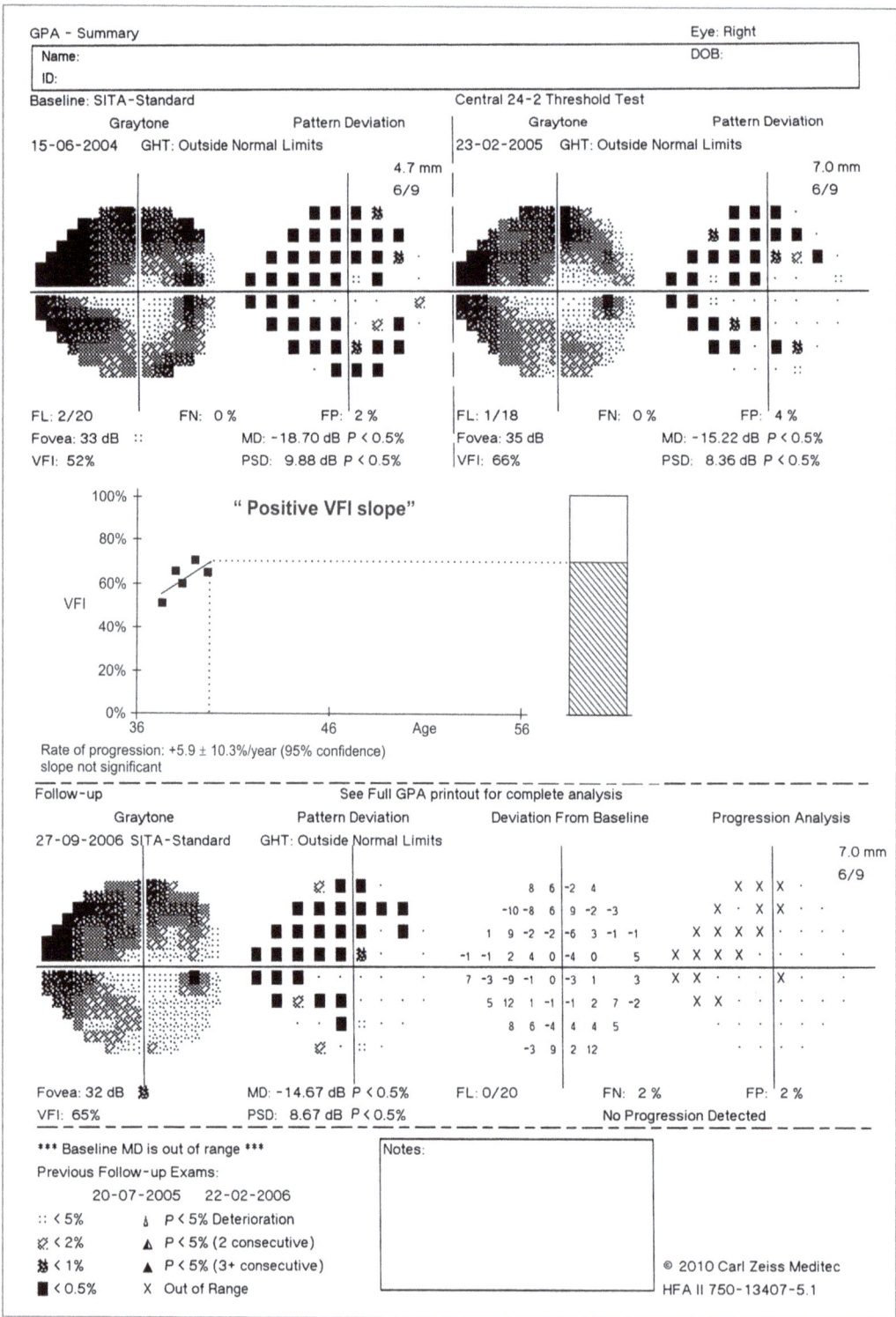

Fig. 10: Positive VFI slope. (GHT: glaucoma hemifield test; GPA II: guided progression analysis; MD: mean deviation; NEG: negative; POS: positive; PSD: pattern standard deviation; VFI: visual field index)
Courtesy: Carl Zeiss Meditec© (2010).

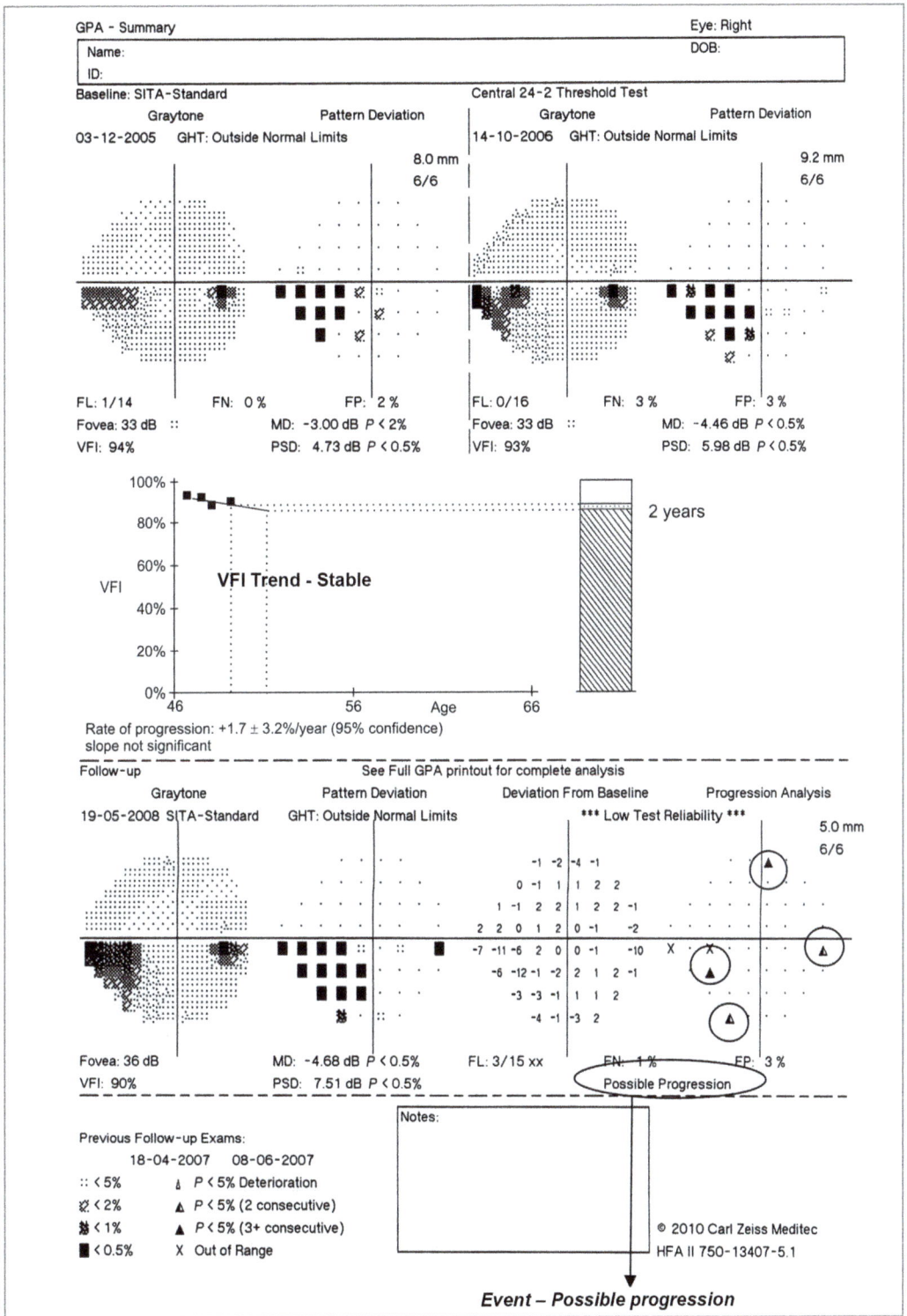

Fig. 11: Possible progression on event analysis with stable VFI trend. (GHT: glaucoma hemifield test; GPA II: guided progression analysis; MD: mean deviation; PSD: pattern standard deviation; VFI: visual field index)
Courtesy: Carl Zeiss Meditec© (2010).

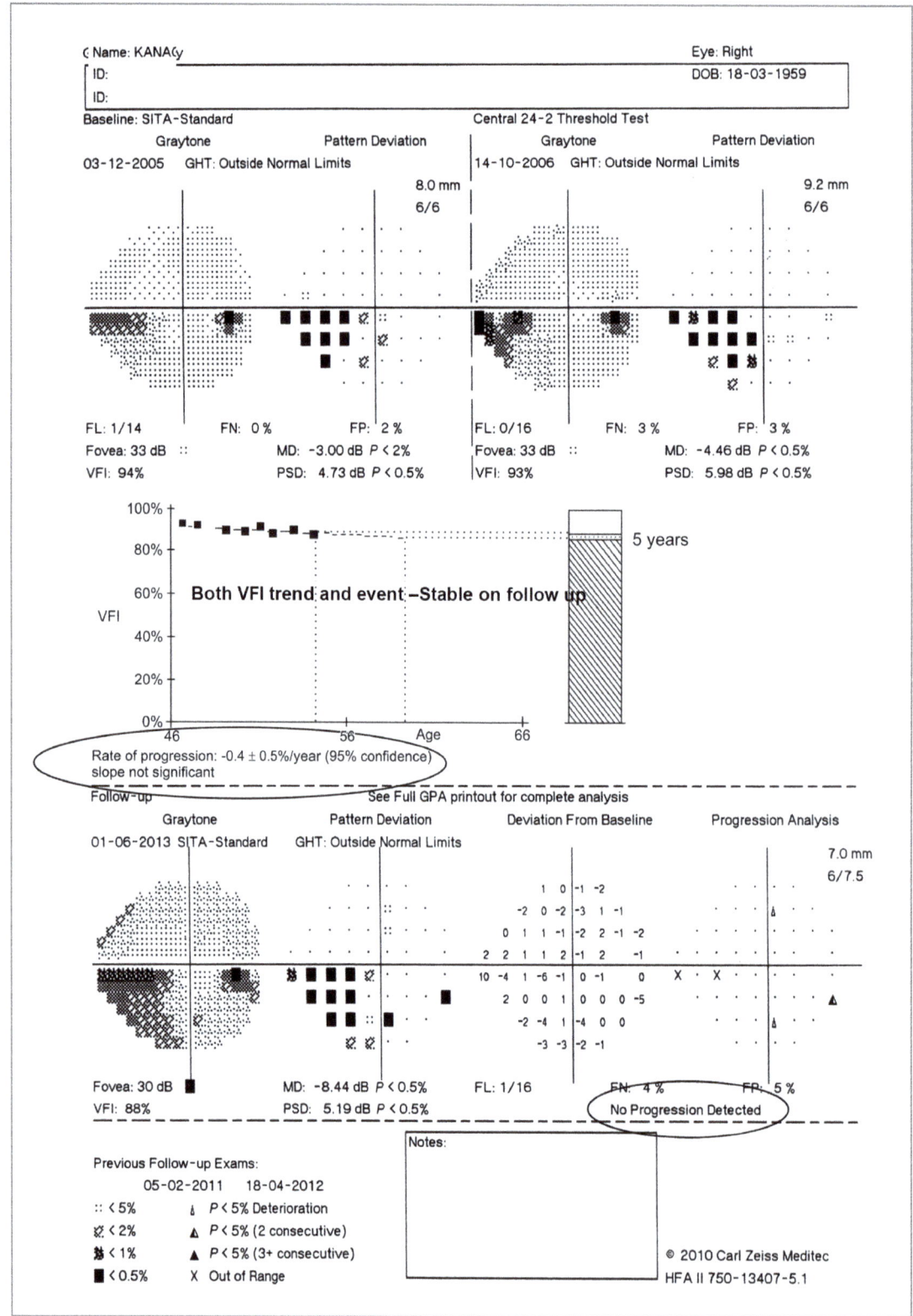

Fig. 12: Stable visual field on VFI trend and event analyses. (GHT: glaucoma hemifield test; GPA II: guided progression analysis; MD: mean deviation; PSD: pattern standard deviation; VFI: visual field index)
Courtesy: Carl Zeiss Meditec© (2010).

b. This patient **(Fig. 13)** has a very early cecocentral defect. The event showed a PP message with a stable VFI trend. The trend would not have detected progression since it is a very early defect that showed hardly any changes in the VFI. The points that showed progression in event analysis are the paracentral point and a few mid-peripheral points. Considering the location of progression points, we need to closely

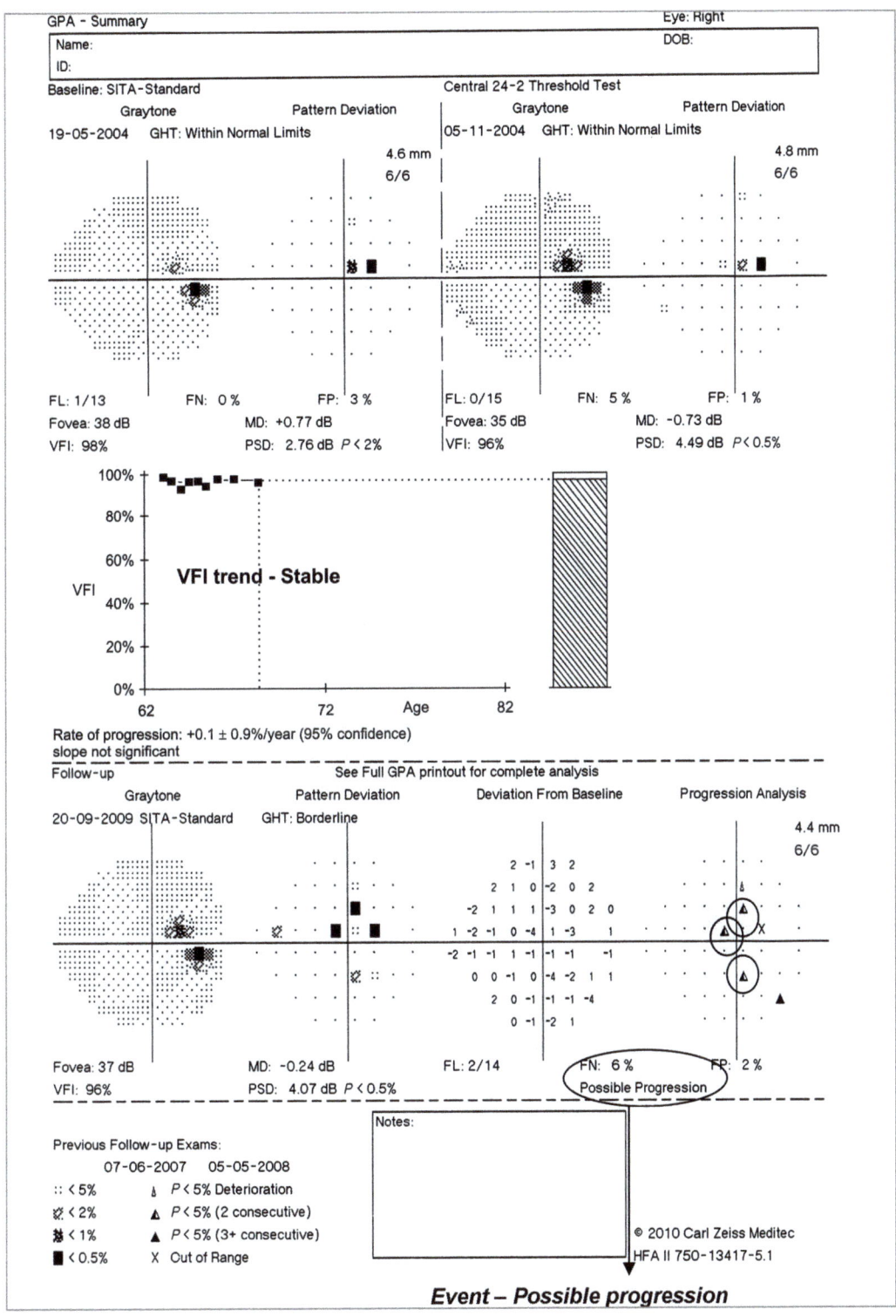

Fig. 13: No progression seen in VFI trend. (GHT: glaucoma hemifield test; GPA II: guided progression analysis; MD: mean deviation; PSD: pattern standard deviation; VFI: visual field index)
Courtesy: Carl Zeiss Meditec© (2010).

monitor this patient. We can consider performing other central threshold programs like 10-2 or macular threshold to monitor the progression.

c. In this case **(Fig. 14)** of a complete superior arcuate defect sparing the two paracentral points in the superotemporal quadrant, both the VFI and event showed stability. When we actually look into the progression analysis of the event, it warrants progression (half-filled triangle) in the two paracentral points.

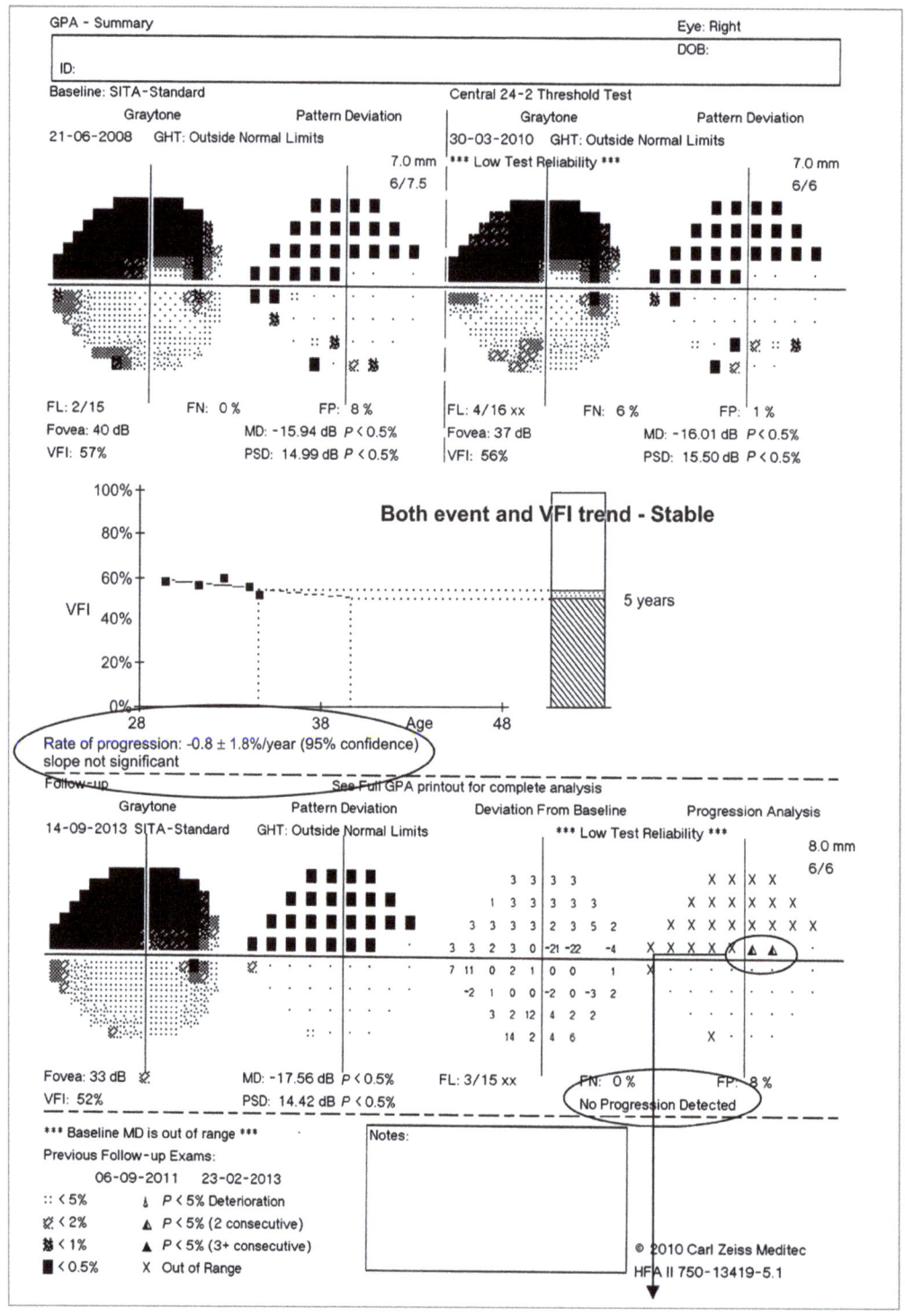

Fig. 14: Progression seen in paracentral points. (GHT: glaucoma hemifield test; GPA II: guided progression analysis; MD: mean deviation; PSD: pattern standard deviation; VFI: visual field index)
Courtesy: Carl Zeiss Meditec© (2010).

From these examples, one can infer that sometimes the progression message given by software might actually mask/mimic change in VF. Using subjective analysis of the change in VF along with the help of software and clinical presentation, one can categorize the VF as progressed/nonprogressed and accordingly plan the treatment regimen for each patient.

3. *Significance of reestablishing the baseline:* The VF threshold is not a stable quantity and fluctuation is found to be greater in the glaucomatous VF. The changes in VF are likely due to a learning curve/fluctuation or a true change due to disease progression. The selection of the baseline report should reflect the true VF status of the patient. Poor selection of baseline can overestimate or underestimate the progression rate of VF deterioration.

   a. This is a case **(Fig.15)** where this patient gradually progressed from normal fields to superior arcuate defects over almost 8 years of follow-up. By having the normal fields as the baseline, both the event and

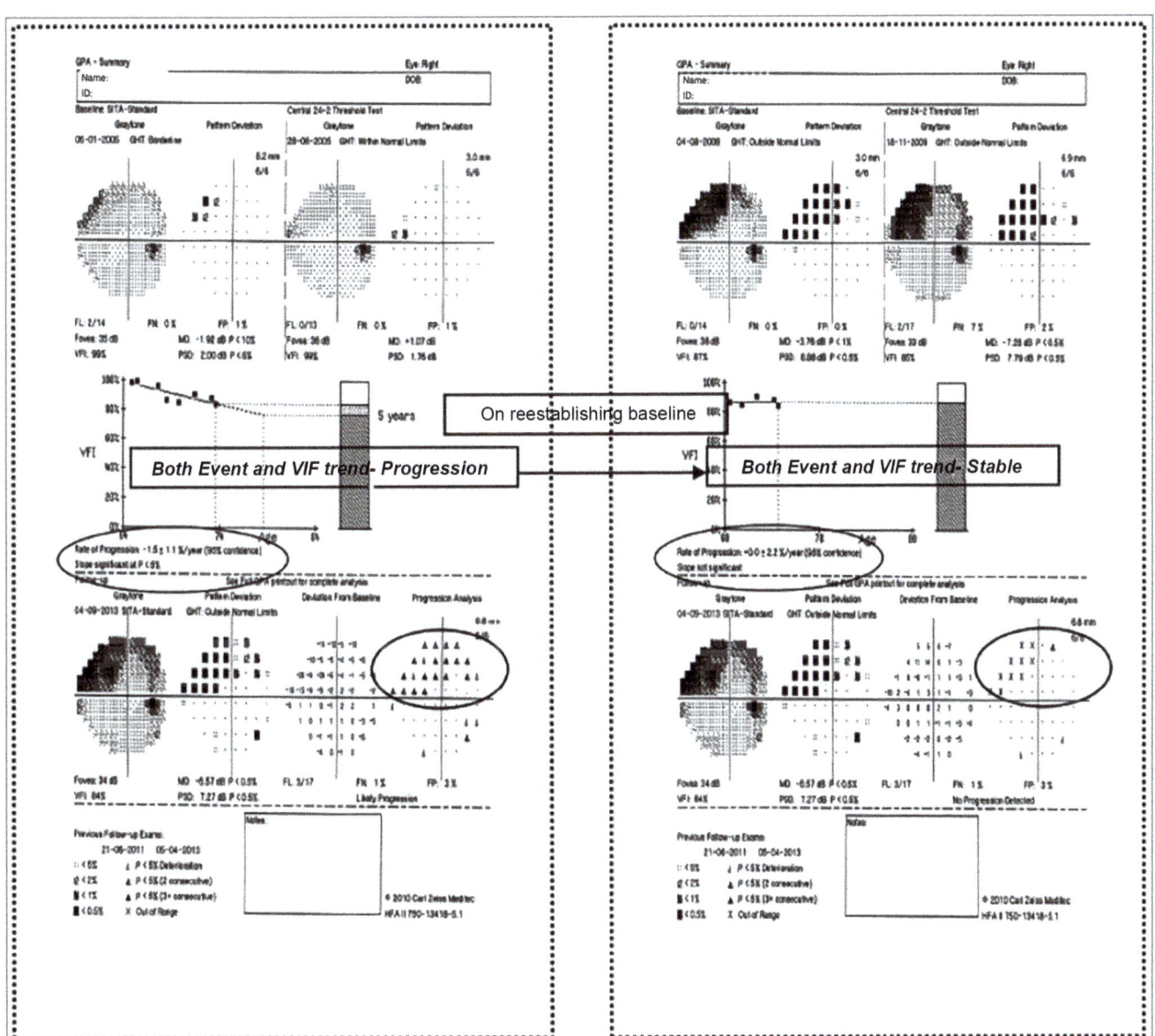

Fig. 15: Reestablishing baseline. (VFI: visual field index)

trend analyses showed progression. We probably do not need software to confirm the progression in the current VF status as compared to its normal baseline fields. Definitely, it is not required and the baseline does not represent the true VF status of the patient. The patient acquired a VF defect in the year 2008. After reestablishing the baseline, the VF is almost stable from the year 2008 to 2013 with a VFI ROP of +0.00% ± 2.2%/year.

b. In this example **(Fig. 16)**, the patient initially presented with superonasal defects that progressed to biarcuate defects with the intervention of trabeculectomy after the fourth visit. Having the superonasal defect as the baseline, both the event and trend showed progression. From the VFI trend, it is clearly visible that the patient VF gradually progressed from the first four visits and later became almost stable followed by trabeculectomy. Having changed the baseline followed by trabeculectomy, the event looked stable with an improved VFI trend slope presenting ROP of −2.2% ± 2.2%/year.

4. *Dealing with multiple VF visits/follow-ups:* Any trend analysis picks up progression earlier than the event if they have more number of VF visits. Here we present three examples, where VFI picked up progression in early, moderate, and severe VF loss.

a. This is a case of a very early superonasal defect **(Fig. 17)** where both event and trend picked up

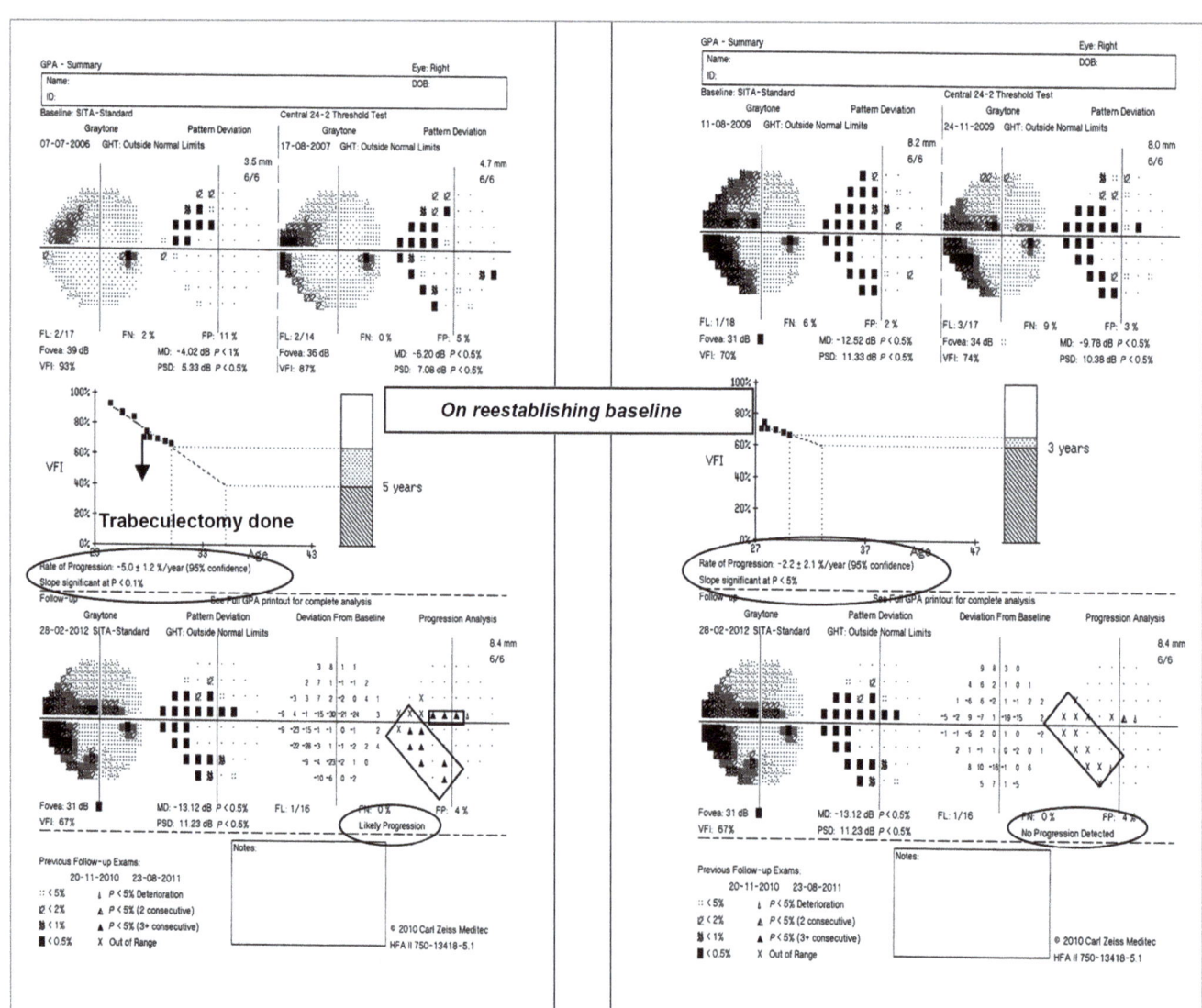

Fig. 16: Resetting baseline after trabeculectomy. (GHT: glaucoma hemifield test; FL: fixation losses; FN: false negative; FP: false positive; MD: mean deviation; PSD: pattern standard deviation; VFI: visual field index)
Courtesy: Carl Zeiss Meditec© (2010).

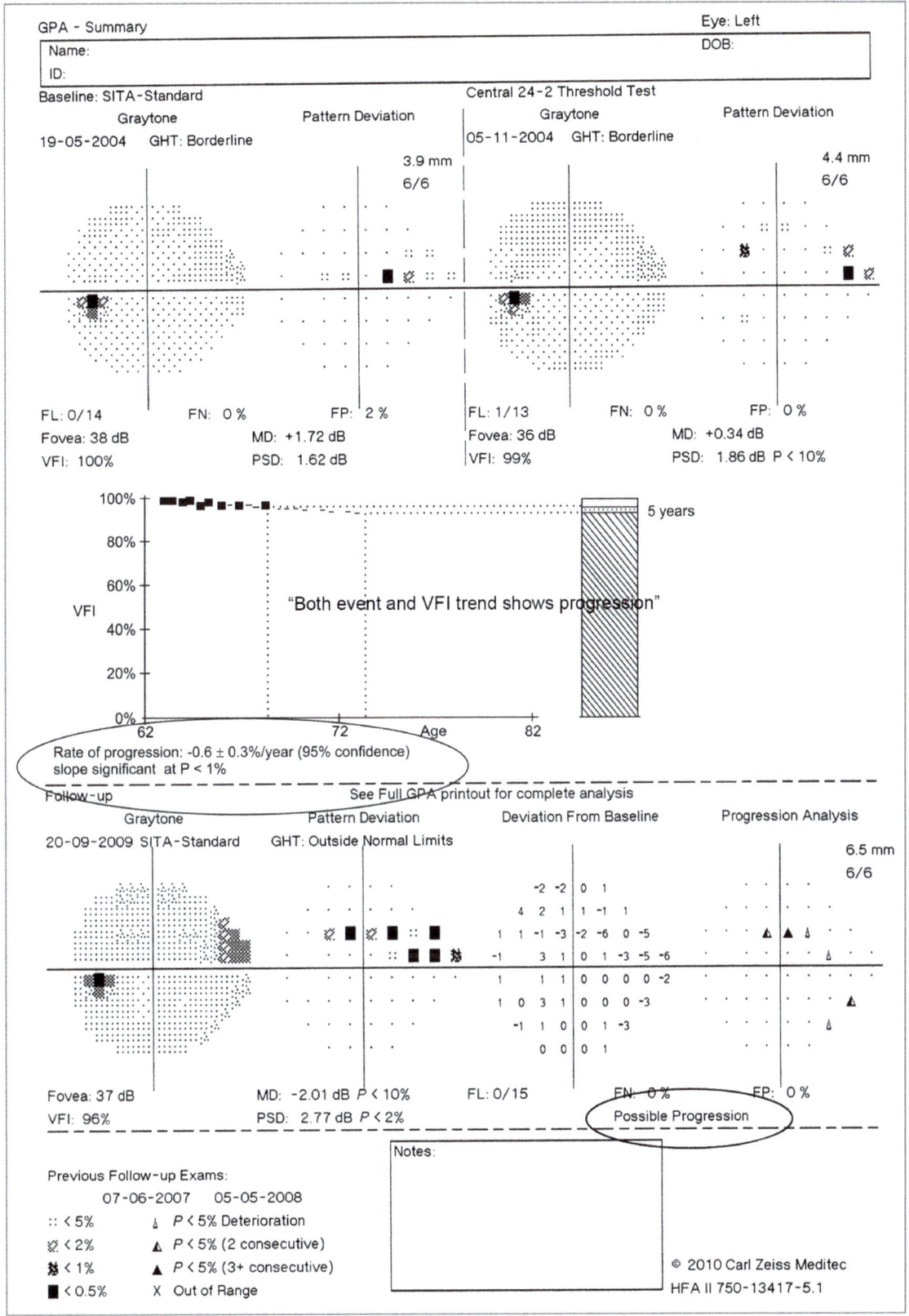

Fig. 17: Progression on both event and VFI trend. (GHT: glaucoma hemifield test; FL: fixation losses; FN: false negative; FP: false positive; MD: mean deviation; PSD: pattern standard deviation; VFI: visual field index)
Courtesy: Carl Zeiss Meditec© (2010).

progression. It is known that the event is likely to pick up progression earlier in an early VF defect as it does point-by-point analysis with the baseline report. The VFI trend requires a noticeable difference in the global index of VFI to warrant progression. With more follow-up fields, trend analysis can pick up the progression as well as the event.

b. This is a case of moderate VF loss where the patient presented with a superior arcuate defect in the year 2004 and maintained a stable defect pattern until 2009 with 15 VF visits. Both the MD trend and event **(Fig. 18)** analyses of the GPA I showed stable VF. The VFI trend picked up progression with ROP slope significant at $p < 1\%$ **(Fig. 19)**.

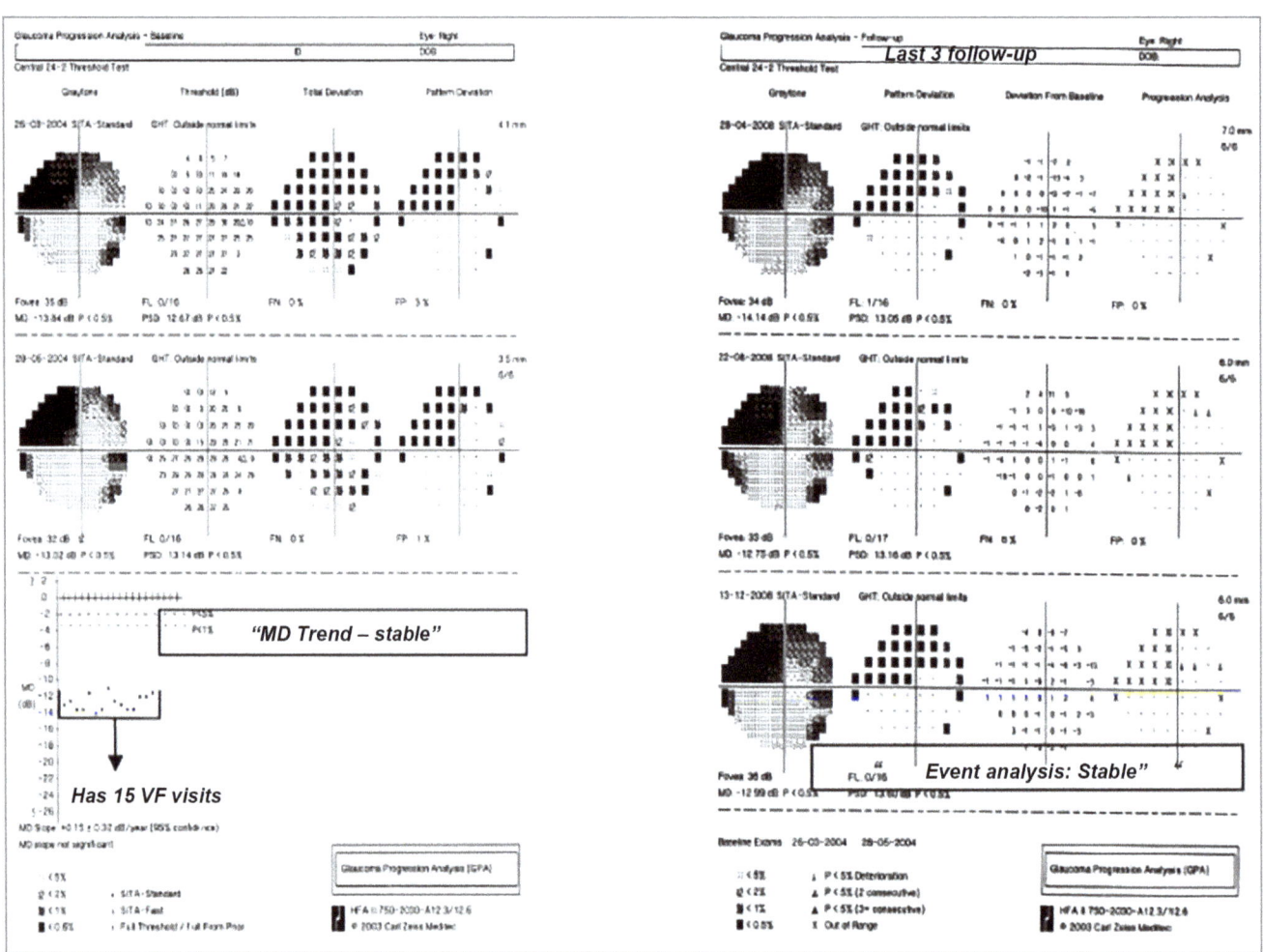

Fig. 18: Stable MD trend and event analyses. (MD: mean deviation; VF: visual field)

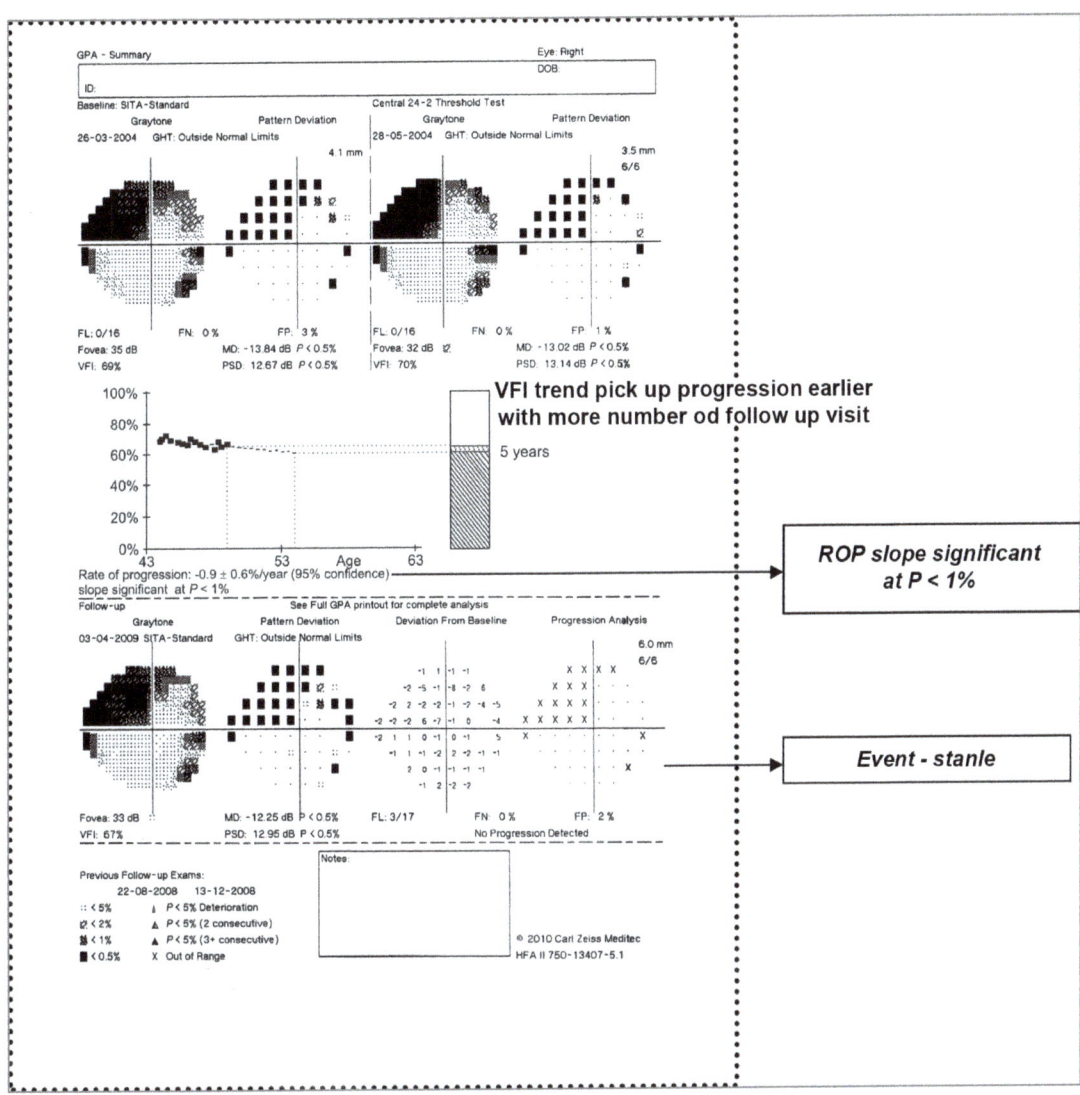

Fig. 19: VFI trend showing earlier progression. (GHT: glaucoma hemifield test; FL: fixation losses; FN: false negative; FP: false positive; MD: mean deviation; PSD: pattern standard deviation; ROP: rate of progression; VFI: visual field index)
Courtesy: Carl Zeiss Meditec© (2010).

c. This patient's VF **(Fig. 20)** progressed significantly from an inferior arcuate (2001) to advanced field loss (2013). The event analysis is not shown as the VF is severely depressed (> –20 dB). The VFI trend analysis shows progression at the rate of 4-6%/year with a slope significant at $p > 0.1\%$. Having changed the baseline from the initial inferior arcuate to a dense biarcuate defect, the VFI trend still detected ongoing progression almost leading to blindness in next 3 years.

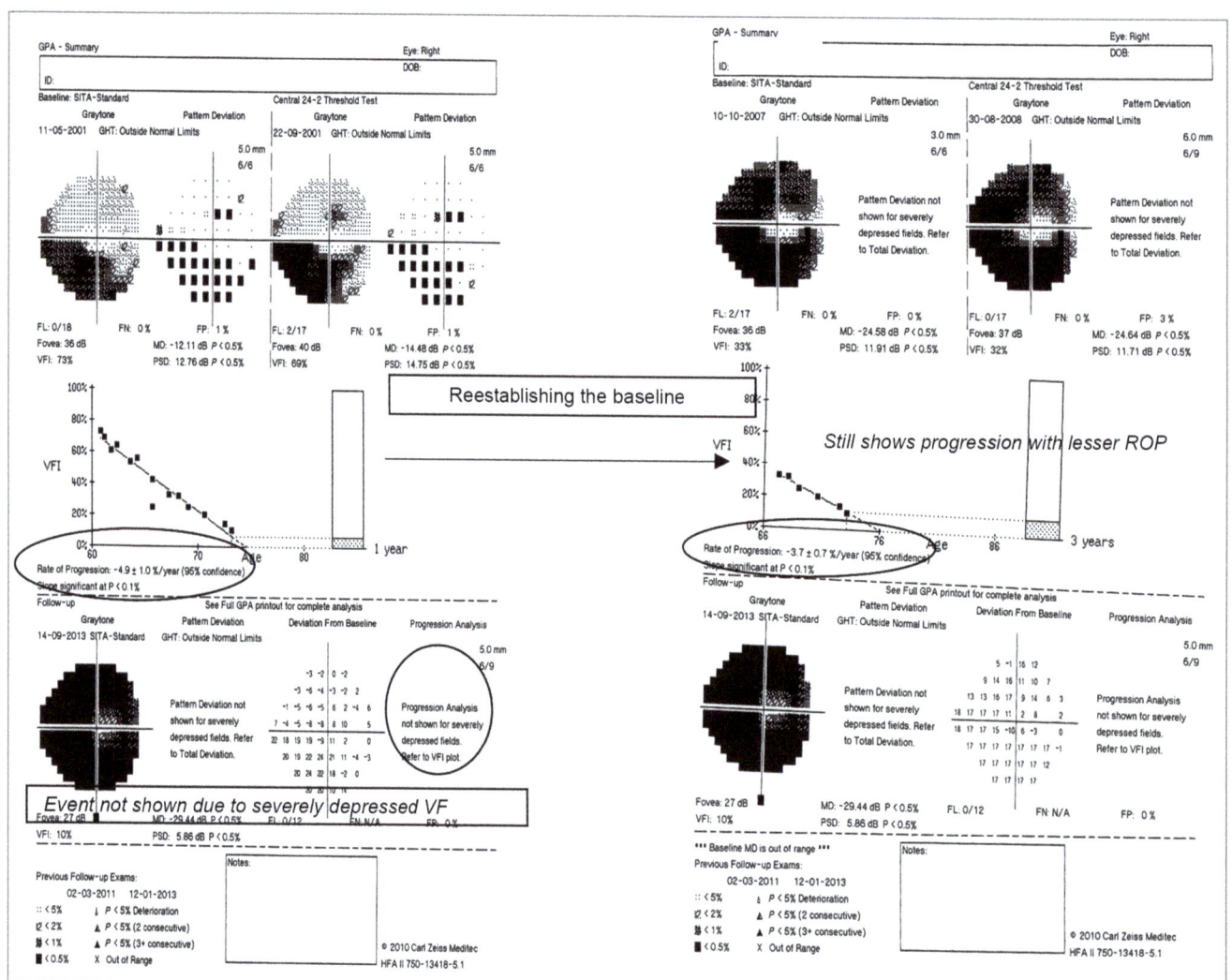

Fig. 20: Significant progression seen even after resetting the baseline. (GHT: glaucoma hemifield test; FL: fixation losses; FN: false negative; FP: false positive; MD: mean deviation; PSD: pattern standard deviation; ROP: rate of progression; VFI: visual field index)
Courtesy: Carl Zeiss Meditec© (2010).

VISUAL FIELD PROGRESSION ON 10-2 PROTOCOL

In addition to the assessment of VF progression using the standard protocol measuring the central 24° of the VF (24-2 program), we can evaluate progression on the 10-2 program too. This is beneficial in all cases with central defects, especially when the 24-2 GPA II shows progression involving the paracentral points.[23] In such cases, 24-2 based assessments fail to detect any further decline in thresholds because of the fact that the majority of the peripheral points are possible to have touched their "floor level." Here, GPA II based on the central VF program offers a greater resolution and can be relied upon **(Fig. 21)**.

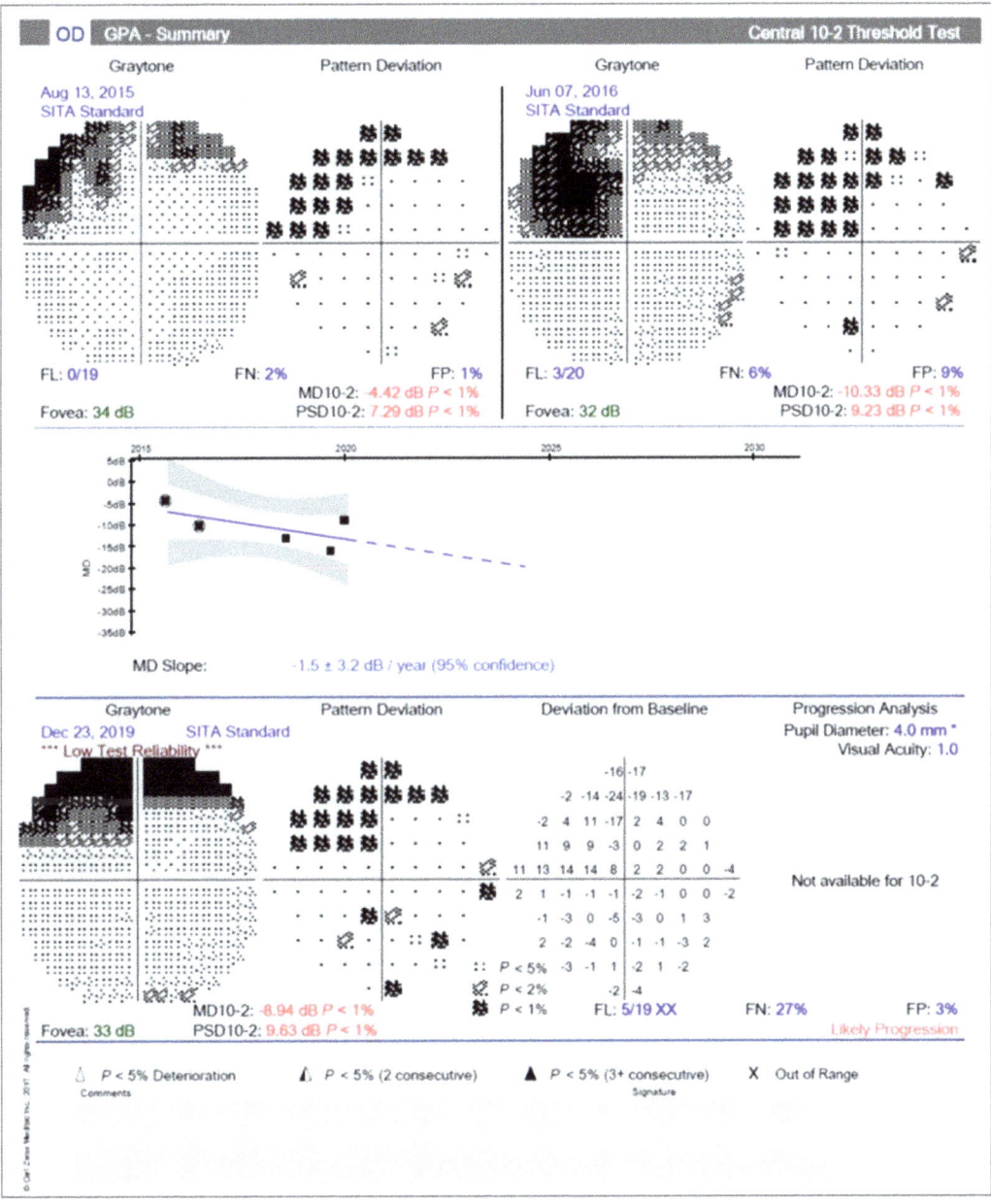

Fig. 21: 10-21 VFI trend showing likely progression. (GPA II: guided progression analysis; FL: fixation losses; FN: false negative; FP: false positive; MD: mean deviation; PSD: pattern standard deviation; VFI: visual field index)

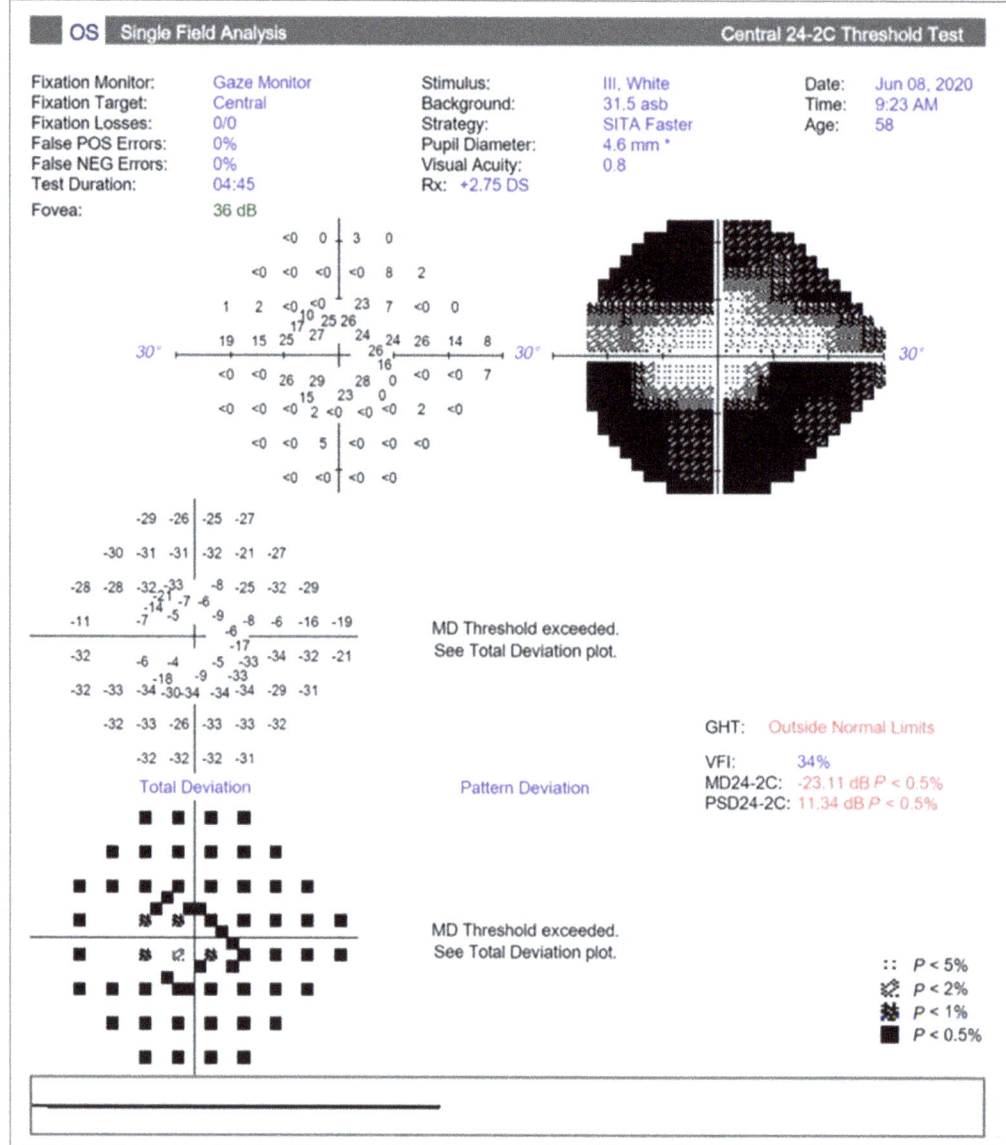

Fig. 22: 24-2C report. (GHT: glaucoma hemifield test; MD: mean deviation; NEG: negative; POS: positive; PSD: pattern standard deviation; VFI: visual field index)

In addition to 24-2 and 10-2 protocols, HFA is also equipped with a new 24-2C grid, which is basically the 24-2 grid but with 10 additional central 10° test points **(Fig. 22)**. These tests can also be incorporated in the progression analysis.

CONCLUSION

It is important to understand the principles of VF testing and the strategies employed in detecting VF defect progression. However, while interpreting a report, it is essential to pay attention to all the information presented and to not focus only on a single parameter in order to accurately interpret patient data that we come across in our routine clinical practice.

REFERENCES

1. Mikelberg FS, Drance SM. The mode of progression of visual field defects in glaucoma. Am J Ophthalmol. 1984;98:443-5.
2. Boden C, Blumenthal EZ, Pascual J, McEwan G, Weinreb RN, Medeiros F, et al. Patterns of glaucomatous visual field progression identified by three progression criteria. Am J Ophthalmol. 2004;138:1029-36.
3. Sample PA, Johnson CA. Functional assessment of glaucoma. J Glaucoma. 2001;10:S49-52.
4. Johnson CA. Psychophysical measurement of glaucomatous damage. Surv Ophthalmol. 2001;45:S313-8.
5. Turalba AV, Grosskreutz C. A review of current technology used in evaluating visual function in glaucoma. Semin Ophthalmol. 2010;25:309-16.
6. Jampel HD, Singh K, Lin SC, Chen TC, Francis BA, Hodapp E, et al. Assessment of visual function in glaucoma: A report by

the American Academy of Ophthalmology. Ophthalmology. 2011;118:986-1002.
7. Heijl A, Lindgren A, Lindgren G. Test-retest variability in glaucomatous visual fields. Am J Ophthalmol. 1989;108:130-5.
8. Heijl A, Asman P. Pitfalls of automated perimetry in glaucoma diagnosis. Curr Opin Ophthalmol. 1995;6:46-51.
9. Gonzalez de la Rosa M, Pareja A. Influence of the "fatigue effect" on the mean deviation measurement in perimetry. Eur J Ophthalmol. 1997;7:29-34.
10. Hutchings N, Wild JM, Hussey MK, Flanagan JG, Trope GE. The long-term fluctuation of the visual field in stable glaucoma. Invest Ophthalmol Vis Sci. 2000;41:3429-36.
11. Nordmann JP. How to assess the stability of glaucoma? Visual field. Fr Ophthalmol. 2006;29:22-6.
12. Tattersall CL, Vernon SA, Menon GJ. Mean deviation fluctuation in eyes with stable Humphrey 24-2 visual fields. Eye (Lond). 2007;21:362-6.
13. Susanna R Jr. Unpredictability of glaucoma progression. Curr Med Res Opin. 2009;25:2167-77.
14. Fogagnolo P, Sangermani C, Oddone F, Frezzotti P, Iester M, Figus M, et al. Long-term perimetric fluctuation in patients with different stages of glaucoma. Br J Ophthalmol. 2011;95: 189-93.
15. Gardiner SK, Crabb DP. Frequency of testing for detecting visual field progression. Br J Ophthalmol. 2002;86:560-4.
16. Ernest PJ, Schouten JS, Beckers HJ, Hendrikse F, Prins MH, Webers CA. The evidence base to select a method for assessing glaucomatous visual field progression. Acta Ophthalmol. 2012;90(2):101-8.
17. Spry PG, Johnson CA. Identification of progressive glaucomatous visual field loss. Surv Ophthalmol. 2002;47: 158-73.
18. Thomas R, George R. Interpreting automated perimetry. Indian J Ophthalmol. 2001;49:125-40.
19. Brusini P, Johnson CA. Staging functional damage in glaucoma: Review of different classification methods. Surv Ophthalmol. 2007;52(2):156-79.
20. Bengtsson B, Heijl A. Visual field index for calculation of glaucoma rate of progression. Am J Ophthalmol. 2008;145:343-53.
21. Chauhan BC, Garway-Heath DF, Goñi FJ, Rossetti L, Bengtsson B, Viswanathan AC, et al. Practical recommendations for measuring rates of visual field change in glaucoma. Br J Ophthalmol. 2008;92(4):569-73.
22. Shaarawy TM, Sherwood MB, Hitchings RA, Crowston JG (Eds). Glaucoma, 2nd edition. United Kingdom: Saunders Ltd.; 2014. p. 128.
23. Rao HL, Begum VU, Khadka D, Mandal AK, Senthil S, Garudadri CS. Comparing glaucoma progression on 24-2 and 10-2 visual field examinations. PLoS One. 2015;10(5):e0127233.

Visual Field Progression Analysis with Octopus Perimetry

CHAPTER 7

Mohana Sinnasamy, Murali Ariga, Jayasudha Roopesh, Niranjana Balasubramaniam

INTRODUCTION

Early detection of progression is essential in glaucoma care. When progression occurs, a new lower target intraocular pressure is to be set, and pressure-lowering treatment needs to be intensified.[1] However, since aggressive treatment is associated with an increased risk of medical and surgical complications, true progression needs to be identified from nonglaucomatous field changes due to the progression of cataracts, higher long-term fluctuations, or decreased sensitivity in uncooperative patients. Poor accuracy, disagreements among experts, excessive time consumption, and the inability to assess the rate of progression make the subjective comparison of serial visual field (VF) reports unacceptable for determining progression. When the rate of glaucomatous progression is at 1.0 decibel (dB)/year, an eye with a mild VF defect of 5.0 dB mean defect (MD) value at baseline will eventually progress to severe VF loss in 10 years, with minimal subjective symptoms. Thus, determination of the rate of progression early in the follow-up with software-guided analysis enables prompt intervention and better restoration of vision-related quality of life.

SELECTION OF ADEQUATE VISUAL FIELDS FOR PROGRESSION ANALYSIS[2,3]

Baseline Fields

A good baseline of reliable VFs is essential to monitor progression. In patients with a low–moderate lifetime risk of visual disability, at least two reliable VFs are optimal in the first 6 months. For those who already have advanced damage, where the lifetime risk of visual disability is high, three baseline VFs may be necessary.

Follow-up Fields

The higher the number of reliable cross-sectional fields used for progression analysis, the more reliable becomes the calculated progression slope. The frequency of follow-ups should be based on the risk of clinically significant progression in terms of the extent of damage and life expectancy.

Initial 2 years: To avoid misinterpretation of the results, using at least six reliable tests within the first 2 years of follow-up are recommended.

After 2 years: In low-risk and clinically stable patients VF should be one field per year, and in high-risk patients, subsequent VF frequency should be two VFs per year. As a rule, VF should be repeated sooner if clinical or event-based progression is identified.

Pay Attention to Quality and Threshold Strategy

Unreliable tests and tests made in the perimetric learning period must not be included in the analysis. Since different test strategies [normal, dynamic, and tendency-oriented perimetry (TOP) strategies] provide somewhat different sensitivity and defect values, only tests done with the same strategy are to be selected for progression analysis. EyeSuite progression analysis offers trend calculations only on tests that have been done with the same test pattern, stimulus, and background characteristics.

PROGRESSION ANALYSIS FUNCTIONS OFFERED BY THE OCTOPUS EYESUITE SOFTWARE[4,5]

Event analysis detects whether the change from baseline is greater than a predefined threshold. This threshold is based on test–retest variability (according to the level of damage). Trend analysis determines the rate of change over time. This significance is determined by the variability of the measurement and the magnitude of change. Rate-based analyses are used later in the follow-up when a greater number of VFs over a sufficient period are available to measure the rate of progression.

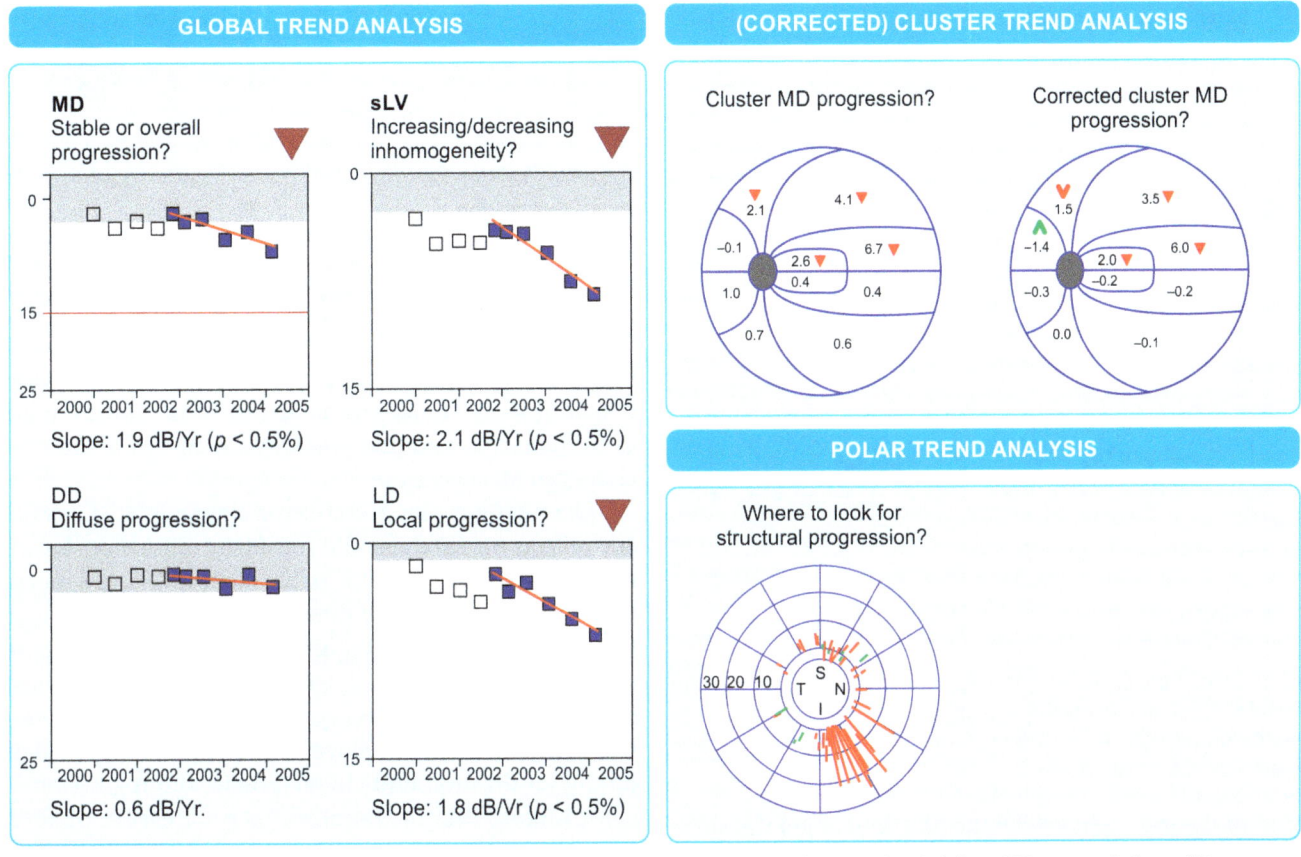

Fig. 1: Progression analysis tools with the Octopus EyeSuite software. (DD: diffuse defect; LD: local defect; MD: mean defect; sLV: square root of loss variance)
Source: Adapted from Racette L et al.[5]

In Octopus perimetry, a 15-dB MD value reflects a severe decline in vision-related quality of life. Also, localized defects in the paracentral area with lesser MD values can cause a similar decline in vision-related quality of life. Progressions of both small paracentral and larger scotomas within the 30° central VF can cause a clinically significant decline in the vision-related quality of life. However, the progression of these two types of deterioration cannot be optimally investigated with the same method. Thus, both the global and the individual cluster progression parameters need to be evaluated and clinically considered for decision-making. EyeSuite progression analysis of Octopus perimeter offers three types of progression analysis to assess VF change over time as shown in **Figure 1**.
1. Global trend analysis (GTA)
2. Cluster trend analysis (CTA) and corrected cluster trend analysis (CCTA)
3. Polar trend analysis (PTA)

Global Progression Analysis with the Octopus EyeSuite Software

The global progression analysis measures long-term change and statistically classifies it as global indices, namely mean defect (MD), diffuse defect (DD), local defect (LD), and square root of loss variance (sLV). The parameters analyzed for progression have been defined earlier in this book. The results of a global progression analysis are shown in **Figure 2**. It evaluates whether a series of VFs are stable or show a significant change. It also provides quantitative information about the rate of change in dB/year and on the local, diffuse, or combined nature of progression. The operator can select the individual tests for inclusion in progression analysis thus enabling ophthalmologists to exclude technically incorrect tests. In the progression analysis report, tests that are not used for the current analysis are represented with empty boxes, and those that are analyzed for progression are indicated with blue boxes.

For all plots, the zero value is given on the top of the Y-axis together with the corresponding normal range (gray zone), and the positive values (in dB) increase downward. The test date is plotted on the X-axis. Below each graph, the steepness of the corresponding progression slope (in dB/year) and its statistical significance are given along with the corresponding long-term fluctuation (in dB) and its statistical significance. When a progression slope shows a statistically significant worsening, filled red downward arrow (at $p < 1\%$) or a red downward arrow (at $p < 5\%$) is

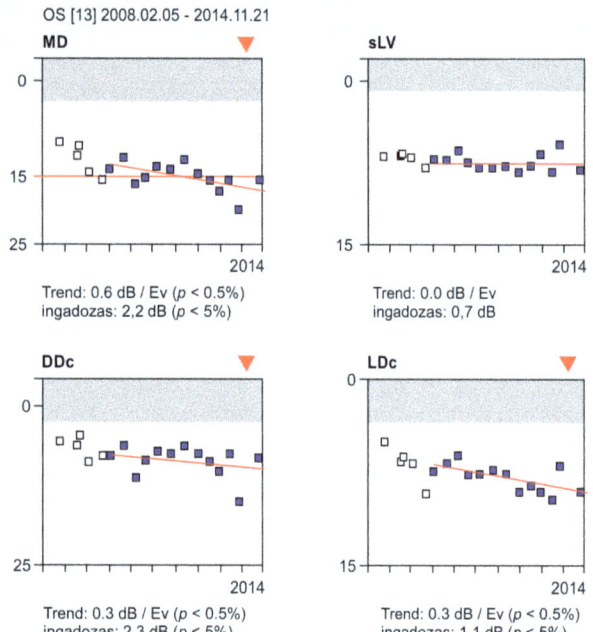

Fig. 2: Global progression analysis with the Octopus EyeSuite software. A detailed explanation is given in the text. (DDc: diffuse defect change; LDc: local defect change; MD: mean defect; sLV: square root of loss variance)

added to the top right side of the plot, and when the slope shows a statistically significant, improvement, a filled green arrow (at $p < 1\%$) or a green arrow (at $p < 5\%$) is added at the similar position. In advanced glaucoma, the overall loss of sensitivity in visual field series is frequently more than 20 dB. In such advanced disease states, it may not be possible to determine the stability or progression through the visual field series and is referred as floor effect.

It is important to note that these easy-to-use symbols reflect significant mathematical directions and not always clinical worsening or improvement. For example, relatively homogeneous field indicated by low sLV (green arrow) can be seen in normal visual field series and in advanced glaucoma, when all test points with some maintained sensitivity keep losing sensitivity and therefore become similar to the other test points and each other.

The top left plot is the MD slope. The change of the MD slope reflects the sum effect of all conditions and diseases that cause sensitivity reduction (e.g., cataracts, glaucoma, diabetic retinopathy, and age-related macular degeneration). For this reason, the MD slope is most important when the vision-related quality of life is investigated, but has limited usefulness when the progression of glaucoma is measured. In short, MD change is a good index to track overall VF change.

Interpretation of red trend line: If the line is flat, then the VF series is stable, if the line is sloping upward, then the field series is improving, and if the line is sloping downward, then the series is worsening. The red line at 15 dB MD as in

TABLE 1: Different situations reflecting progression in global trend analysis.

	MD	sLV	DD	LD
Stable				
Diffuse progression	▼		▼	
Local progression	▼	▼		▼
Diffuse and local progression	▼	▼	▼	▼

(DD: diffuse defect; LD: local defect; MD: mean defect; sLV: square root of loss variance)

Figure 2 indicates the level of a significant decline in vision-related quality of life. The steepness of the line is referred to as the slope, and this provides a measure of the rate of change in MD over time.

The top right plot presents the slope of the sLV change. sLV reflects on the threshold sensitivity differences between test points, for the given 24° or 30° central VF. It is a measure of the inhomogeny of the VF. No symbol is described if there is no change as in **Figure 2**. Increasing inhomogeneity is indicated by the red downward arrows and increasing homogeneity is indicated by the green upward arrows. On the other hand, the sLV slope does not provide information on the localization and characteristics of progression. sLV can progress due to the onset or progression of several other diseases with focal sensitivity losses (e.g., active chorioretinitis, vitreous floaters, or progression of diabetic retinopathy).

To overcome the limitations of the sLV plot, the bottom two plots evaluate the diffuse or local component of the defect. The bottom left is the diffuse defect change (DDc) plot, which determines whether there is diffuse field change independent of the LD. DDc represents the magnitude of the DD and reflects mainly on cataract progression, except for end-stage glaucoma where the final glaucomatous decline is diffuse.

The bottom right plot shows the nondiffuse (local) change of the cluster defects [local defect change (LDc)] independent from the presence or absence of a DD. A significant increase of LDc reflects on retinal nerve fiber bundle-type progression, which is typical of glaucomatous progression. In progressing end-stage glaucoma, the LDc progression slope, similar to the sLV progression slope, may decrease or remain unchanged. **Table 1** shows the trend of global indices in GTA as seen in four stages of disease progression—stable, diffuse progression, local progression, and diffuse and local progression.

Cluster Progression Analysis with the Octopus EyeSuite Software[6-8]

A separate progression analysis can also be made for each of the 10 VF clusters. The advantage of this analysis is that it enables ophthalmologists to detect and quantify

CHAPTER 7: Visual Field Progression Analysis with Octopus Perimetry

TABLE 2: Progression symbols, and their explanations used in cluster trend analysis (CTA) and corrected cluster trend analysis (CCTA).

Arrow marks	Probability (p)	Inference
∨	Worsening p <5 %	Likely worsening
▽	Worsening p <1%	Highly likely worsening
∧	Improvement p <5 %	Likely improving
△	Improvement p <1 %	Highly likely improving
◇	Fluctuation <5%	Likely fluctuating
◆	Fluctuation <1%	Highly likely fluctuating
⌐	Floor effect	Assessment of progression or stability cannot be done due to an advanced disease state with more than 20dB sensitivity loss

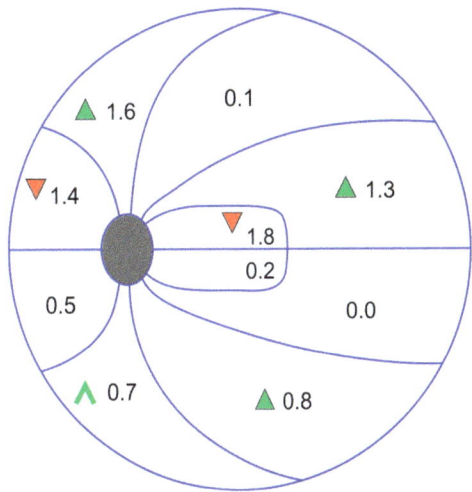

Fig. 4: The Corrected Trend Analysis wherein the changes due to diffuse defects are eliminated and reflects the local defects that correlate well with those due to glaucomatous changes.

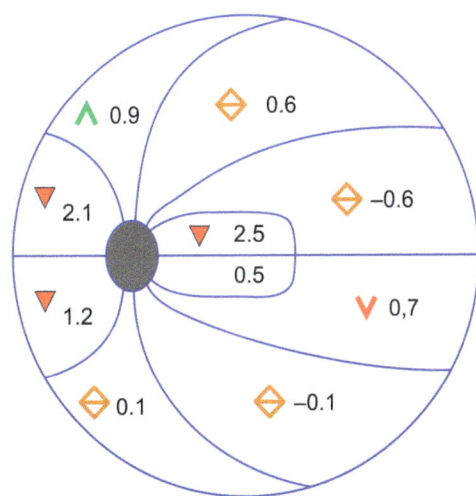

Fig. 3: The Cluster Trend Analysis showing the 10 clusters of VF that correlate with retinal nerve fiber layer spatially. This analysis includes both diffuse and local defects.

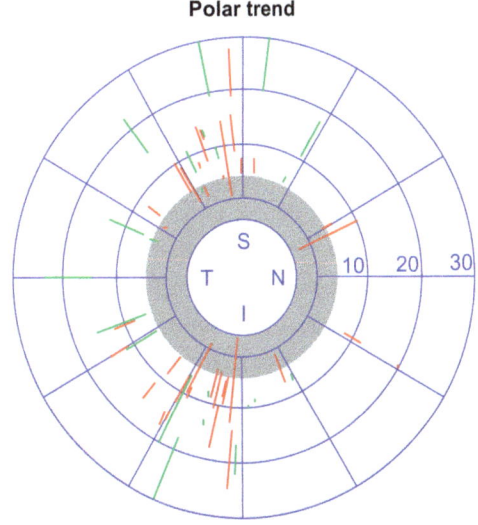

Fig. 5: Polar trend analysis for the eye and follow-up period shown in **Figures 3** and **4**.

the progression in dB/year for each cluster, separately. In CTA, the cluster defect is analyzed without any correction, wherein the influence of diffuse component (e.g., cataract) is eliminated in CCTA, thus, it reflects only glaucomatous progression. The progression symbols, and their explanations used in CTA and CCTA are shown in **Table 2**. **Figure 3** shows the results of CTA, and **Figure 4** shows the results of CCTA for the same eye. The differences between the corresponding cluster progression values of CTA and CCTA illustrate the usefulness of the removal of the diffuse progression component from the analysis when glaucomatous progression is evaluated.

Progression Analysis with the Polar Trend Analysis Function of the Octopus EyeSuite Software

The cross-sectional polar graph report is explained in detail in Chapter 4. PTA performs individual point-wise trend analysis to determine the trend line at each VF test location, where the corresponding retinal nerve fiber bundles arrive at the margin of the optic nerve head.[9] For test points with worsening sensitivity values, the change is indicated with red bars; for test points with improving sensitivity values, the change is indicated with green bars (**Fig. 5**). It does not give the quantity of change numerically, though the approximate change of each defect in dB can be identified on the graph.

This enables ophthalmologists to identify optic disc and retinal nerve fiber layer areas where structural progression is expected. Confirmation and objective measurement of the true structural change, however, is to be made with structural measurement methods such as disc photographs, optical coherence tomography, or scanning laser tomography. PTA is useful for the combined evaluation of the structural and functional progression as it correlates well with structural progression data.

SUMMARY OF THE CLINICAL UTILITY OF DIFFERENT PROGRESSION ANALYSIS METHODS

Both global and cluster progression need to be investigated when a decision on VF progression or stability is made. The following are different scenarios emphasizing the importance of considering all the progression parameters before making any therapeutic decision.

Scenario 1: No significant progression of the MD, sLV, DDc, and LDc slopes. This reflects disease stability.

Scenario 2: Progression of the MD and DDc slopes with no significant sLV and LDc slopes. This reflects isolated cataract progression or in some end-stage glaucoma cases where the final progression is a diffuse sensitivity loss.

Scenario 3: A significant isolated progression of the sLV and LDc slopes reflects on nerve fiber bundle-type progression (glaucomatous progression) without cataract progression.

Scenario 4: Both the MD and DDc slopes and the sLV and LDc slopes progress in a significant manner. This signifies combined glaucomatous and cataract-related progression as seen in many cases.

Scenario 5: When sLV progresses but LDc does not progress, the change is not due to a nerve fiber bundle-type progression. This is seen in nonglaucomatous conditions with focal sensitivity loss such as chorioretinitis and diabetic retinopathy.

To evaluate the impact of the localized progression (e.g., progression in a paracentral or inferior cluster) on the patient's quality of life, CTA and CCTA values need to be investigated. With the assistance of PTA, ophthalmologists can check if measurable structural progression is present in locations that spatially correspond to the rapidly progressing VF clusters. The presence of a functionally corresponding structural progression strengthens the indication for additional therapeutic intervention.

REFERENCES

1. European Glaucoma Society. Terminology and Guidelines for Glaucoma, 5th edition. Br J Ophthalmol. 2021;105(Suppl 1): 1-169.
2. Chauhan BC, Garway-Heath DF, Goñi FJ, Rossetti L, Bengtsson B, Viswanathan AC, et al. Practical recommendations for measuring rates of visual field change in glaucoma. Br J Ophthalmol. 2008;92(4):569-73.
3. Weinreb RN, Garway-Heath DF, Leung C, Crowston JG, Medeiros FA; World Glaucoma Association. WGA Consensus Series 8: Progression of Glaucoma. Amsterdam: Kugler Publications; 2011.
4. Rangaraj NR, Ariga M. Octopus Perimetry: A Synopsis. Diagnosis and Management of Glaucoma. New Delhi: Jaypee Brothers Medical Publishers (P) Ltd.; 2013. p. 219.
5. Racette L, Fischer M, Bebie H, Holló G, Johnson C, Matsumoto C (Eds). Visual Field Digest. A guide to perimetry and the Octopus perimeter, 6th edition. Köniz, Switzerland: Haag-Streit AG; 2016.
6. Aoki S, Murata H, Fujino Y, Matsuura M, Miki A, Tanito M, et al. Investigating the usefulness of cluster-based trend analysis to detect visual field progression in patients with open-angle glaucoma. Br J Ophthalmol. 2017;101(12):1658-65.
7. Naghizadeh F, Holló G. Detection of early glaucomatous progression with octopus cluster trend analysis. J Glaucoma. 2014;23(5):269-75.
8. Gardiner SK, Mansberger SL. Detection of functional deterioration in glaucoma by trend analysis using comprehensive overlapping clusters of locations. Sci Rep. 2020;10(1):18470.
9. Holló G, Naghizadeh F. Evaluation of Octopus Polar Trend Analysis for detection of glaucomatous progression. Eur J Ophthalmol. 2014;24(6):862-8.

8 Visual Fields—An Overview

Ankur Sinha, Gitanjali Sharma

DEFINITION

Visual field is defined as a part of space in which the objects are visible while keeping the focus of the eye fixed at a point, which can be of one eye (called as monocular field of vision) or both eyes (called as binocular field of vision).

To experience and understand this, when one closes both the eyes, the person experiences darkness or lack of vision. Now when, one opens an eye, and fixes the focus to a particular object, he or she is able to see other objects around the point of fixation in the space. This is what is the visual field. When both eyes are open the visible area or the field of vision increases.

The horizontal and vertical extent (two dimensions) of visual field can be easily perceived and charted. When the retinal sensitivity or the ability to perceive stimulus is also added as the third dimension, it forms a three-dimensional hill-like structure, which was described by Traquair[1] as "an island of vision or hill of vision surrounded by a sea of blindness".

Here, the peak of the hill corresponds with the fovea (maximum retinal sensitivity),[2] as one moves away, the retinal sensitivity drops sharply from 0 to 3°, then a little gradually from 3 to 30° and again falls sharply from 30° degrees and beyond. It should be borne in mind that every point in retina has a representation in the visual field. However, as the image formed on retina is upside down and side by side inverse, a point nasal to fovea, will be represented in the temporal field and vice versa.

ASSESSMENT AND MEASUREMENT OF VISUAL FIELD

When we talk of visual field assessment and measurement, there are some pertinent terms that should be kept in mind for better understanding.

Field of Vision

As described previously, the horizontal and vertical extent of visual field can be easily perceived and understood, however, the visible area or the visual field increases as the object moves away from the eye as a result the size of the object decreases. Hence, it is pertinent to express the visual field in such a way that "the distance factor" is negated, so the visual fields are expressed in degrees from the center of fixation. Similarly, the apparent size of the stimulus plays an important role, e.g., 1.00 mm spot at 33 cm will look similar in size to a 2.00 mm spot at 1 meter or a 6.0 mm spot at 2 meter.

For each eye, the nasal and superior boundary of the field is approximately 60°, (limited by the nasal bridge and the brow and supraorbital margin, respectively), temporal visual field boundary is 100°, and inferior extent is 70° (limited by the cheek).

Assessment of visual field requires measurement of the outermost boundary and the degree of retinal sensitivity (or the visual function) at each point within the boundary.

Scotoma

It is a measure of visual field abnormality in terms of visual field defects. For simpler understanding, it can be considered as a complete nonseeing area (area of no vision or zero retinal sensitivity) surrounded by a seeing area called as absolute scotoma. Or it may be areas of relatively less vision (with diminished or reduced sensitivity as compared age-matched normal population) known as relative scotoma.

Luminance

Luminance is the degree of brightness of a stimulus. A brighter stimulus or more intense light would be easily perceived as compared to dimmer or less intense light. There are various measurement systems used to measure intensity of light. In current day perimeters, it is measured in apostilbs (it corresponds to 1 lumen of total emittance per square meter of illuminated surface). The maximum stimulus intensity of Humphrey perimeter is 10,000 apostilbs, while that of Octopus or Goldmann perimeter is 1,000 asb.

Retinal Sensitivity

It is an objective measure of visual function at a particular retinal point. Dimmest or the weakest stimulus seen at a particular point is said to be the retinal sensitivity of that point. The retinal ability to detect the weakest point/spot of light depends on the color of stimulus, size of stimulus, luminous intensity of stimulus, background illumination, and movement of stimulus (Riddoch phenomenon, i.e., moving targets are more easily visible).

In current perimeters, the maximum intensity of light is attenuated or reduced with help of neutral density filters. This attenuation of light is measured in logarithmic units or decibels (dB). A 0 dB stimulus has no reduction from maximum intensity, hence blind spot's sensitivity would have value of 0 dB, i.e., even the brightest stimulus is not visible. Higher the retinal sensitivity, weaker the stimulus visible or seen, greater is the attenuation or the decibel reading, which in turn, means the stimulus intensity is lower (apostilbs). Therefore, a point with sensitivity of 20 dB is more sensitive than a point with sensitivity of 10 dB. As dB is not a linear but a log scale, one log unit attenuation equals to 10 dB, which in turn reduces the stimulus intensity of one-tenth of maximum. Decibel and apostilbs are inversely proportional. As mentioned earlier, the maximum stimulus intensity of Octopus and Humphrey are different. A 10 dB stimulus on Octopus perimeter would not be equal to 10 dB stimulus on Humphrey perimeter.

Background Illumination

It is standardized at 31.5 apostilbs for both the Goldmann perimeter and the Humphrey field analyzer (HFA).

Isopter

It is the line connecting points of the same retinal sensitivity. It is a concept associated with kinetic perimetry as described later.

Threshold

As described previously, every retinal point has different sensitivity, hence its own threshold intensity of light seen. With fixed stimulus size and background illumination, the weakest stimulus seen on at least 50% times it is presented is called as threshold stimulus. It is defined as "the luminance of a given test stimulus at which it is seen on 50% of the occasions, it is presented". It is highest at fovea and decreases progressively toward the periphery. A stronger stimulus than threshold is called suprathreshold and a weaker is called as infrathreshold stimulus. Humphrey takes into account the weakest stimulus seen, while octopus takes into account average of weakest seen and strongest not seen.

TABLE 1: Goldman's notation for stimulus size in mm sq and degrees.

Size	mm² at 30 cm	Average diameter
O	0.0625 (1/16)	0.05°
I	0.25 (1/4)	0.11°
II	1	0.22°
III	4	0.43°
IV	16	0.86°
V	64	1.72°

Stimulus Size

The retinal sensitivity also depends on the apparent size of stimulus. To standardize this, the diameter of cupola of visual field and the size of stimulus is standardized and expressed as Goldmann's notation as shown in the **Table 1**.

METHODS OF ASSESSMENT OF VISUAL FIELD

For assessing the gross outermost boundary at the bedside or in the office, the fastest and easiest method used is confrontation visual fields. In this method, the observer compares his/her visual field with that of subject. It is useful for moderate to advanced sensitivity losses, but it does not pick up subtle defects.

Broadly speaking, there are two methods of assessment of visual field—(1) Static perimetry and (2) Kinetic perimetry.

Static Perimetry

It is the most commonly performed and easily available form of perimetry.

The name "static" refers to the stimulus being stationary, however, its intensity and stimulus size may be varied. In a typical static perimeter program, the stimulus size remains fixed for one examination, the intensity may be changed. The basic format of testing is to ascertain the minimal intensity perceived at a particular fixed retinal point and compare it with the age-matched normative database. To accomplish this the intensity of light is increased until it is just seen (threshold) or reduced until it is no longer seen.

As it is standardized and reproducible, it brings out subtle visual field defects, however, it is operator dependent. Static perimetry is an important part of glaucoma evaluation as, in glaucoma one needs to find out how much retinal sensitivity is lost at a particular point.

Humphrey field analyzer HFA and the Octopus® perimeter are the most common perimeters under this category. Kinetic programs are also available on these but not used commonly.

Kinetic Perimetry

As the name suggests, in this method, the stimulus is kinetic, i.e., moved (at a constant speed 2–4° per second) from a nonseeing area to a seeing area until it is just perceived. These points, perceived by the subject, are marked along various meridians, and then joined. The lines thus created are called isopters. The overall result is equivalent to contour lines on the hill of vision. When the isopter lines are crowded it means there is a steep scotoma. It should be noted that is no change in the intensity or size of the stimulus for one isopter.

The most common kinetic perimeter is the Goldmann perimeter. Although it is easier to comprehend and perform, it is sparingly used in clinical practice due to dependency on the performance of the perimetrist. It does not provide numerical data and is also not reproducible from institution to institution.

Kinetic perimetry plays more role in neurological defects, as here it is important to ascertain pattern of visual field loss, which may help in localizing the lesion, in visual pathway.

AUTOMATED STATIC THRESHOLD PERIMETRY

Static perimetry, as mentioned earlier, involves stationary test points. The testing stimulus could be of two types—(1) Suprathreshold and (2) Threshold.

Suprathreshold testing involves testing with a stimulus of intensity above the threshold for age-matched control population, to assess whether it is seen by the subject or not. It is a rapid test and its use is limited to screening purposes.

Threshold perimetry, on the other hand, is used for detailed visual field assessment, where the exact threshold at each point is determined by presenting stimulus of increasing intensity at the point it is first seen, and then reducing its intensity to reach the threshold. This is automated,[3,4] i.e., it is age-matched and points are projected randomly and at somewhat varied time interval to eliminate patient anticipation. Data is presented as grayscale symbols and numerical sensitivity values in decibels. The standard protocol is white-on-white (white target on white background) stimuli with default Goldmann size III target. For advanced defects, the target size may be increased up to a size V, however, the normative database may not be available for nonstandard parameters. In order to detect, defect early, blue on yellow (blue target in yellow background) or short-wavelength automated perimetry may be used.

Test Strategies and Type of Program

There are various strategies and programs on a given perimeter.

In Humphrey perimeter, the available test strategies are full threshold, FASTPAC and Swedish interactive threshold algorithm (SITA) strategy.[5-7] SITA can further have standard, fast and faster strategies, or algorithms.

In full threshold strategy, to begin with, a stimulus is presented at a test location. If the subject responds by click of the button, then it is gradually reduced in intensity by 4 dB, if not, then the stimulus intensity is increased by 4 dB. Once the subject responds, the stimulus is then decreased by 2 dB till the subject fails to respond. The last seen stimulus is taken as the threshold for the test point. This staircase strategy or bracketing is used at all the test points.

In the FASTPAC program, a fixed 3 dB step size to ascertain the retinal sensitivity.

In SITA program, complex mathematical models are used to ascertain the retinal threshold. SITA programs have standard, fast, and faster strategies (as the name suggest, fast and faster are respectively less time consuming).

Perimeters have 30-2, 24-2, and 10-2 as common glaucoma programs to choose from.[8] The number "–2" in all the above programs signifies that the test points are on either side of midline vertically as well as horizontally, such that no point falls on the midline. 30-2, 24-2, and 10-2 test the central 30°, 24°, and 10° of fields with 76, 54, and 68 test points, respectively. While 30-2 and 24-2 are routinely used for glaucoma screening and diagnosis, 10-2 along with macular program (with central 16 points) is used for advanced glaucoma. The newer Humphrey perimeters have 24-2C program available from early 2019, where 10 additional points (asymmetric in arrangement) are added to 24-2 program, to detect early central defects.

INTERPRETATION OF A HUMPHREY FIELD ANALYZER TEST REPORT

Once the perimeter has finished testing the patient, it provides a printed report for single field. It is important to methodically analyze the report. For the ease of understanding the single field printout can be divided into eight parts, the details are given here (**Fig. 1**):

1. At the top is the procedure information and the patient data. It provides patient's name, hospital ID, date of birth, the eye examined, the date and time of examination, the strategy used, stimulus size, visual acuity, refractive correction, and the pupil diameter. One should always check each information, as this ensures correctness of the fields with respect to patient and the eye, date of examination, etc. It also helps in checking the defects due to small pupil size, poor vision, or incorrect glasses placed in the lens holder. It is advisable to use the same strategy for each follow-up. Date of birth should be entered correctly as the data is compared with age-matched control population **(Fig. 2)**.

2. Just below it, on the right corner are the reliability indices:[9]
   i. *Fixation monitor:* To monitor the fixation, Humphrey perimeter utilizes the physiological blind spot of the patient, the blind spot is mapped early in the course of field testing.
   ii. *Fixation target:* Fixation target is the target given to the patient during the course of perimetry. It is usually the central yellow light; however, it can be changed in cases with poor vision or specific types of tests being performed.
   iii. *Fixation losses:* It is a measure of how steadily the subject is looking at the point of fixation. They are determined by Heijl-Krakau method where intermittently stimulus is presented at the blind spot and if the subject responds positively, it is measured as a fixation loss. A maximum of 20% fixation losses are acceptable.
   iv. *False positive:* As the name suggests, they are positives (reported "seen" by the patient) erroneously. It signifies that the patient has reported seeing a stimulus without the presentation of stimulus, such patients are called as "trigger-happy". The upper limit of acceptable false positives is 15%. With high false positives, there would be abnormally high thresholds of the first few points, with high mean deviation (MD) and abnormally lengthy testing. The glaucoma hemifield test (GHT) would show "abnormal high sensitivity" and there would

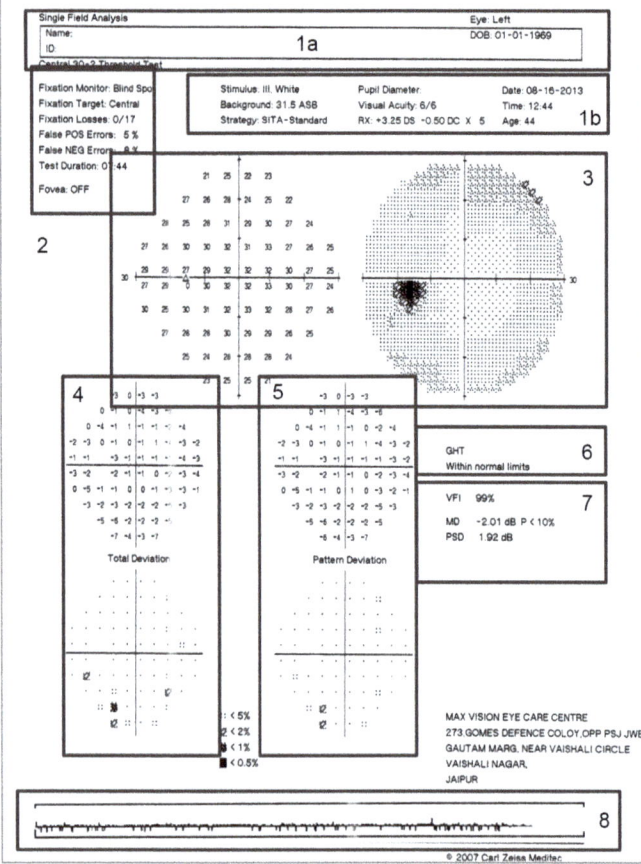

Fig. 1: Division of single field print out of Humphrey in various parts for analysis. 1a and 1b: Procedure information and patient data, 2: Reliability indices, 3: Raw numeric data and grayscale, 4: Total deviation numeric and probability plot, 5: Pattern deviation numeric and probability plot, 6: Glaucoma hemi field test, 7: Global indices and visual field index (VFI), 8: Gaze tracker.

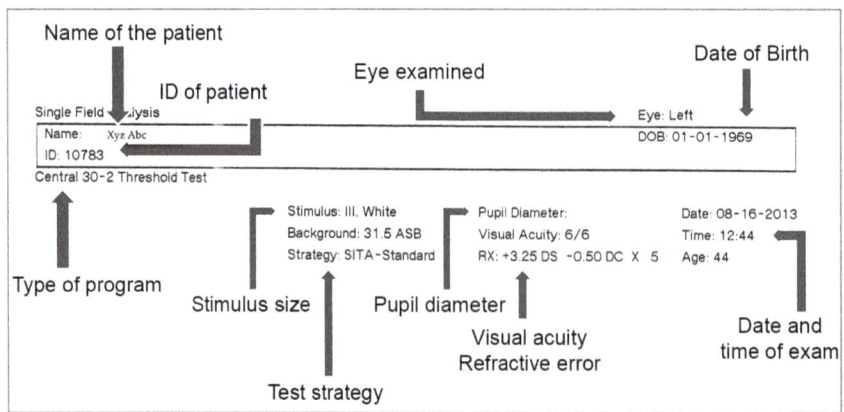

Fig. 2: The details of patient data and procedure information in a single field print out of Humphrey visual field.

be larger defects in the pattern deviation rather than MD plots.

v. *False negative:* As the name suggests, the responses are erroneously reported "not seen" by the patient, i.e., a presumably visible stimulus (9 dB higher than the previously determined threshold sensitivity) reported by the patient as not seen. This occurs when the patient has lost concentration, is fatigued, or is inattentive, where the patient is not responding to the stimuli. With excessively high false negatives, the MD will show a high negative value along with a high pattern standard deviation (PSD). The usual acceptable limit of false negatives is 20%, however, higher value up to 33% may be accepted in cases with advanced defects due to inconsistencies in testing in the defective areas or due to retinal fatigue due to disease.[10]

vi. *Foveal threshold:* It measures the foveal sensitivity, in a similar fashion to the threshold sensitivity at other points, however, it is done just before the test. A poor foveal threshold, with good visual acuity may point toward early involvement of fovea, while a good foveal threshold with a poor visual acuity may point toward refractive error.

3. *Raw data and grayscale:* The next part of the report is the raw data, which provides the actual value of the retinal sensitivity in decibels at the points tested by the perimeter. Adjacent to it is the grayscale representation of the same. Although, it presents an easily comprehensible light and dark picture based on change in the threshold. It may be useful for patient demonstration and bringing out the common artifacts, however, it should be borne in mind that the difference in the values of two adjacent points should not be judged. Age and media opacities can cause generalized depression, but it is not used for interpretation of glaucomatous defects.

4. *Total deviation numeric and probability plot:* This plot compares the threshold values of the patient with the age-matched normative database at that particular tested location.[11] It is numerically denoted at each test point. Positive number denotes a more sensitive point while a negative number represents a less sensitive point. This plot is center weighted (more importance given to central points) and provides the generalized view of patient hill of vision as compared to normative database. Below the numerical plot is the probability plot which provides the statistical value to each point in terms of being likely normal by denoting a *p* value (<5%, <2%, <1%, and <0.5%).

5. *Pattern deviation numeric and probability plot:* In this plot, the patient's field is corrected for the seventh most sensitive nonedge point.[11] This filters out the generalized field suppression and picks up the localized visual field defects, which may be a typical feature of an early glaucoma. In advanced defects where the whole field is severely depressed, the pattern deviation plot may show "reversal". Pattern deviation symbols absent in total deviation plot are usually false positives.

6. *Glaucoma hemifield test:* This compares five clusters of corresponding areas in the superior and inferior hemifields, as the field defects in glaucoma respect the horizontal meridian. GHT is a sensitive indicator for glaucomatous damage.[12,13] It is displayed as one of these five results:

   i. Within normal limits—no significant difference in the upper and the lower field clusters.

   ii. Outside normal limits—the difference between two zones has a *p* value of <0.01 or difference between two members of any pair of zones has a *p* value of <0.005.

   iii. Borderline—the sensitivity level has a difference that does not reach a statistically significant level.

   iv. General reduction of sensitivity—the test locations are so low in sensitivity levels, as to be seen in only 0.5% of normal subjects, with no significant difference between the zones.

   v. Abnormally high sensitivity—abnormally high sensitive values, as seen in "trigger-happy" patients.

7. *Global indices:* The global indices are also center weighted which are:

   i. *Mean deviation:* It statistically measures, how abnormal is the patient's field with respect to normative database. It takes into account the average of all deviation points on the total deviation numerical plot. MD values lesser than −2 dB should arouse a suspicion of glaucoma. More "minus" the MD, greater is the severity of the field defect.

   ii. *Pattern standard deviation:* It is a measure of how abnormal is the field of vision, it measures the standard deviation of all deviation in total deviation numerical plot. Higher the PSD, greater the focal defects and more is the likelihood of a glaucomatous damage.

   iii. *Visual field index (VFI):* It is a global metric that represents the visual fields as percentage of normal. VFI of 100 signifies a normal visual field and VFI or "0" denotes a perimetrically blind patient.[14] It provides a mixture of event and rate-based progression analysis. The rate of change of VFI (rate of progression), generates a *p* value (on statistical analysis), whether or not the rate of change is significantly different from zero. In the early glaucoma, it utilizes pattern

TABLE 2: The Hodapp–Parrish classification.

	Mean deviation	No of points ≤ 5% level on PD plot	No of points ≤ 1% on PD	Central 5° field
Early	≤ 6 dB	<25% points (18 points)	<10 points	All points with ≥15 dB
Moderate	6–12 dB	<50% points (37 points)	<20 points	• No point with 0 dB/only one • Hemifield with 1 point ≤ 15 dB
Severe	≥ 12 dB	>50% points (>37 points)	>20 points	• At least one point with 0 dB/both • Hemifield with points ≤ 15 dB

deviation plot, while in advanced glaucoma it is derived from MD plot. Like all other indices this is also center weighted.

8. *Gaze tracker:* It is an eye tracking system with a graphical representation of the eye movement during the test. It is displayed as deflections from the horizontal. Upward deviation indicates fixation losses—the patient was not fixating at the target. Large downward deviation indicates the patient closed his lids due to blinking or the eye movement were not traced. Thus, large deflections from the horizontal line should be ruled out before making an inference from the test report. It is found only in SITA.

Now that we have learnt how to read a perimetry report, it is pertinent to understand what a glaucomatous field defect in a perimetry test is.

The Anderson's criteria are helpful to diagnose glaucomatous visual field defect.[2] They include:

- A GHT outside normal limits on at least two fields.
- A cluster of three or more nonedge points on a 30-2 print out in a location typical for glaucoma, all of which are depressed on the pattern deviation plot at a $p \leq 5\%$ level and one of which is depressed at a $p \leq 1\%$ level on two consecutive fields.
- A corrected PSD that occurs in less than 5% of normal fields on two consecutive fields.

One of Anderson's criteria was changed to replace corrected pattern standard deviation (CPSD) with the PSD, as the SITA strategy does not calculate short-term fluctuation.

The glaucomatous visual field defects can further be classified into mild, moderate, and severe based upon the Hodapp–Parrish classification[15] which is given below **(Table 2)**.

EXAMPLES OF VISUAL FIELD DEFECTS

Example 1: Given are the right eye visual fields, optical coherence tomography retinal nerve fiber layer (OCT RNFL), colored fundus picture and red-free fundus picture of right eye. All of the three Anderson's criteria are fulfilled (i.e., GHT outside normal limits, cluster of three nonedge points having a *p* value of <5%, with at least one having a *p* value of <1% and PSD of<5%), so the field probably is glaucomatous. As per the Hodapp–Parrish classification the field is probably moderate to severely affected (as the MD is −7.66 dB, there are 28 points having a *p* < 5%, 16 points having *p* value of <1% and one point is <1 dB in one Hemifield). The OCT RNFL shows thinning superiorly and inferiorly and an inferior notch. The fundus picture shows disc hemorrhage inferiorly and a corresponding nerve fiber layer defect.

Example 2: Given are the left eye visual fields. All the three Anderson's criteria are fulfilled (i.e., GHT outside normal limits, cluster of three nonedge points having a *p* value of <5%, with at least one having a *p* value of <1% and PSD of <5%), so the field probably is glaucomatous. As per the Hodapp–Parrish classification the field is probably mild to moderately affected (as the MD is −5.03 dB, there are 26 points having a *p* < 5%, 16 points having *p* value of <1% and there is no point is <15 dB in central 5°). But, the field does not correspond to the nearly normal looking disc, hence the fields are repeated with lid taping, the fields are better as the defect was an artifact due to dropping of eye lid.

Example 3: Given are the left eye visual fields and OCT RNFL. Note the early glaucomatous defect, nasal step, corresponding to inferior nerve fiber loss in OCT RNFL, in case of open angle glaucoma.

Example 4: Given are the right eye visual fields. Note the early arcuate defect in the superior field and nasal step/early arcuate in a case of moderate combined mechanism glaucoma.

Example 5: Given are the right eye visual fields and OCT RNFL. Note inferior actuate scotoma in a case of open angle glaucoma with right eye showing superior NRR loss in the OCT RNFL.

Example 6: Given are the visual fields and OCT RNFL of both eyes and OCT macula of left eye in a case of bilateral chronic primary angle closure glaucoma (CPACG) with pseudophakia and age-related macular degeneration (AMD). Fields OD suggestive of superior arcuate scotoma, Fields OS suggestive of central defect, which is likely due to AMD rather than glaucoma.

Examples 7A and B: Given are the visual fields of right eye showing white scotoma in case of a trigger-happy patient,

CHAPTER 8: Visual Fields—An Overview

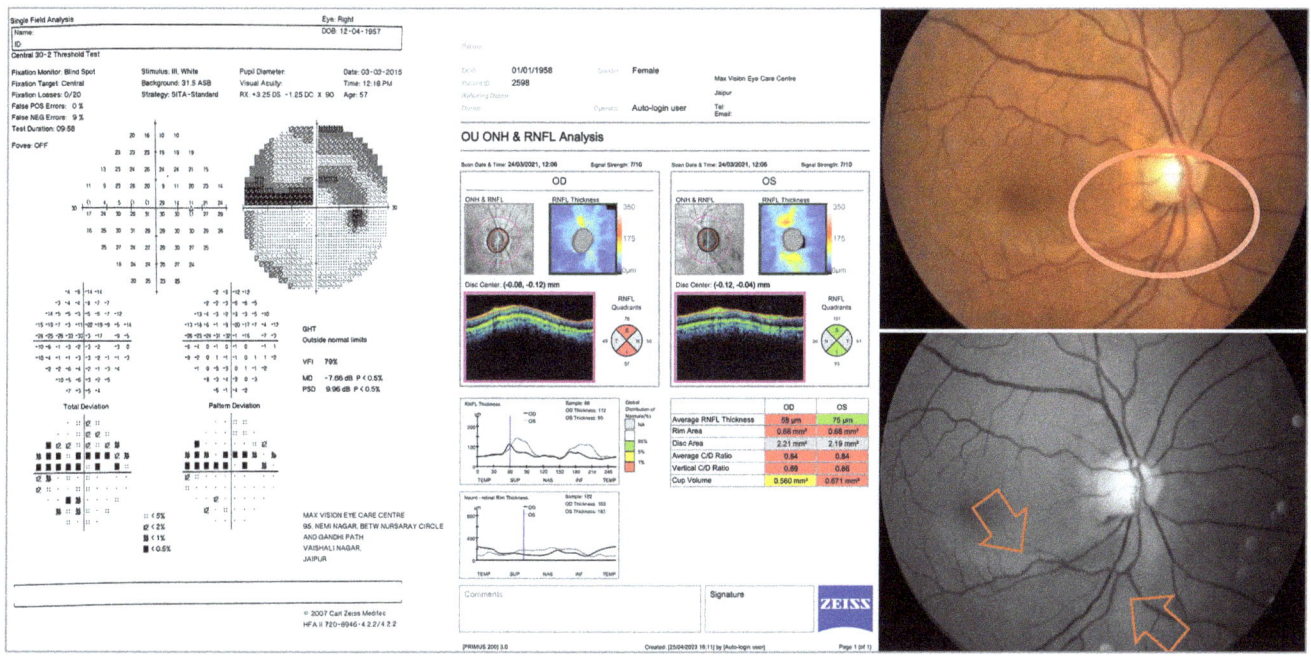

Example 1

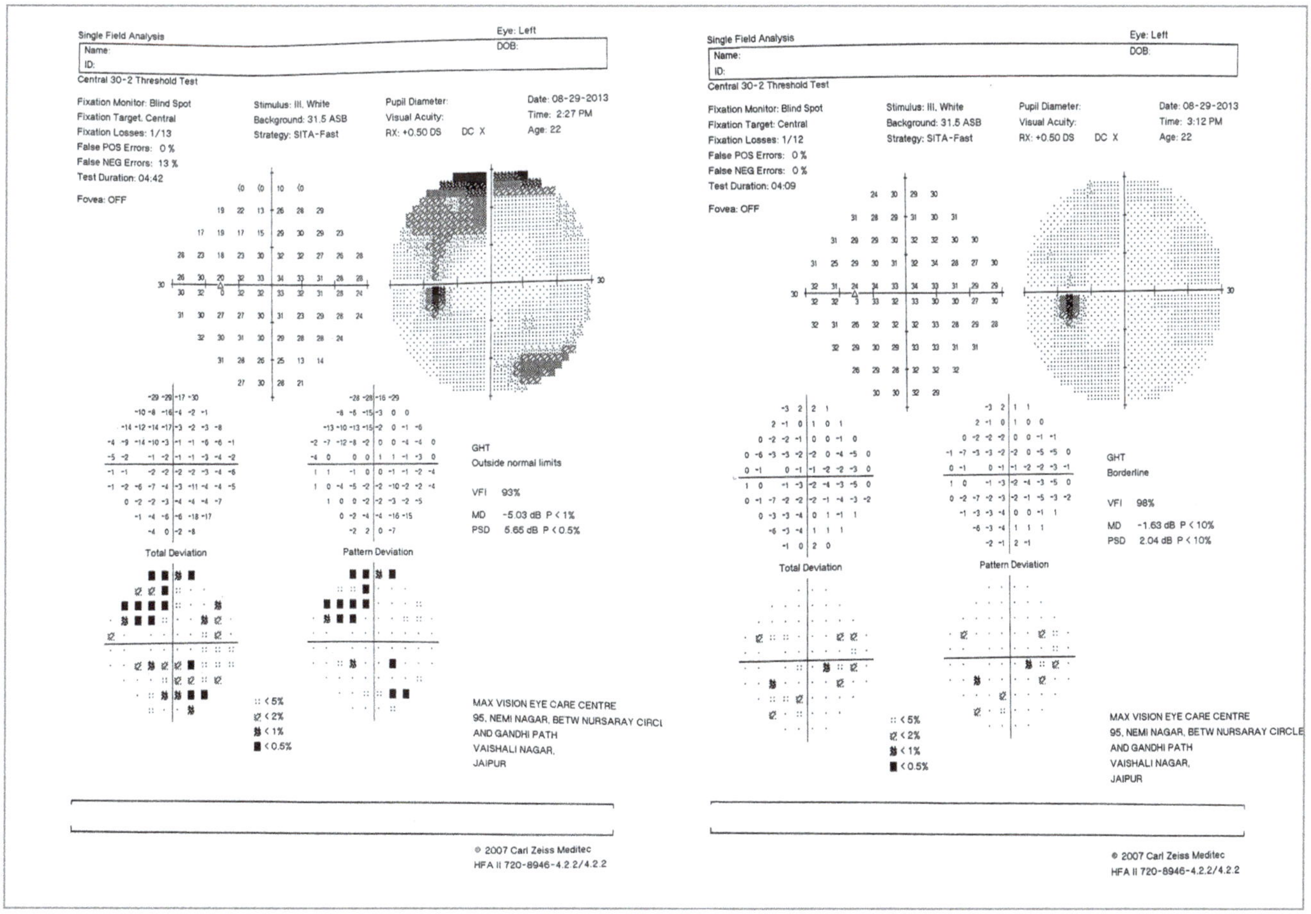

Example 2

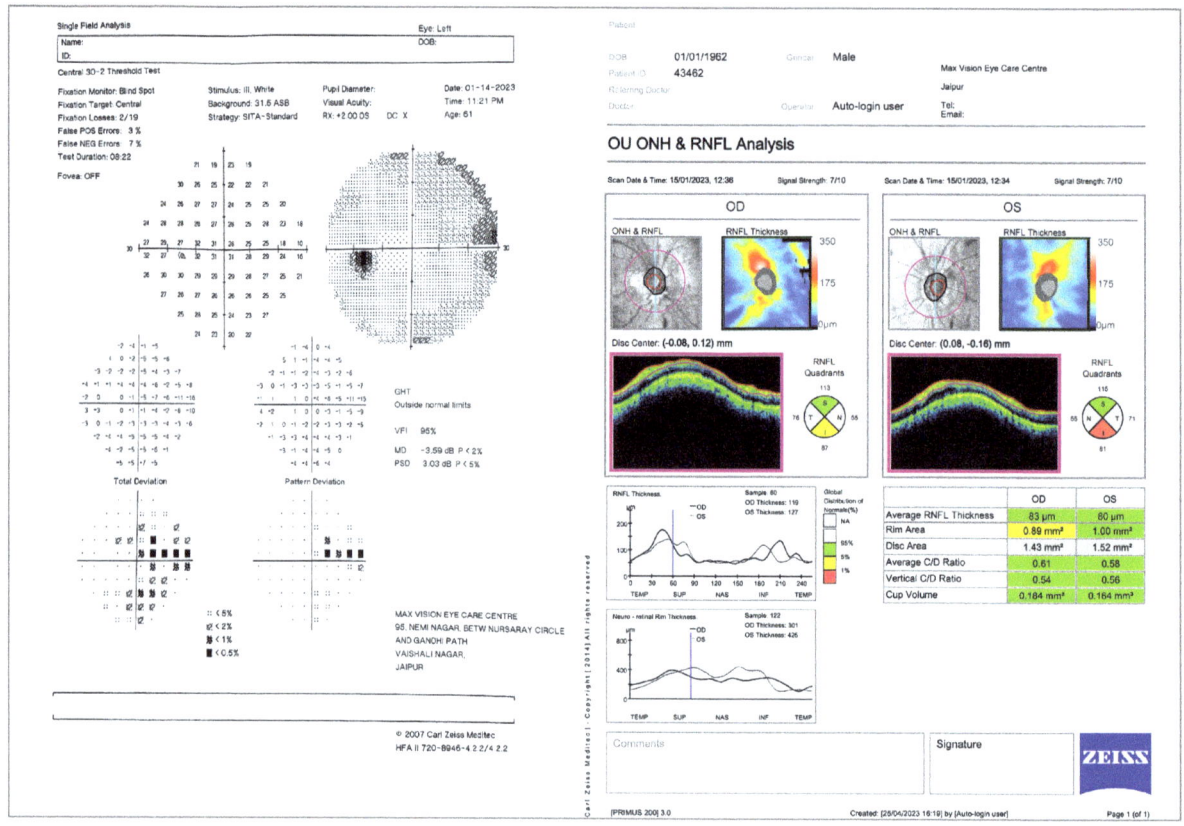

Example 3

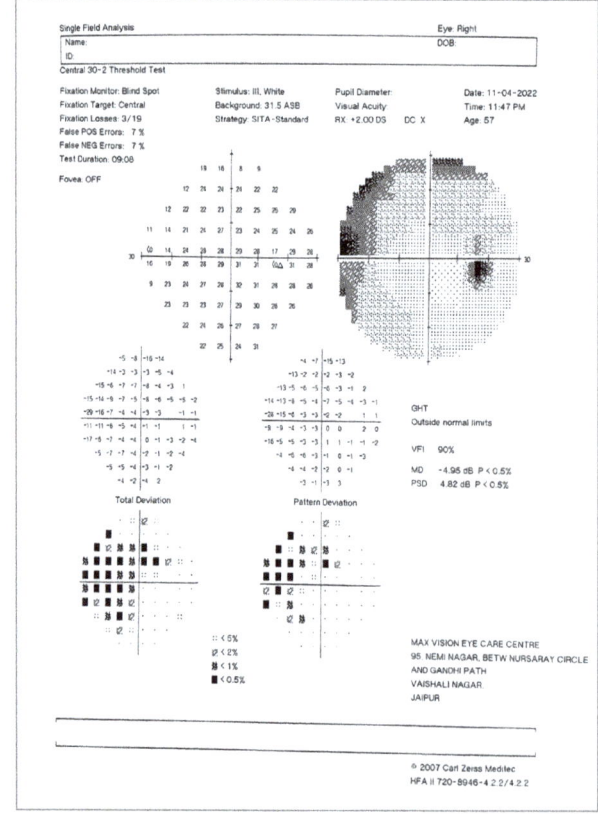

Example 4

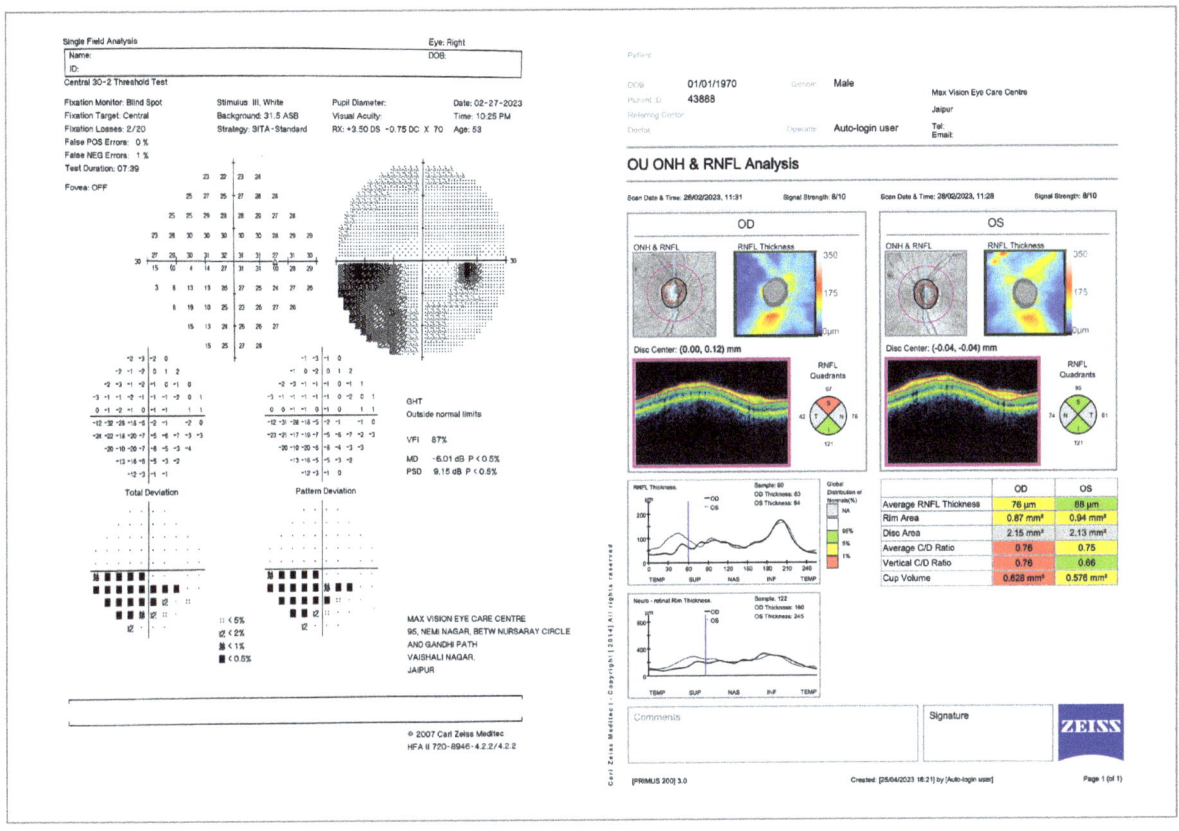

Example 5

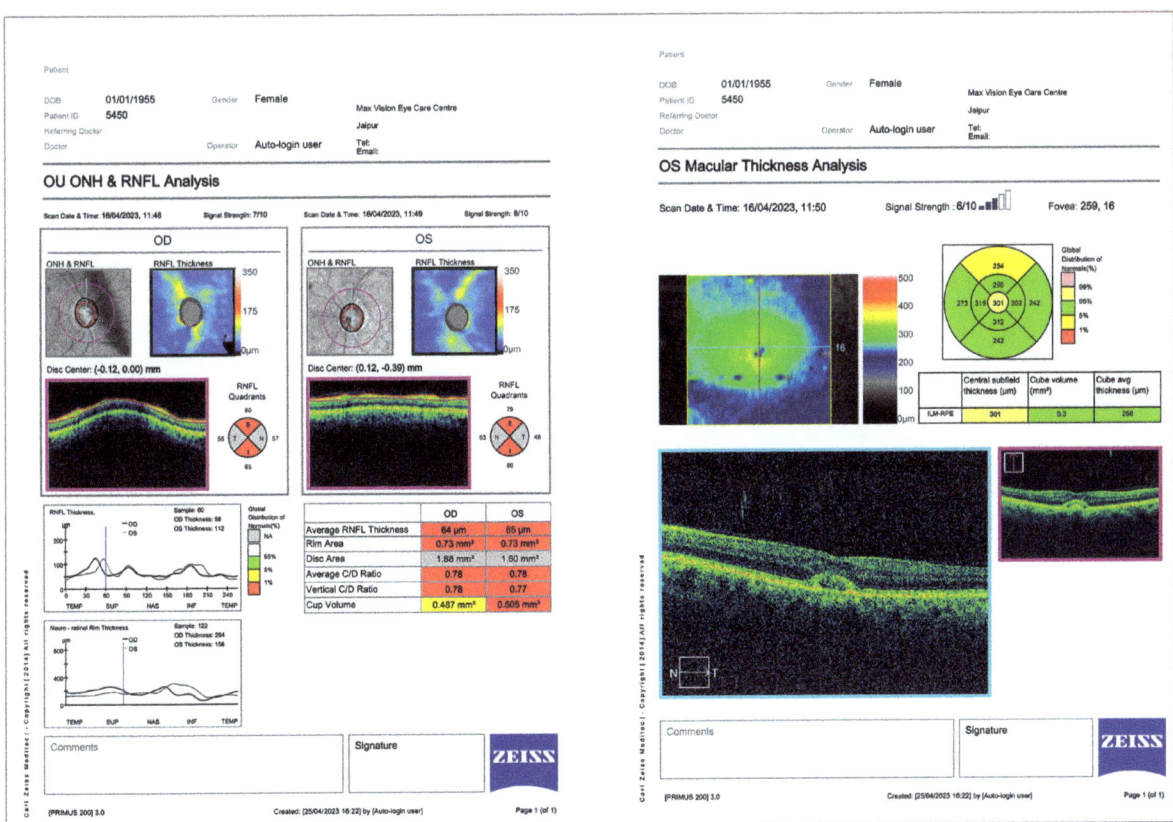

Example 6

Contd...

100 SECTION 2: Visual Field Interpretation

Contd...

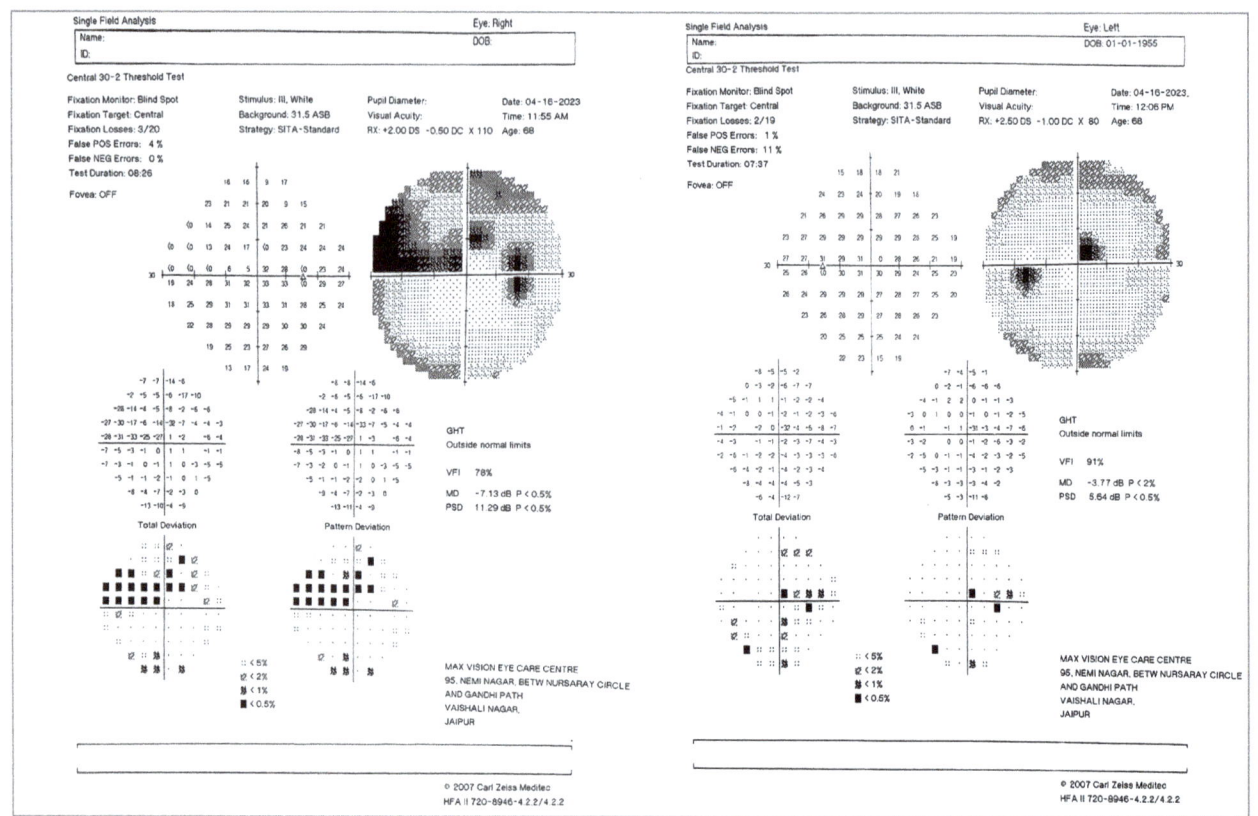

Example 6

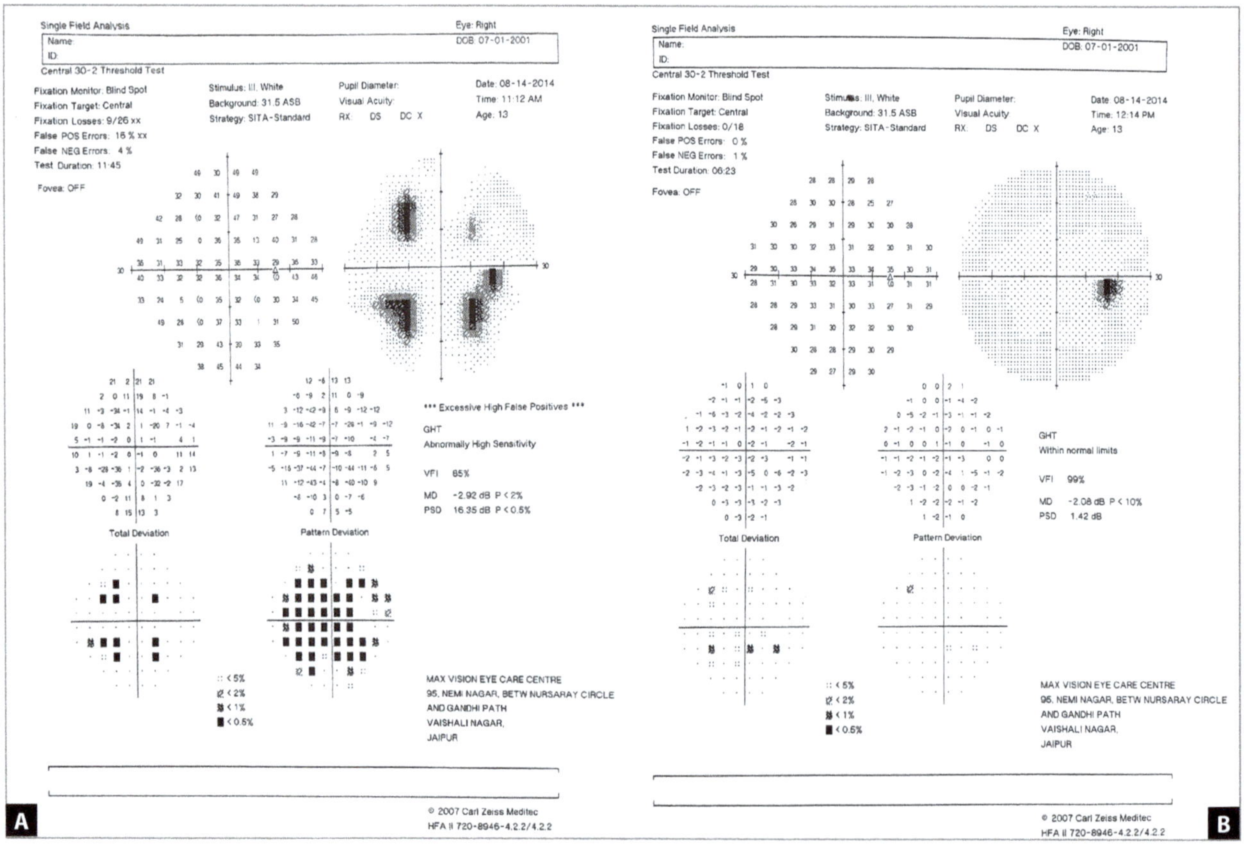

Examples 7A and B

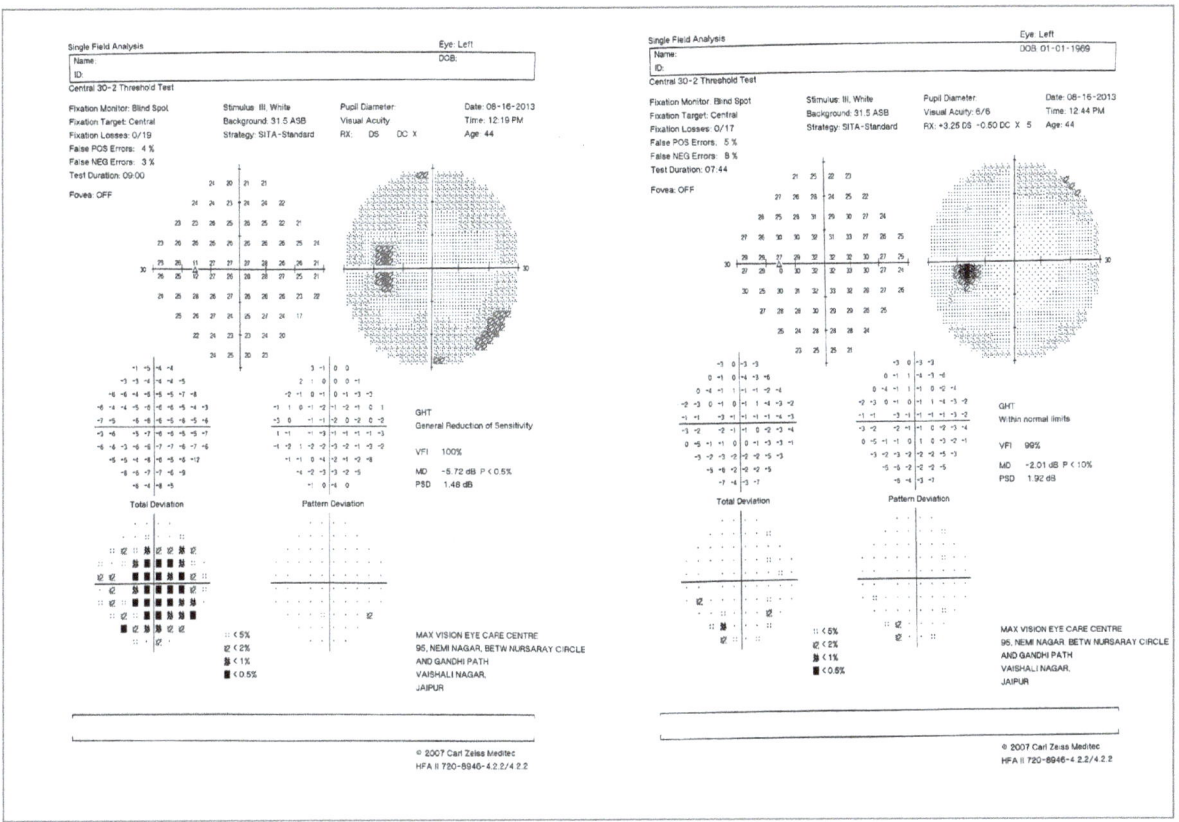

Example 8

leading to excessively high false positives. After the patient is explained the method, the fields turn out to be normal.

Example 8: Given are the visual fields of left eye showing generalized depression due to improper/no lens placement in the lens holder of the perimeter, which gets corrected once the correct lenses are placed.

Example 9: Given are the visual fields of right eye, note the rim artifact due to improper lens holder position.

Example 10: Given are the visual fields of both eyes showing right homonymous hemianopia in a case of left-sided weakness and infarct in left cerebral hemisphere.

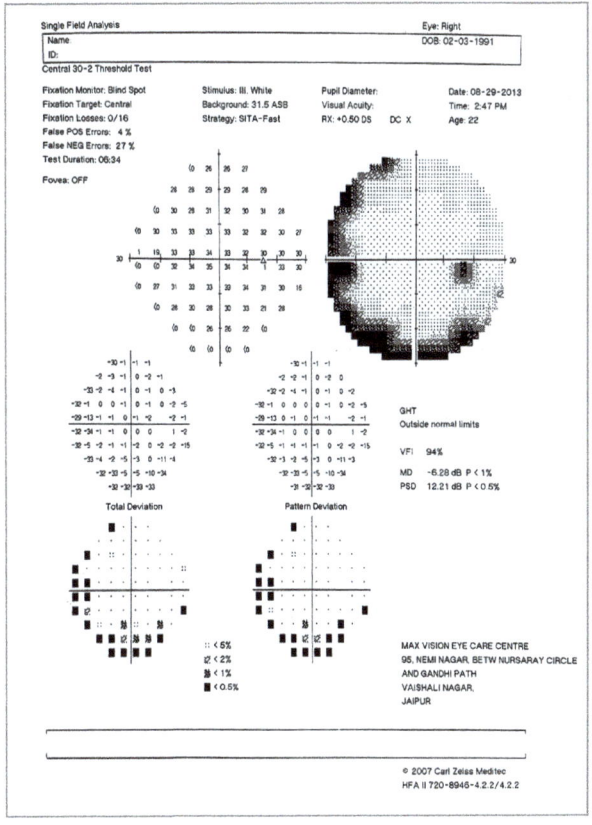

Example 9

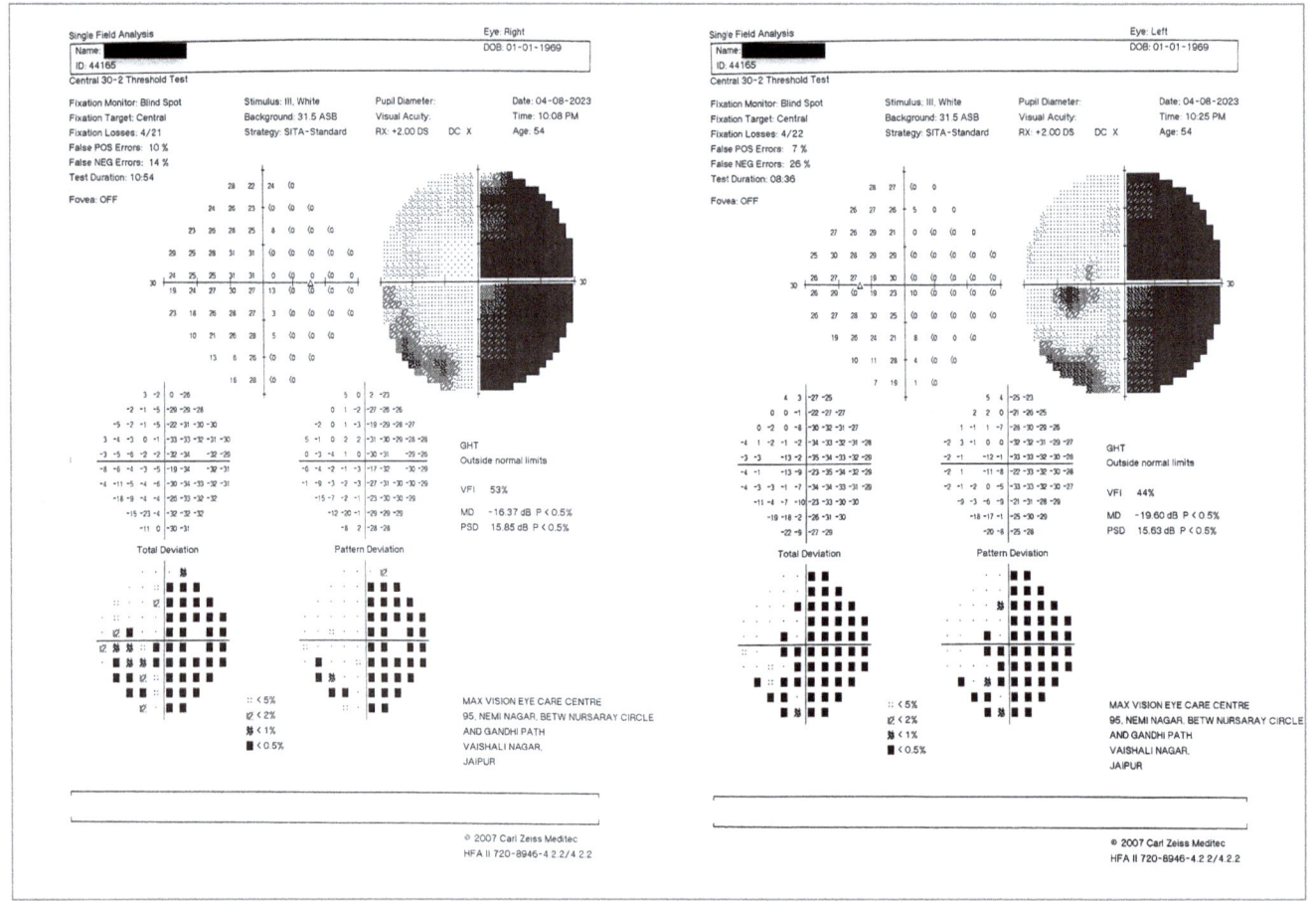

Example 10

REFERENCES

1. Traquair HM. An Introduction to Clinical Perimetry, 5th edition. London: Henry Kimpton; 1946. pp. 1-16.
2. Thomas R, George R. Interpreting automated perimetry. Indian J Ophthalmol. 2001;49(2):125-40.
3. Johnson CA, Keltner JL, Balestrery FG. Suprathreshold static perimetry in glaucoma and other optic nerve disease. Ophthalmology. 1979;86(7):1278-86.
4. Heijl A. Automatic perimetry in glaucoma visual field screening. A clinical study. Albrecht Von Graefes Arch Klin Exp Ophthalmol. 1976;200(1):21-37.
5. Wu Z, Medeiros FA. Recent developments in visual field testing for glaucoma. Curr Opin Ophthalmol. 2018;29(2):141-6.
6. Bengtsson B, Olsson J, Heijl A, Rootzén H. A new generation of algorithms for computerized threshold perimetry, SITA. Acta Ophthalmol Scand. 1997;75(4):368-75.
7. Bengtsson B, Heijl A. SITA Fast, a new rapid perimetric threshold test. Description of methods and evaluation in patients with manifest and suspect glaucoma. Acta Ophthalmol Scand. 1998;76(4):431-7.
8. Bosworth CF, Sample PA, Johnson CA, Weinreb RN. Current practice with standard automated perimetry. Semin Ophthalmol. 2000;15(4):172-81.
9. Lee M, Zulauf M, Caprioli J. The influence of patient reliability on visual field outcome. Am J Ophthalmol. 1994;117(6):756-61.
10. Vingrys AJ, Demirel S. False-response monitoring during automated perimetry. Optom Vis Sci. 1998;75(7):513-7.
11. Heijl A, Lindgren G, Olsson J, Asman P. Visual field interpretation with empiric probability maps. Arch Ophthalmol. 1989;107(2):204-8.
12. Sommer A, Duggan C, Auer C, Abbey H. Analytic approaches to the interpretation of automated threshold perimetric data for the diagnosis of early glaucoma. Trans Am Ophthalmol Soc. 1985;83:250-67.
13. Hart WM, Becker B. The onset and evolution of glaucomatous visual field defects. Ophthalmology. 1982;89(3):268-79.
14. Bengtsson B, Heijl A. A visual field index for calculation of glaucoma rate of progression. Am J Ophthalmol. 2008;145(2):343-53.
15. Hodapp E, Parrish RK II, Anderson DR. Clinical decisions in glaucoma. St Louis: The CV Mosby Co; 1993. pp. 52-61.

SECTION 3

Special Situations

9. **Structural and Functional Correlation in Glaucoma**
   Ganesh V Raman, Mrunali M Dhavalikar, Sunada Subramaniam

10. **Role of Perimetry in Diagnosis and Management of Neuro-ophthalmic Disorders**
    Nikhil S Choudhari, Sirisha Senthil

11. **Role of Perimetry in Diagnosis and Management of Retinal or Macular Disorders**
    Sathidevi AV, Gowri J Murthy, Rajani S Battu, Vinaya Kumar Konana, Supriya Dabir, Padmamalini Mahendradas, Chitralekha De, Priyanka Sudhakar

12. **Frequency Doubling Perimetry**
    Parul Ichhpujani, Shibal Bhartiya, Dewang Angmo, Tanuj Dada

13. **Short-wavelength Automated Perimetry**
    Rengaraj Venkatesh, Palaniswamy Krishnamurthy

14. **Integrating Technologies: Current Status**
    Shibal Bhartiya, Parul Ichhpujani, Oscar Albis-Donado, Faisal TT

15A. **Recent Advances in Perimetry**
    Parul Ichhpujani, Hennaav Dhillon

15B. **Brief Overview of Various Types of Head-mounted Virtual Reality Perimeters**
    Prasanna Venkatesh Ramesh, Shruthy Vaishali Ramesh, Vivek Velumani, Aji Kunnath Devadas

16. **Care and Maintenance of Perimeters**
    Shibal Bhartiya, Parul Ichhpujani

17. **History of Perimetry**
    Harsha L Rao, Zia S Pradhan, Chris A Johnson

9. Structural and Functional Correlation in Glaucoma

Ganesh V Raman, Mrunali M Dhavalikar, Sunada Subramaniam

■ INTRODUCTION

Glaucoma is an ocular disease characterized by progressive and irreversible loss of retinal ganglion cells (RGCs), and intraocular pressure being an important modifiable risk factor. There has been remarkable advances in glaucoma diagnostics till date, which has helped ophthalmologist to detect glaucoma early, treat, and halt its progression. Our concept about this disease is expanding because of the advancement in diagnostic techniques, be it structural or functional. The definition of preperimetric glaucoma is also well established with the current imaging modalities.

Functional tests such as Swedish interactive threshold algorithm (SITA), short-wavelength automated perimetry (SWAP), and frequency doubling technology (FDT) are designed to measure the function of specific subpopulations of RGCs and are often proposed to detect early visual field loss, even when function is normal on standard automated perimetry (SAP). Investigations for detecting structural loss such as stereoscopic fundus photography, optical coherence tomography (OCT), confocal scanning laser ophthalmoscope (CSLO), and scanning laser polarimetry (SLP) are now commonly used to reliably quantify the structural loss in glaucoma.

Glaucoma runs a gamut from suspects to established glaucoma and more often clinical examination alone may not be sufficient to reliably define each of them and is subject to inter and intraobserver errors. The individual variability in structure and function among normal individuals and glaucoma patients, and the errors and drawbacks of each diagnostic technique, limits our decision making based on a single investigational modality. Hence, a combined approach based on investigations and the clinical examination helps us to clearly define normal subjects from glaucoma suspects and patients.

A number of studies evaluated the structure function relationship using one or more of these automated devices, with sometimes conflicting results. The results from these studies suggest that the correlation is stronger if a wide range of individuals is included (from normal subjects to those with advanced disease), and regional correlations are usually stronger than global ones. Studies performed with OCT and SLP correlating RNFL and visual field parameters showed similar pattern of results as the ones performed with CSLO.[1-3] Bowd et al.[1] correlated measures of all three automated imaging devices (CSLO, OCT, and SLP) with visual function SAP in normal subjects, glaucoma suspects, and individuals with glaucoma. The authors showed a significant but weak correlation (maximal R^2 with each device was 0.26, 0.38, and 0.21, respectively) between structural and functional parameters, with little difference between linear and logarithmic associations.

This chapter is an attempt to denote the correlations and discrepancies that exist between fundus photography, perimetry, and OCT for glaucoma evaluation through a series of case scenarios with illustrations (**Figs. 1 to 17**).

Every clinician evaluates neuroretinal rim health according to the appearance of the optic disc, the clinically visible surface of the optic nerve head (ONH). Recent anatomic findings with spectral-domain OCT (SD-OCT) have challenged the basis and accuracy of current rim evaluation. Disc margin-based rim evaluation lacks a solid anatomic basis and results in variably inaccurate measurements for two reasons. First, the clinically visible disc margin is an unreliable outer border of rim tissue because of clinically and photographically invisible extensions of Bruch's membrane. Second, rim tissue orientation is not considered in width measurements.

A four-point paradigm change has been proposed by Chauhan[4] that incorporates new anatomic insights provided by SD-OCT imaging of the ONH into the clinical examination of the optic disc for clinical assessment of the ONH.

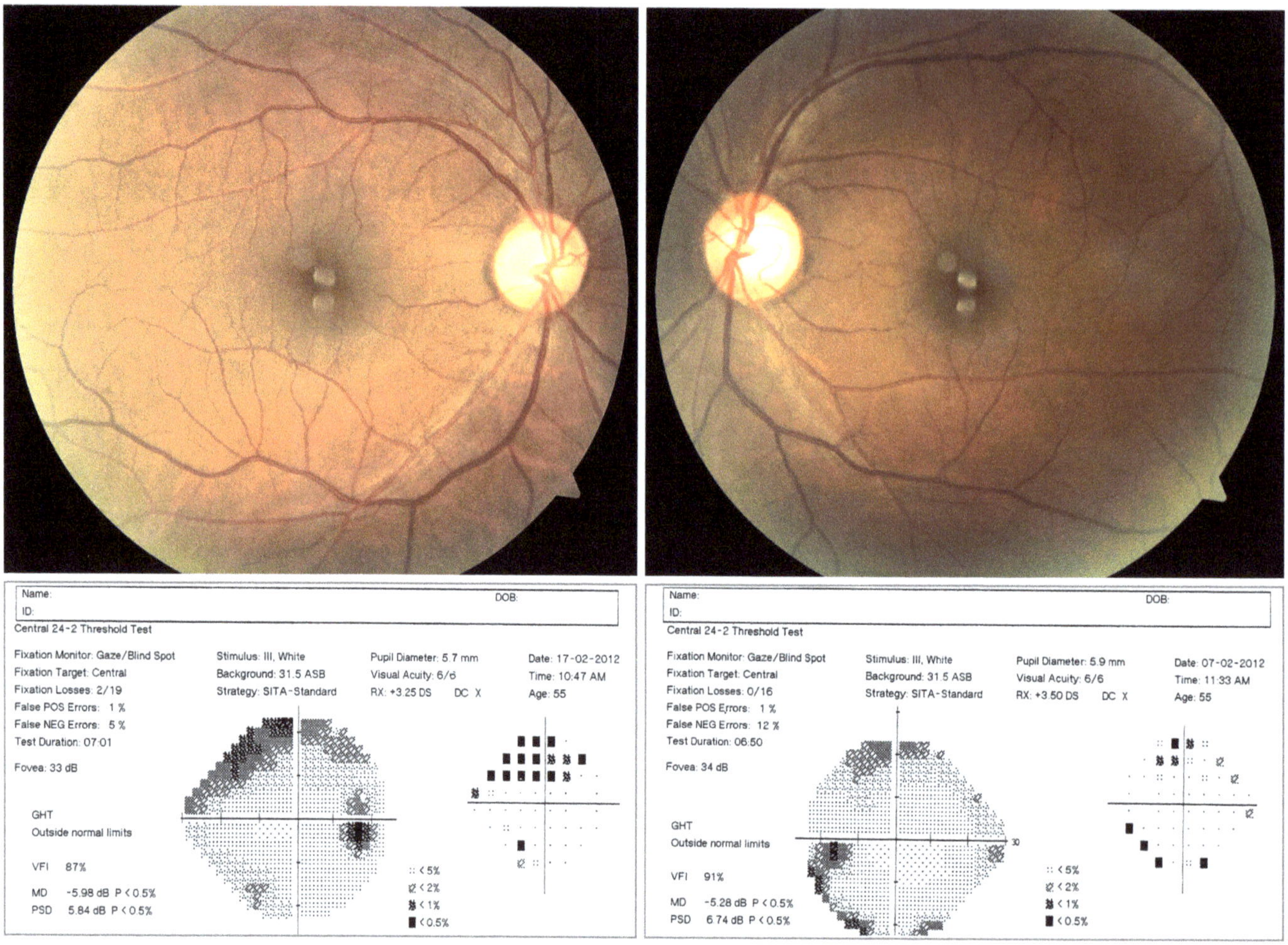

Fig. 1: Fundus photography of this patient shows early wedge defect inferiorly in the right eye with a corresponding field defect superiorly in visual field.

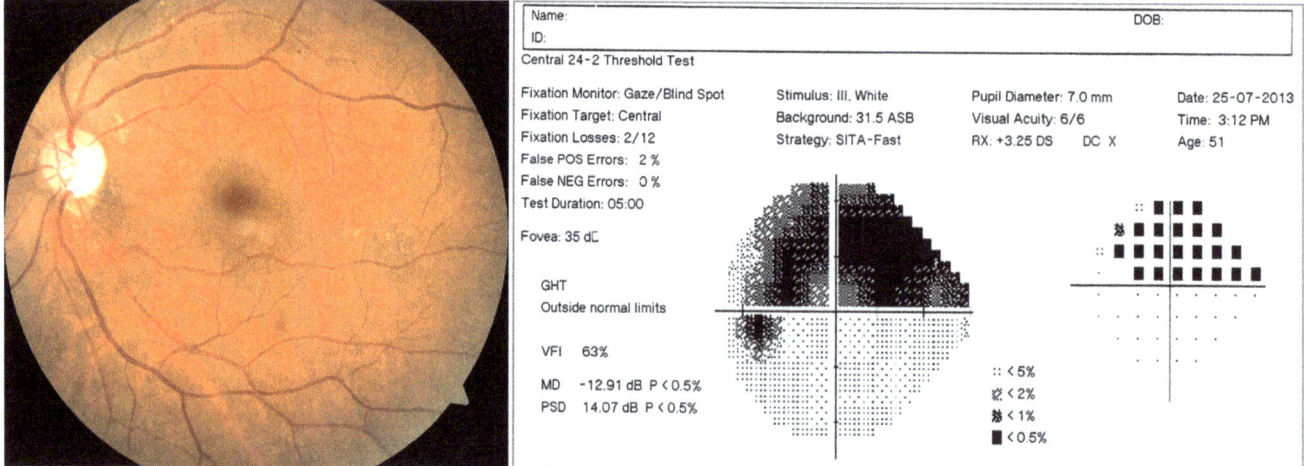

Fig. 2: Fundus photography of left eye of this patient shows an inferior wedge-shaped retinal nerve fiber layer defect and a corresponding superior arcuate scotoma in standard white on white perimetry.

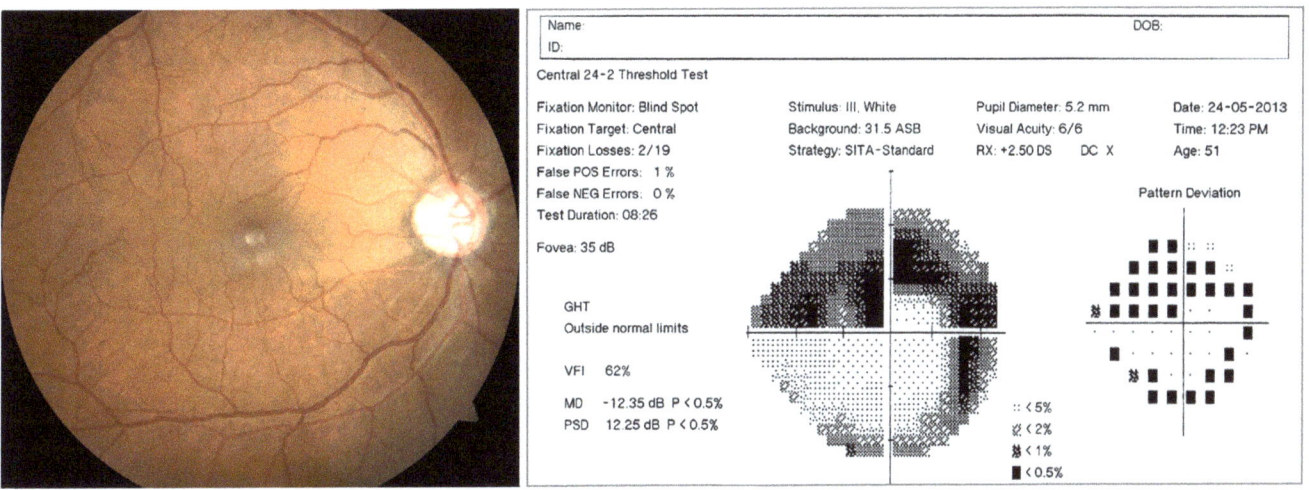

Fig. 3: Fundus photography of this patient showing wedge-shaped retinal nerve fiber layer (RNFL) defect inferiorly with a corresponding superior arcuate scotoma in standard white on white perimetry.

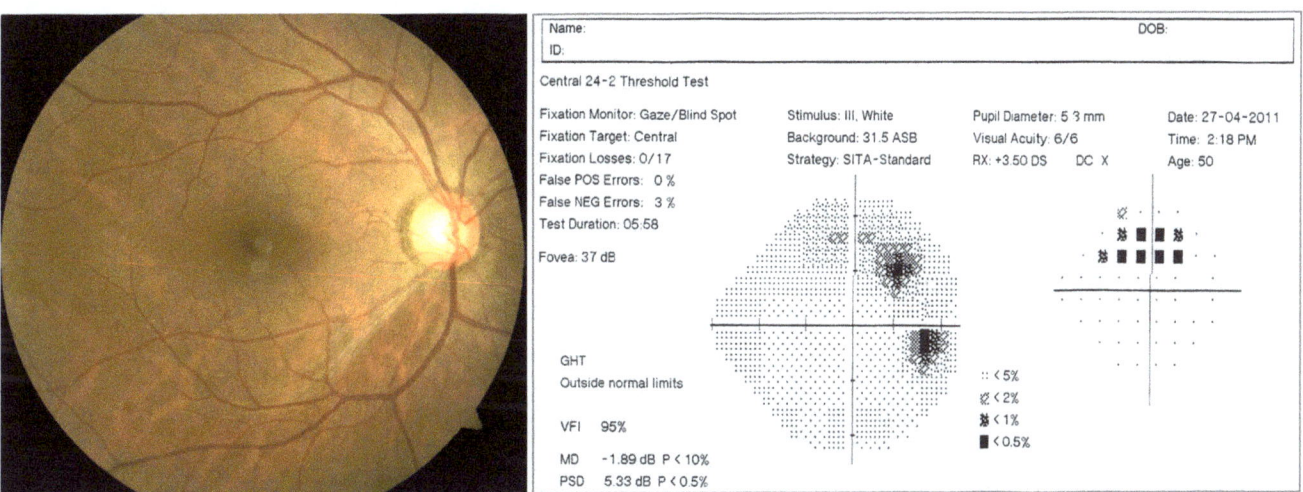

Fig. 4: Fundus photography shows wedge defect inferiorly in the right eye with corresponding superior arcuate scotoma in standard white on white perimetry.

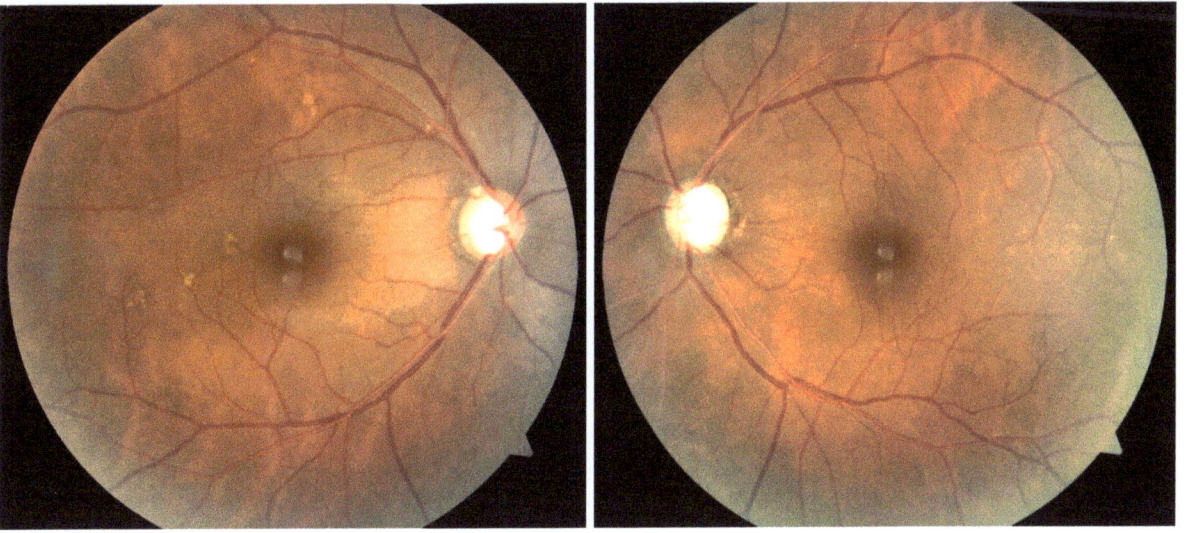

Fig. 5

Contd...

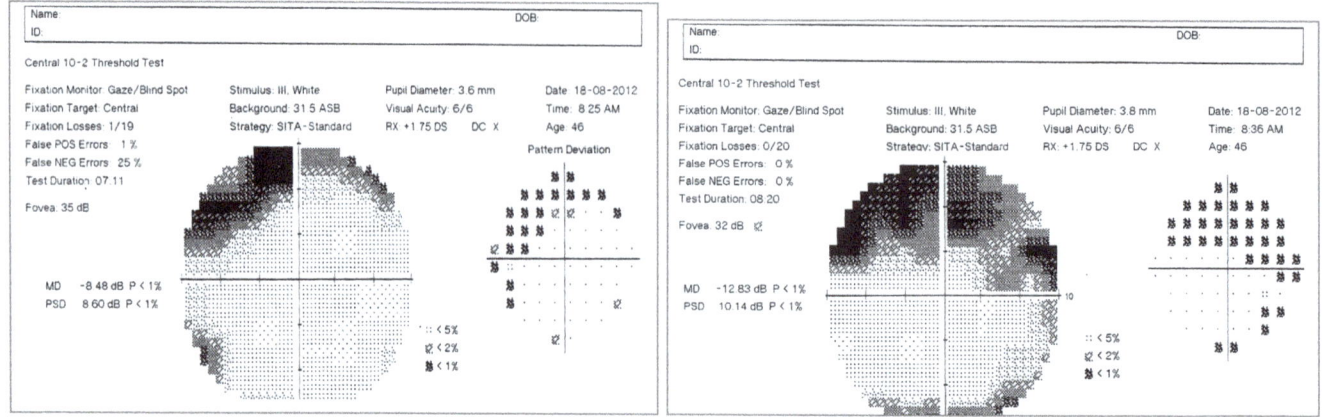

Fig. 5: Fundus photography shows retinal nerve fiber layer (RNFL) wedge defect (inferior > superior) in both eyes, attenuated neuroretinal rim with corresponding superior arcuate scotoma in 10-2 program of standard white on white perimetry.

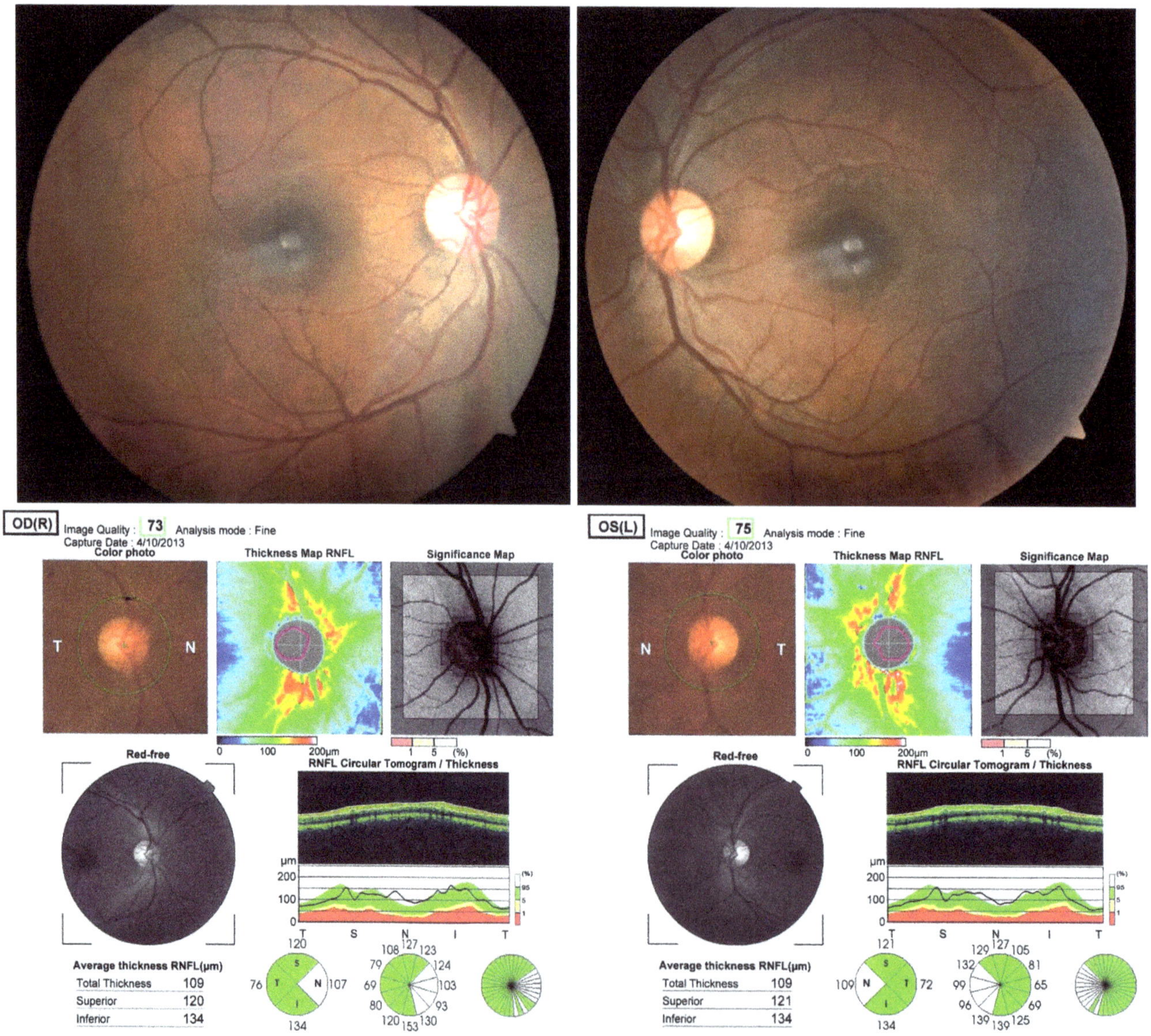

Fig. 6

Contd...

Contd...

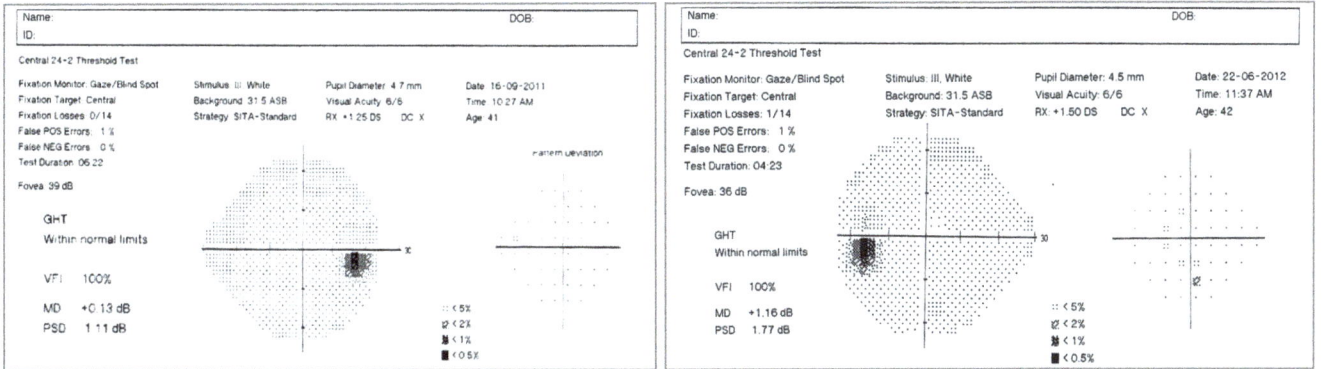

Fig. 6: A fundus photograph image with standard automated perimetry and optical coherence tomography all being normal in this patient.

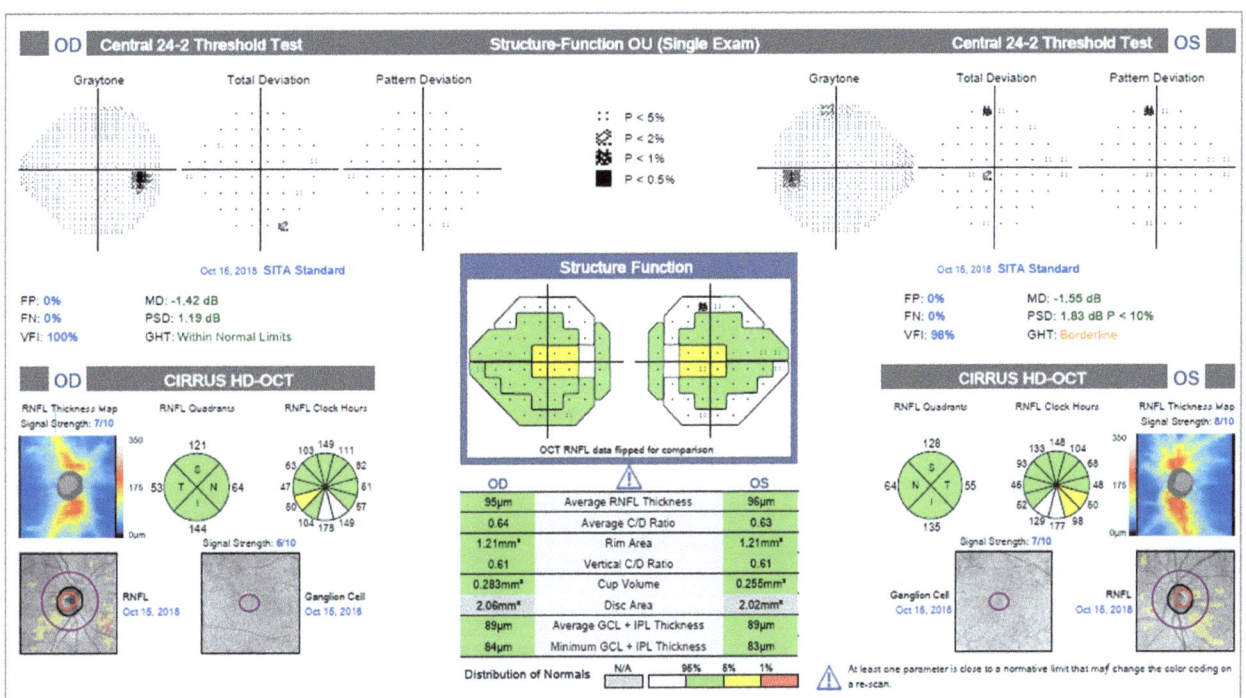

Fig. 7: Structure and function combined reports are useful for assessing the visual field defect and optic nerve head (ONH) parameters at a glance. The lower aspect of the report towards the corners provides the structural content obtained from the optical coherence tomography (OCT). The upper region provides the visual field data. The central area of the report provides the structure and function correlation. Note the healthy retinal nerve fiber layer (RNFL) in both eyes in the OCT heat map. The corresponding visual fields are normal.

The OCT imaging of the optic nerve head should not mimic the clinical examination, instead clinical practice should incorporate knowledge of ONH anatomy detected by SD-OCT into the clinical examination. In a given eye, the clinically examined disc margin may be different from the Bruch membrane opening (BMO) through which the axons pass out of the eye. The SD-OCT image of the optic nerve head should be utilized to understand the anatomy of the ONH rather than to quantify optic nerve head anatomy which may in-turn lead to errors when rim width assessment is done.

Currently, BMO is the most consistent SD-OCT-detected outer border of the neuroretinal rim and a stable landmark that is visible readily in all but a few exceptional B-scans. The minimum distance from BMO to the internal limiting membrane represents the geometrically correct width of the neuroretinal rim [BMO—minimum rim width (MRW)]. Automated algorithms are available which detect BMO and internal limiting membrane. Region-wise neuroretinal rim width can be detected in the future.

The angle between the fovea and the BMO center relative to the horizontal axis as per the fundus image known as

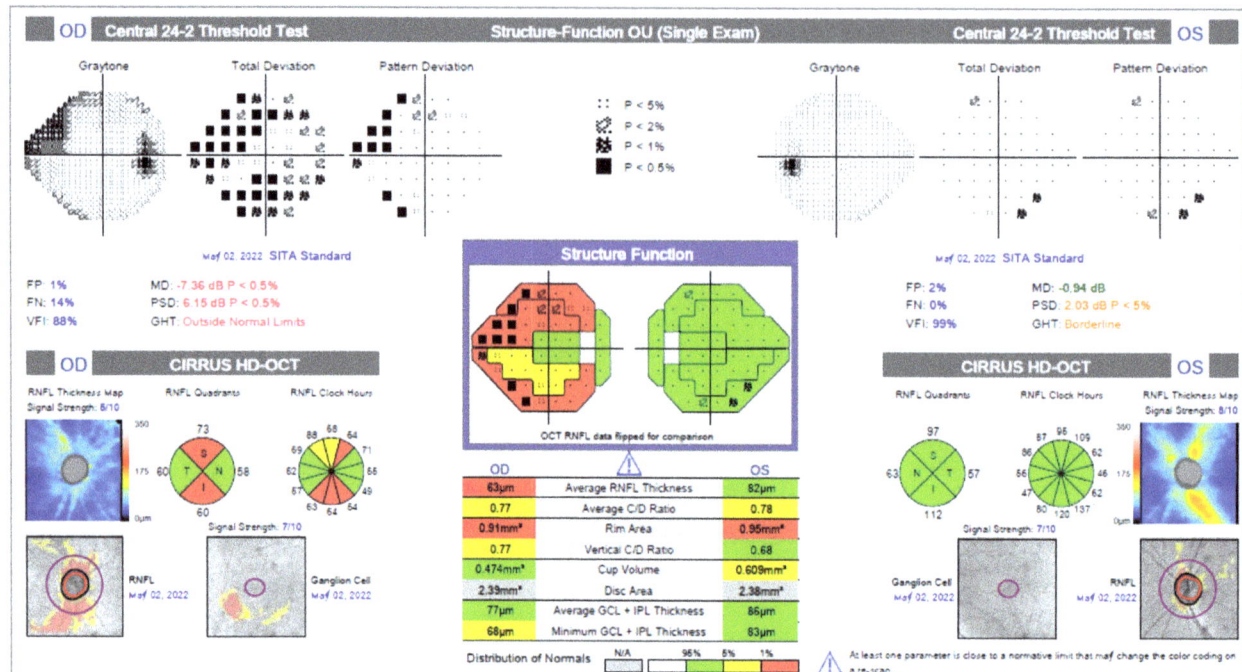

Fig. 8: In this patient with primary open angle glaucoma, there appears in the Left eye mild superonasal retinal nerve fiber layer (RNFL) thinning which is documented in the deviation map below; the clock hour and sectoral RNFL maps appear normal and the corresponding visual field is also normal. In the right eye, extensive visual field defects are present and the correspond the RNFL defect depicted in the optical coherence tomography (OCT) report. As can be seen in the structure and function map, although the structural damage is extensive the functional damage does not correspond proportionately.

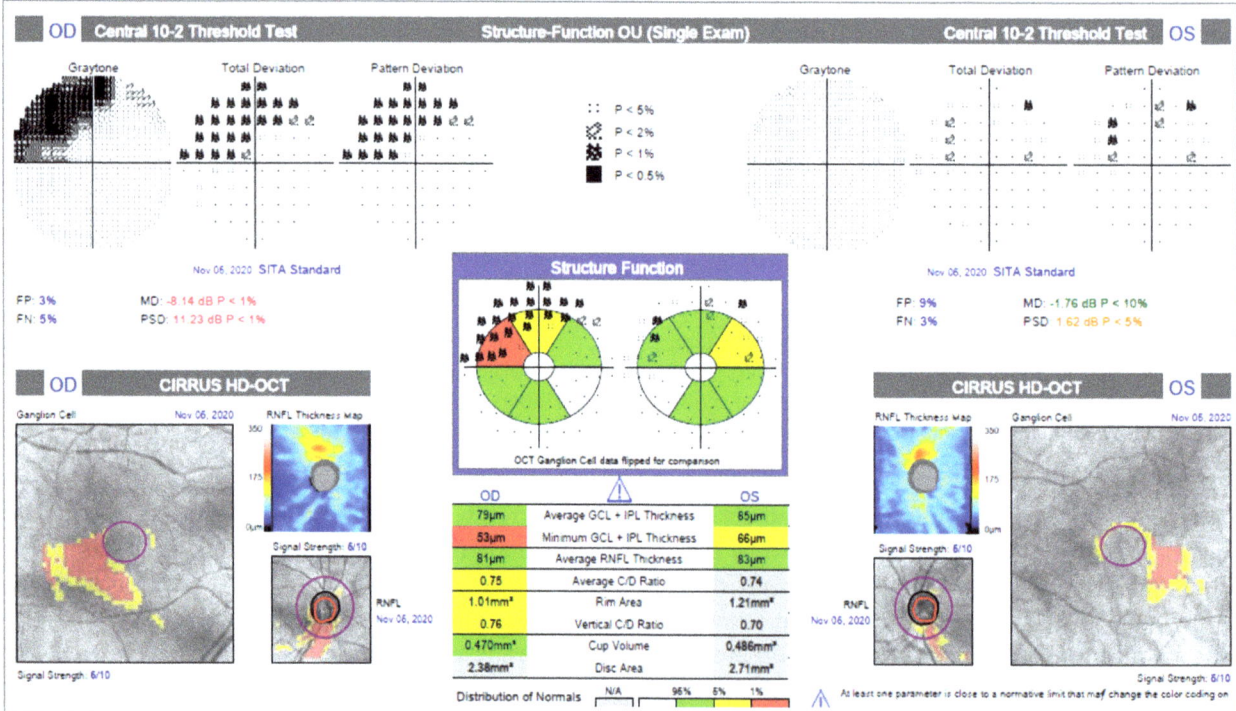

Fig. 9: In advanced stage of the disease, the macular ganglion cell inner plexiform layer (GC-IPL) complex and the central 10° of the visual field can be used to derive structure and function correlation. In the right eye of the patient there is extensive retinal nerve fiber layer (RNFL) loss which may have approached the floor effect. The GC-IPL complex appears reduced with areas of significant loss marked as red and which reflect in the superior arcuate defect in the visual field. In the left eye with minimal GC-IPL thinning the visual fields appear without scotoma in this central field.

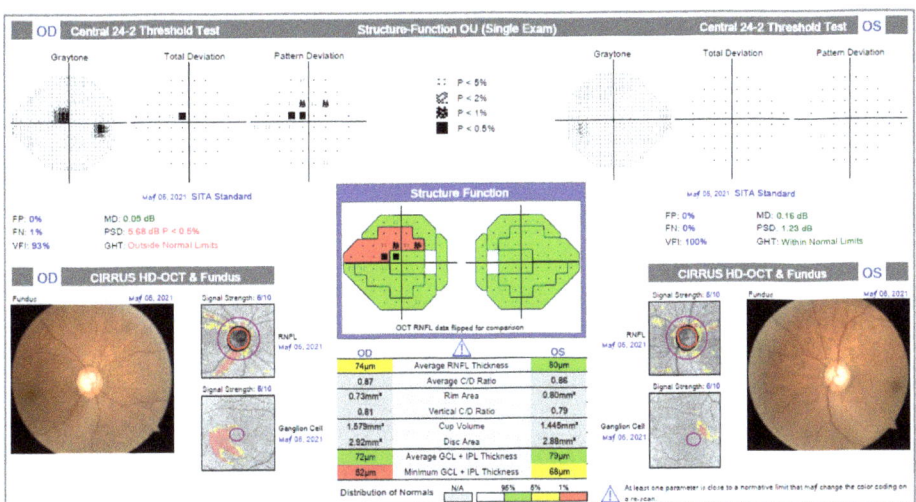

Fig. 10: This is a structure and function report of a patient with normal pressure glaucoma. In the right eye, note the inferior retinal nerve fiber layer (RNFL) defect with ganglion cell inner plexiform layer (GC-IPL) loss and corresponding field defect close to the fixation. The left eye has early glaucoma and mild RNFL defect and the visual field is normal. The visual field is divided into eight region representing the RNFL around the optic disc. In the left eye as the RNFL is healthy, all the eight regions are shaded green to show good structure and function. In the right eye, the region-shaded red corresponds to the region of inferior RNFL defect.

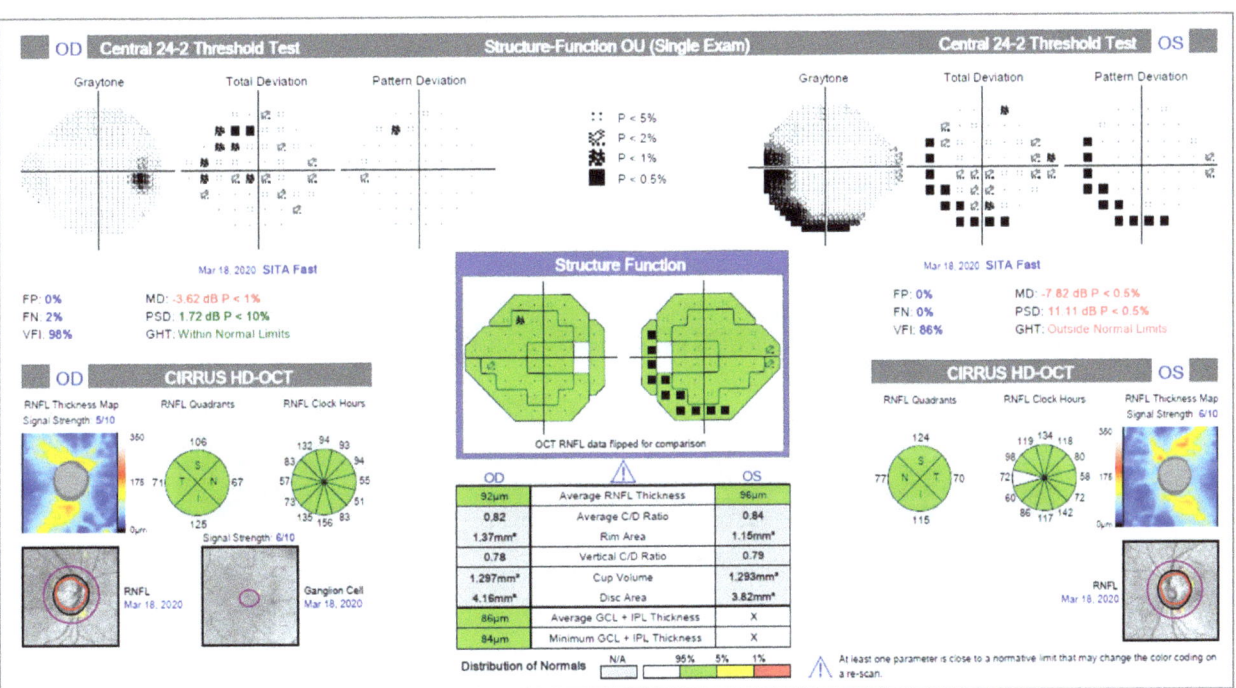

Fig. 11: This is a structure and function report of a glaucoma suspect due to large size of the optic nerve head. Note the normal retinal nerve fiber layer (RNFL) pattern in both eyes. The structure and function map is shaded green denoting good RNFL pattern corresponding to the visual field. There are few scotoma in the right eye and a rim scotoma in the left eye which appears to be marching behind the blind spot. Note the size of the optic nerve head (ONH), 4.16 mm^2 in the right eye and 3.82 mm^2 in the left eye.

the fovea-BMO center axis varies as much as 23°, mean being −7°, i.e., fovea being 7° below the horizontal axis. Such wide variation can occur within the same eye of the same individual and also between eyes of an individual because of cyclotorsion. Therefore, sectoral and regional neuroretinal rim width, RNFL peripapillary, and macular thickness analysis can vary widely. Thus, it is advisable to determine fovea-BMO center axis in each eye followed by data acquisition relative to this.

Optical coherence tomography imaging of the ONH should enhance rather than replace the clinical optic disc examination. Clinical examination helps to characterize

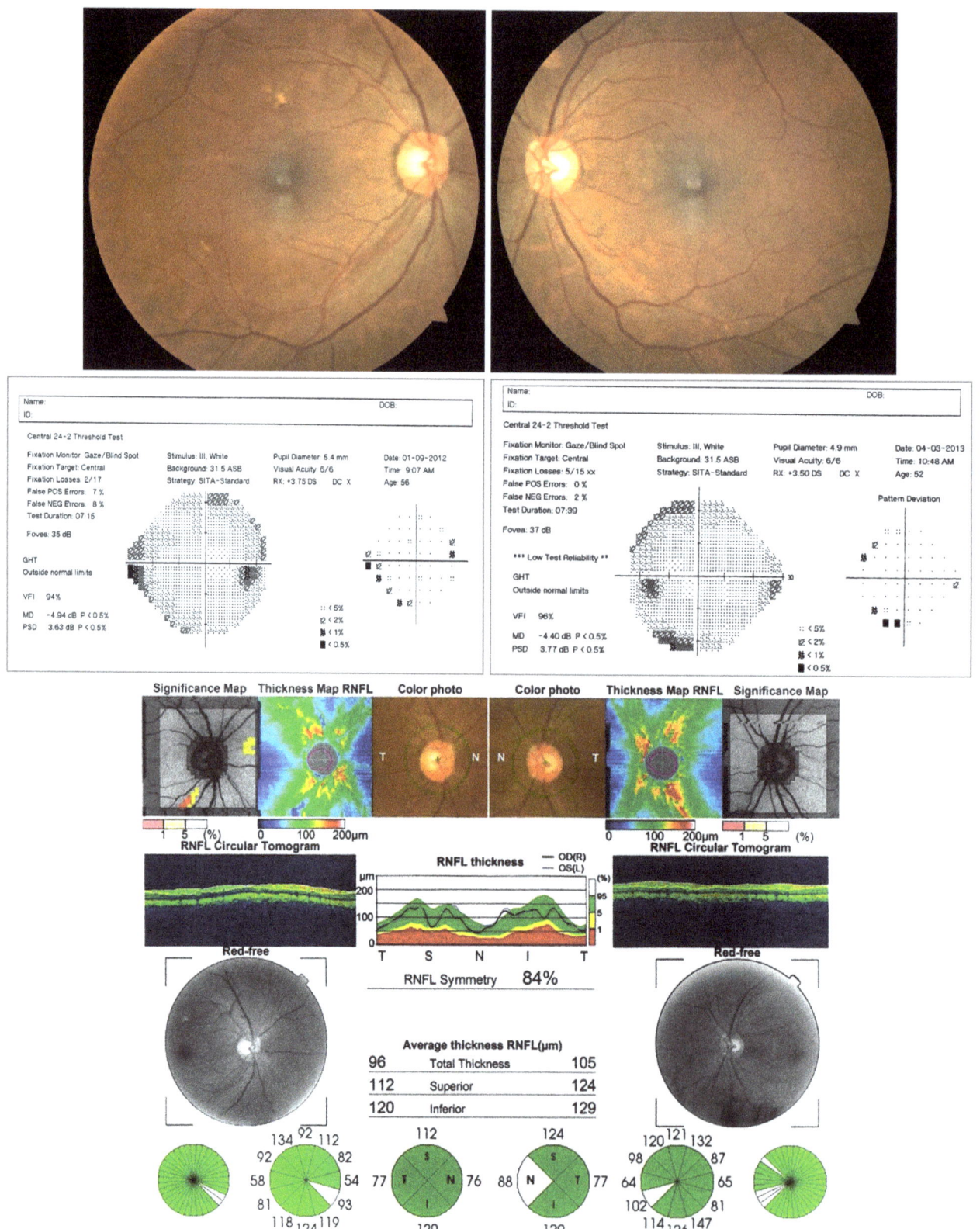

Fig. 12: Fundus photography of this patient shows a slit retinal nerve fiber layer (RNFL) defect in the right eye which correlates with the dipping of the optic disc (OD) RNFL contour line in the superior region of the TSNIT graph. A similar dipping of the OD RNFL contour line occurs in the superior region which is not appreciable in fundus image. The optical coherence tomography (OCT) significance map and the thickness map reflect the inferior RNFL thinning. There is no corresponding defect in the standard white on white perimetry. Such findings suggest close monitoring of the condition for progression. The image quality was 79 and 89 in the right and left eyes, respectively.

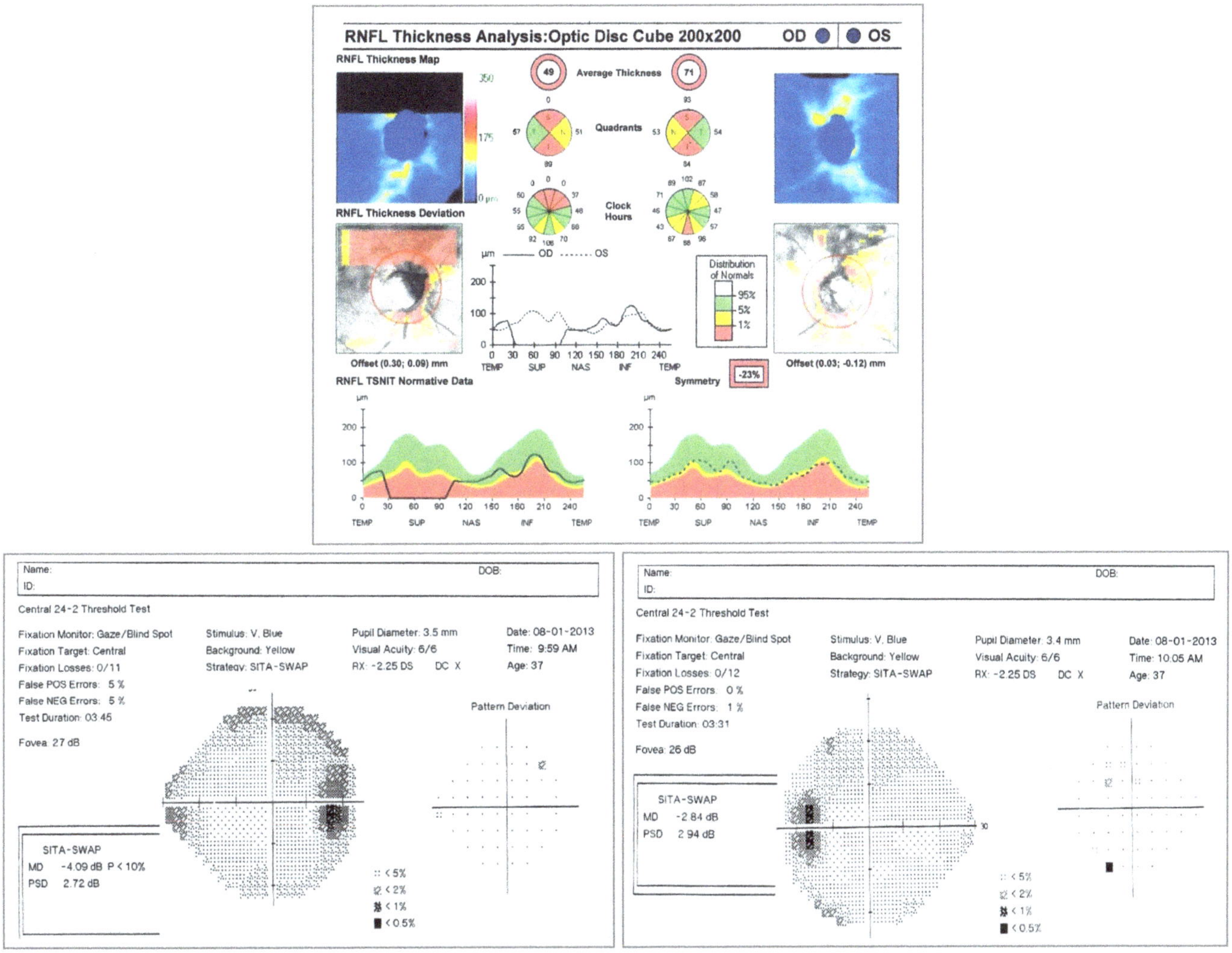

Fig. 13: Optical coherence tomography (OCT) of this patient shows a reduced average and superior, inferior quadrant-wise RNFL thickness, however, the HFA SITA SWAP shows a normal finding. The OCT thickness map of right eye shows an artifact superiorly during image acquisition, which leads to false low RNFL thickness report. The signal strength is 3 for both eye images, rendering the report unreliable. (HFA: Humphrey visual field; SITA: Swedish interactive threshold algorithm; SWAP: short-wavelength automated perimetry; RNFL: retinal nerve fiber layer)

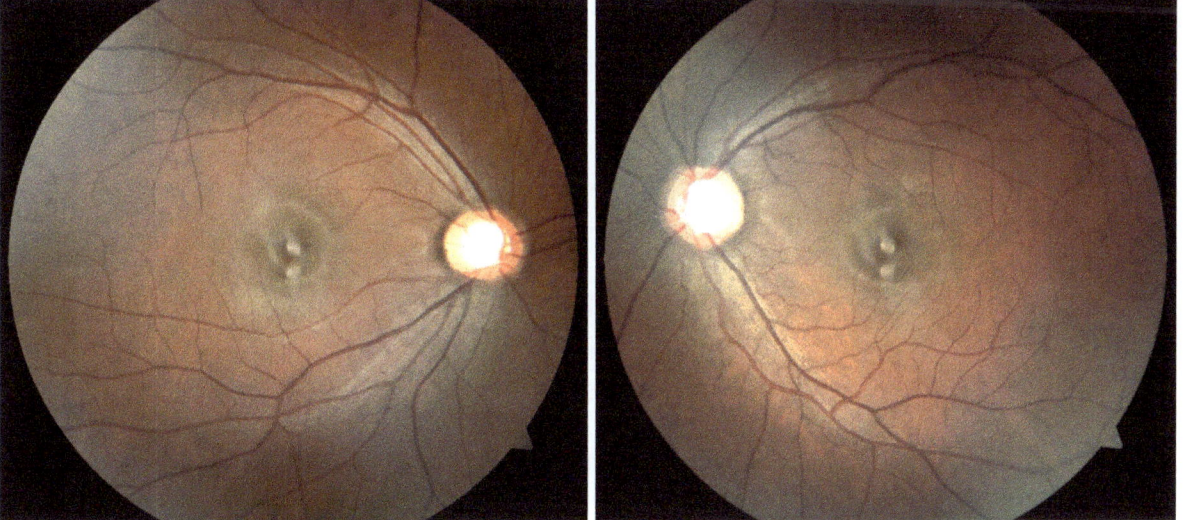

Fig. 14

Contd...

Contd...

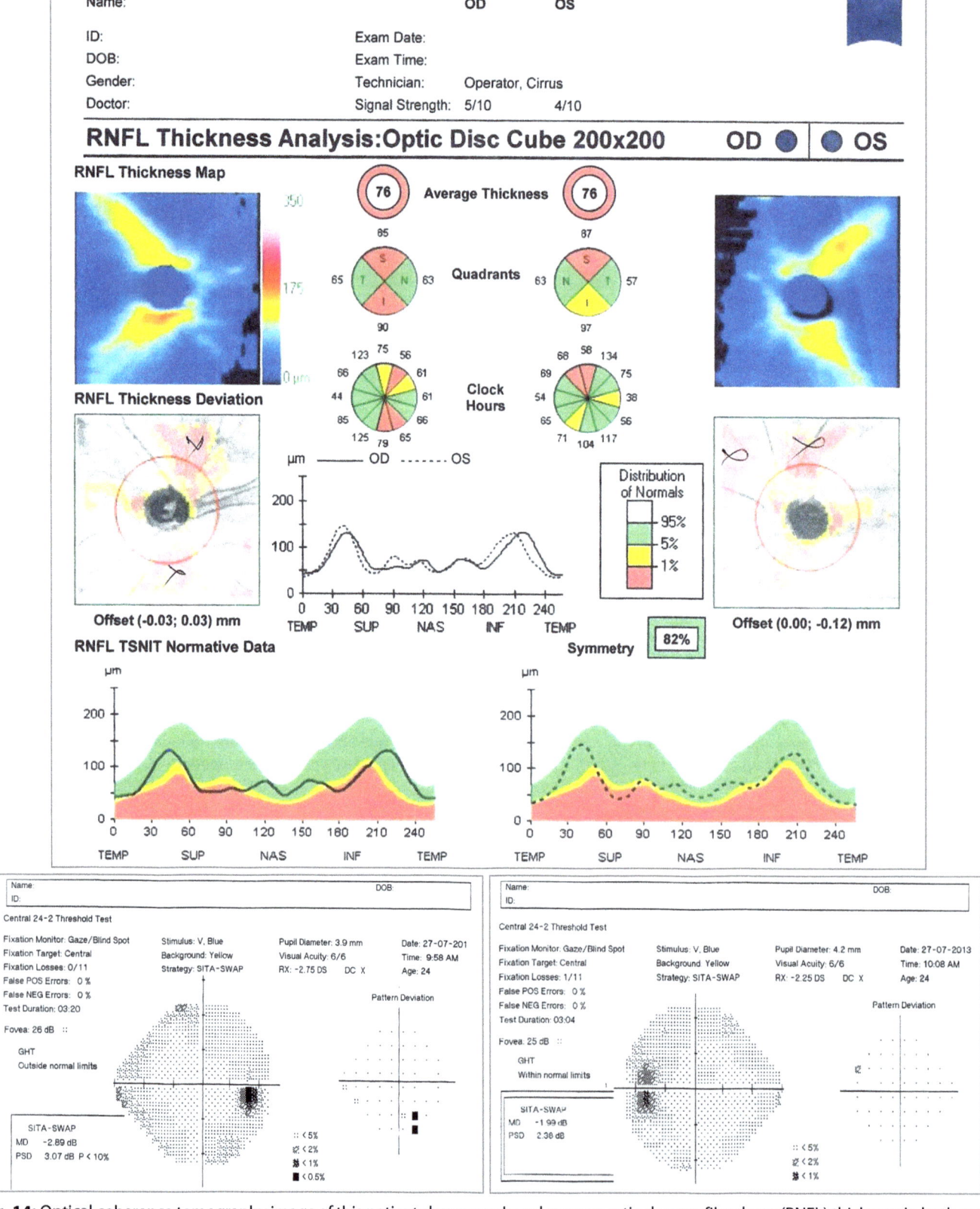

Fig. 14: Optical coherence tomography image of this patient shows a reduced average retinal nerve fiber layer (RNFL) thickness in both eyes. The RNFL is thinner in the superonasal and inferonasal regions of the temporal-superior-nasal-inferior-temporal (TSNIT) graph in both eyes. A fundus photograph with optic nerve head at the center and a 30-2 program of the automated visual field analyzer is the recommended to detect the corresponding field defect.

CHAPTER 9: Structural and Functional Correlation in Glaucoma

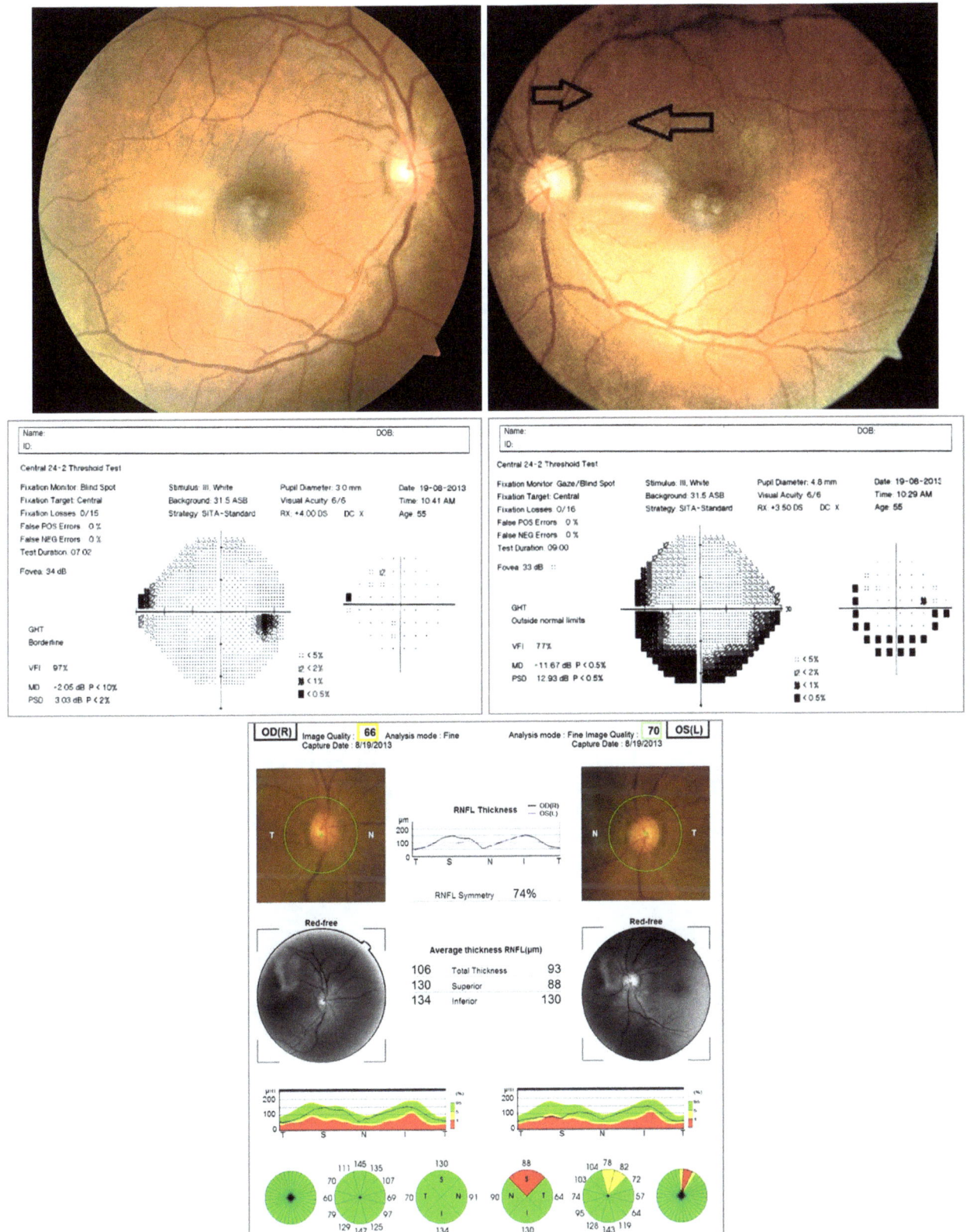

Fig. 15: The fundus image of the right eye is normal, whereas there appears a superior retinal nerve fiber layer (RNFL) defect in the left eye. The defect is made out with difficulty in the fundus photograph, but in the fundus image acquired by the optical coherence tomography (OCT), it is surprisingly quite clear. Correspondingly the standard white on white perimetry reveals an inferior arcuate defect and there appears a dipping of the contour line in the superior region of the temporal-superior-nasal-inferior-temporal (TSNIT) graph in the left eye. Note that the disc is not well centered in the scanned image captured by the OCT in the right eye.

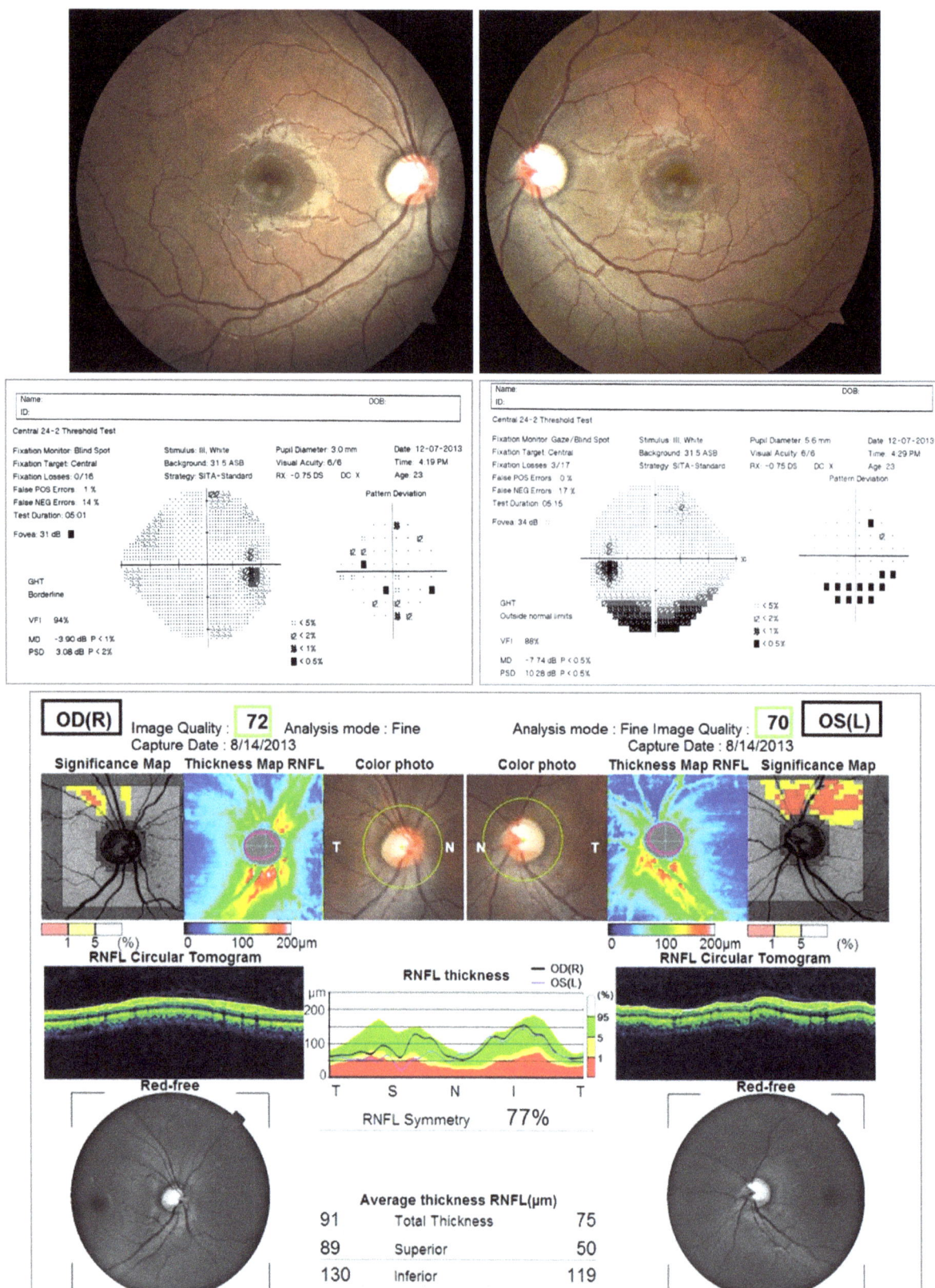

Fig. 16: The fundus photograph shows bilateral superior neuroretinal rim thinning with slit defects of the nerve fiber layer (more so in the left eye). The standard white on white automated perimetry reveals a corresponding inferior arcuate defect in the left eye. The thinned out retinal nerve fiber layer (RNFL) layer is reflected in the RNFL thickness temporal-superior-nasal-inferior-temporal (TSNIT) graphs of both eyes in the Optical coherence tomography (OCT) printout.

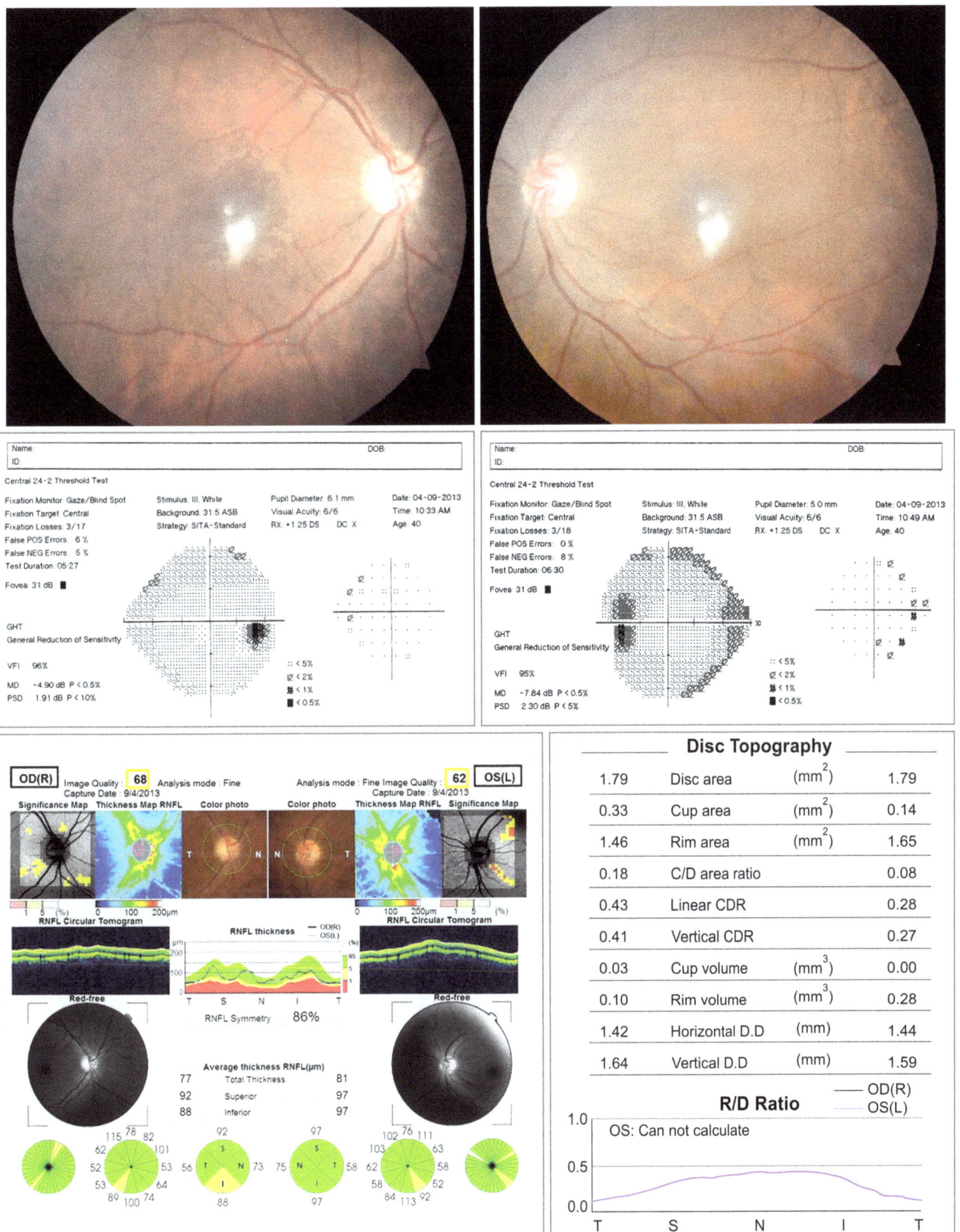

Fig. 17: Optical coherence tomography, fundus photography shows normal findings and Humphrey field analyzer (HFA) shows nonspecific findings due to learning defect.

qualitatively numerous ONH parameters which cannot be detected by OCT. Color of the optic disc, health of the neuroretinal rim regionally, pallor, bowing, excavation of the ONH surface, disc hemorrhages, and peripapillary RNFL defects should be assessed clinically for better structure and function correlation.

REFERENCES

1. Bowd C, Zangwill LM, Medeiros FA, Tavares IM, Hoffmann EM, Bourne RR, et al. Structure-function relationships using confocal scanning laser ophthalmoscopy, optical coherence tomography, and scanning laser polarimetry. Invest Ophthalmol Vis Sci. 2006;47:2889-95.
2. Reus NJ, Lemij HG. Relationships between standard automated perimetry, HRT confocal scanning laser ophthalmoscopy, and GDx VCC scanning laser polarimetry. Invest Ophthalmol Vis Sci. 2005;46:4182-8.
3. Ajtony C, Balla Z, Somoskeoy S, Kovacs B. Relationship between visual field sensitivity and retinal nerve fiber layer thickness as measured by optical coherence tomography. Invest Ophthalmol Vis Sci. 2007;48:258-63.
4. Chauhan BC, Burgoyne CF. From clinical examination of the optic disc to clinical assessment of optic nerve head: A Paradigm Change. Am J Ophthalmol. 2013;156:218-27.

CHAPTER 10

Role of Perimetry in Diagnosis and Management of Neuro-ophthalmic Disorders

Nikhil S Choudhari, Sirisha Senthil

■ INTRODUCTION

Visual field testing forms an important functional element in the evaluation of the lesions affecting the visual pathway. Visual field can be assessed by several techniques, such as confrontation, tangent screen, Goldmann kinetic perimetry, and automated static perimetry.

The expectations of visual field testing are different in glaucoma and neuro-ophthalmology. In glaucoma, the emphasis is on finding the earliest visual field change due to the disease or to detect smallest progression that is significant. On the other hand, the emphasis is on determining the pattern of visual field defect in order to indicate the site of visual pathway involvement in neuro-ophthalmology. In general, the requirement in neuro-ophthalmology is a good qualitative field except in certain situations, e.g., threatened optic nerve compression while quantitative needs prevail in glaucoma.[1]

A significant number of patients with neurological disease cannot cooperate with visual field testing. In Goldmann kinetic perimetry, the perimetric stimulus presentation is done by a human, and a good perimetrist-patient interaction can bring out meaningful information in such patients. The kinetic perimetry is more appropriate for neuro-ophthalmic disorders for few more reasons as well. The test point locations can be customized by the perimetrist during Goldmann perimetry unlike the fixed, 6º spaced grid of conventional automated perimetry. The ability to use specific exploration strategies for individual concerns allows for much more accurate mapping of defect shape. This can be invaluable for the topographic localization of visual field defects. Nevertheless, manual kinetic perimetry has limitations. It is less sensitive than conventional automated perimetry and is more time consuming. Getting trained as a perimetrist is difficult. On the other hand, automated perimetry does not depend much on the examiner, is faster, reproducible, and has the advantages of a computerized system for storage and comparison to normative data. Moreover, the output can be incorporated into the electronic medical record system. Therefore, standard automated perimetry enjoyed rapid acceptance after it became available and has replaced manual kinetic perimetry at most centers.[1,2] Therefore, the treating ophthalmologist should be familiar with understanding of the strengths and weaknesses of automated perimetry in neuro-ophthalmic conditions.

Perimetry fulfills diagnostic and monitoring functions in neuro-ophthalmology. It can reveal involvement of the visual pathway and the pattern of visual field defect helps in localizing the site of the lesion. Visual fields can monitor either resolution or progression and recurrence of disease processes affecting the visual pathway. Visual fields also help planning rehabilitation strategies.

■ HOW VISUAL FIELD INTERPRETATION IS DIFFERENT IN NEURO-OPHTHALMOLOGY THAN THAT IN GLAUCOMA?

The pattern of visual field defect has more emphasis than the light sensitivity at individual test locations in neuro-ophthalmic disorders.[1] Therefore, one should give sufficient attention to the gray scale in the perimetry printout. Having more categories than the probability plots, the gray scale may better reveal denser areas within a scotoma or a field defect that can subsequently be confirmed by looking at the numeric plot **(Fig. 1)**. Many patients with neuro-ophthalmic diseases are young and have clear ocular media. The pattern deviation plot in their visual fields can be misleading. The Anderson's criteria and various available statistical analytical packages, e.g., Guided Progression Analysis Software (GPA) are designed to detect glaucomatous visual field defects and to follow them over time.[3,4] In fact, no comparable statistical package is available for neuro-ophthalmic applications. An

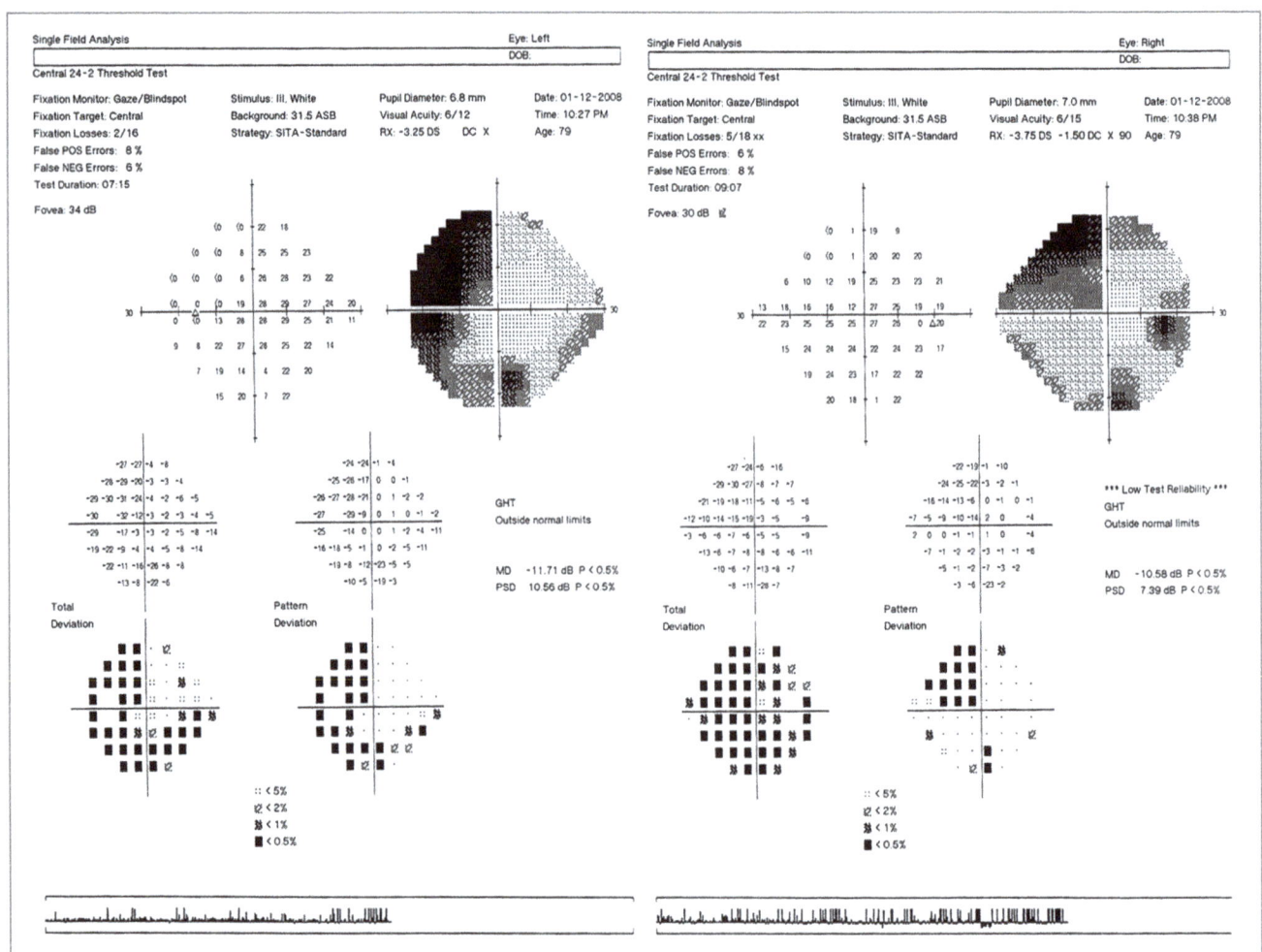

Fig. 1: This 79-year-old diabetic and hypertensive gentleman was diagnosed to have primary open angle glaucoma and was put up on antiglaucoma medication elsewhere. His intraocular pressure was normal in both eyes even after discontinuing the antiglaucoma medication and he had large optic discs with physiological cupping. When the visual fields are seen individually, right eye field can be stated to have an incomplete superior arcuate scotoma and the left field to have an incomplete biarcuate scotoma. However, when the fields are aligned as shown, left incongruous hemianopia that is more dense in the superior half (look at gray scales) is apparent. His magnetic resonance imaging (MRI) brain revealed an infarct involving the right optic tract.
Courtesy: Sankara Nethralaya

overview printout in Humphrey perimeter may ease the assessment of serial fields.

The visual field defects in glaucoma respect the horizontal meridian. On the other hand, careful attention to the vertical meridian is necessary to detect chiasmal and retrochiasmal lesions **(Fig. 2)**. Since the gray scale interpolates the threshold values between measured points, the numeric plot should always be scrutinized for a vertical step. Each threshold value on one side of the vertical meridian should be compared with the corresponding value on the other side of the vertical meridian. The most important comparisons involve the pairs of the thresholds immediately adjacent to the vertical meridian, but should also include the pairs from the second column. At least all three vertically adjacent points should have higher threshold on one side of the vertical meridian and the lower thresholds on the other to suggest a significant vertical step.[1]

The visual field printouts of both the eyes should be simultaneously evaluated in patients with neuro-ophthalmic diseases. Lesions at or behind the optic chiasm produce a visual field defect in the fellow eye as well that usually also shows alignment along the vertical meridian **(Figs. 3A and B)**. Some patients have visual field defects in the fellow eye that do not respect the vertical meridian such as blindness or a central scotoma, but have localizing value to the anterior chiasm. The neuro-ophthalmic visual field defects, e.g., hemianopias are named depending upon how the patient experiences the world. Therefore, visual field printout of the left eye should be kept on the left side and visual field printout of the right eye should be kept on the right side

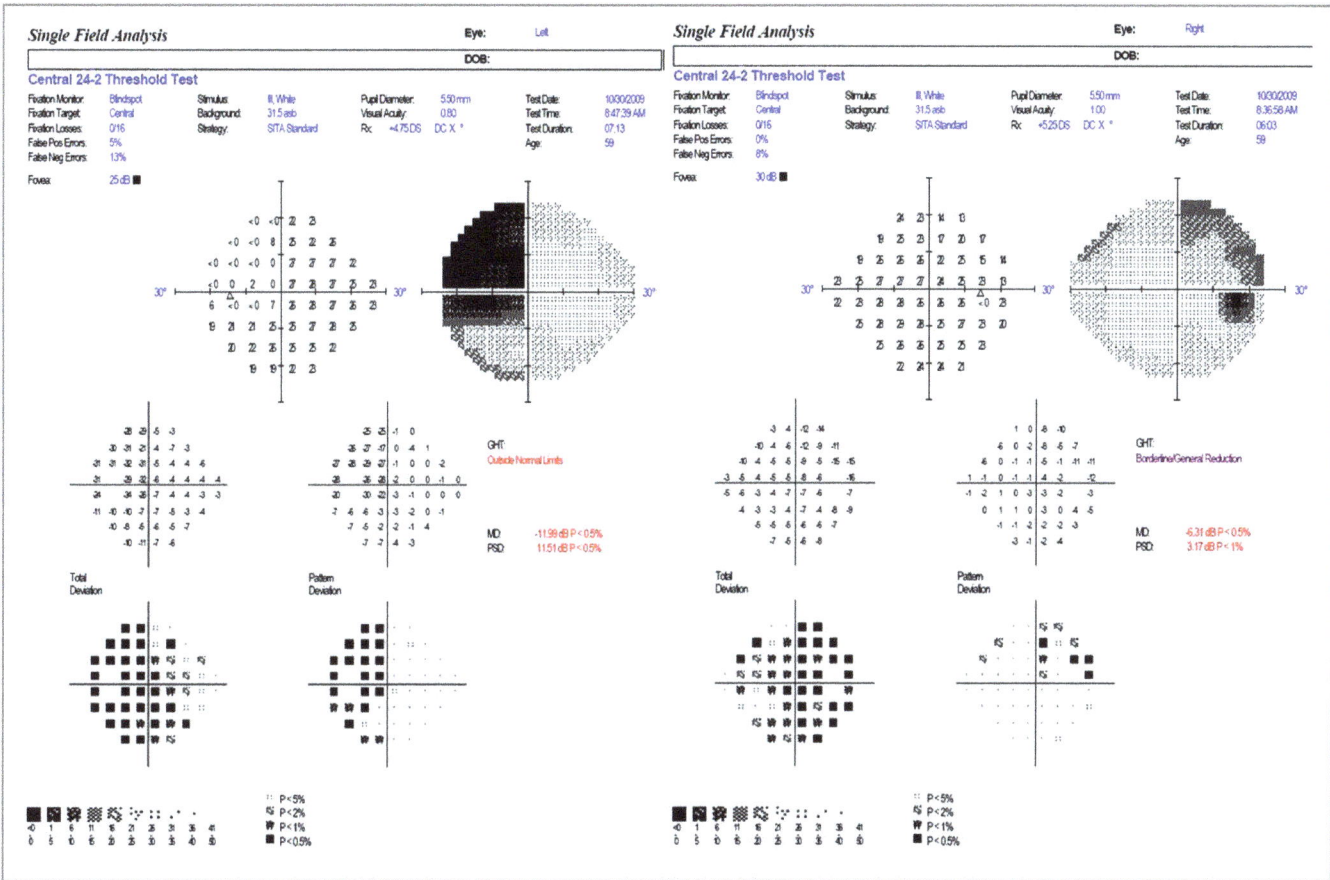

Fig. 2: This is an asymmetric bisuperotemporal scotoma. This patient was a professor who complained of a recent-onset visual difficulty while writing in the upper left corner of the black board. Visual acuity, including color test was normal. The optic discs appeared normal on clinical examination. The field defect was a tip off for neuroimaging which picked up a pituitary adenoma compressing the chiasm.

while simultaneously evaluating printouts of both the eyes of a patient (*see* **Fig. 1**). A bitemporal hemianopia can appear binasal if this rule is not followed!

SELECTION OF AN AUTOMATED VISUAL FIELD TEST IN NEURO-OPHTHALMOLOGY

For patients who are not fully cooperative, a suprathreshold screening test can be a more appropriate choice. Because multiple stimulus presentations at each point are not used, the suprathreshold static testing method is quite fast and at the same time can produce qualitative information which can help in detection and localization of a visual pathway lesion **(Fig. 4)**.

Most visual field defects of neuro-ophthalmic significance manifest within the central 30°. Hemianopic defects may be more obvious in the periphery, but they also demonstrate vertical meridian-respecting central visual field defects. But in rare situations, peripheral visual field testing might be warranted to diagnose a neuro-ophthalmic condition **(Figs. 5A to D)**.

The clinical appearance of the optic disc and the pattern of the visual field defect often do not correlate in neuro-ophthalmic diseases, unlike in glaucoma **(Figs. 6 and 7)**. Nevertheless, management decisions in neuro-ophthalmic conditions should be based on the total clinical picture and the results of the appropriate investigations put together and not solely on one or two pieces of information.[5]

Visual Fields to Diagnose Neuro-Ophthalmic Disorders

Perimetry can find afferent visual pathway loss that may not be apparent to the patient **(Fig. 2)**. Alterations in central visual function are often symptomatic. Peripheral vision loss, on the other hand, can often go unnoticed, especially if it is gradual and monocular.

Perimetry can help to diagnose a neuro-ophthalmic condition when clinical assessment is difficult or patient's symptoms and the examination findings do not correlate e.g., visual pathway lesions in patients in whom the optic disc is difficult to interpret clinically such as a myopic optic

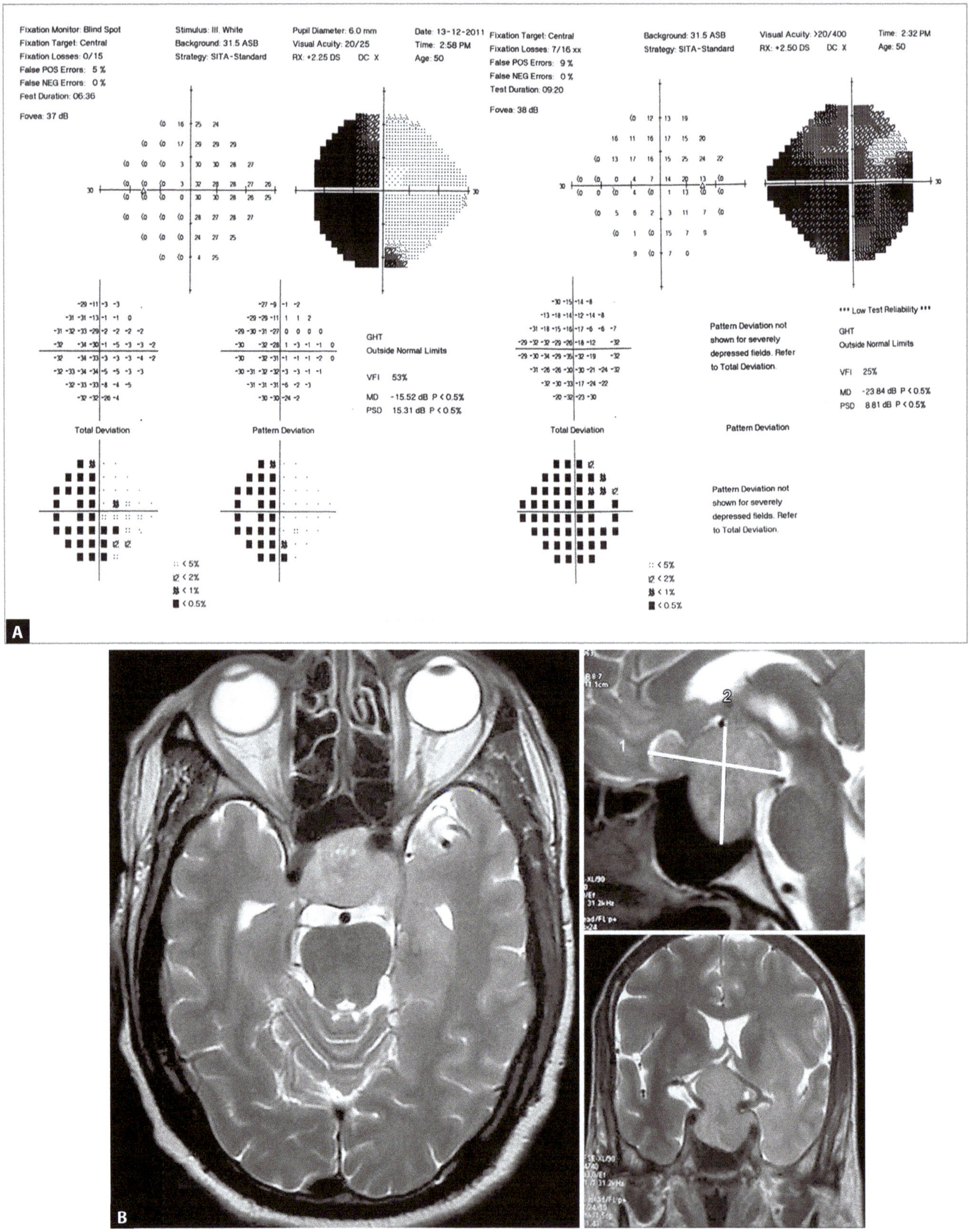

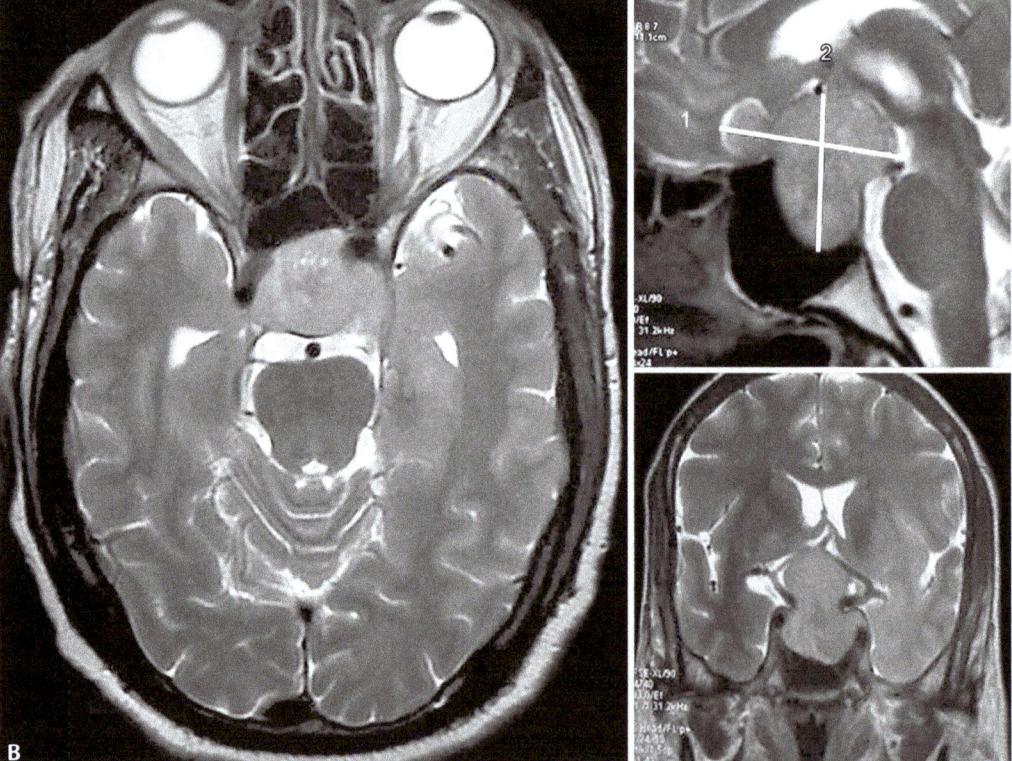

Figs. 3A and B: (A) The visual field of the right eye has a diffuse depression. But the field defect in the fellow eye respects the vertical meridian; (B) This was the indication for neuroimaging which revealed chiasmal compressive lesion suggestive of a craniopharyngioma.

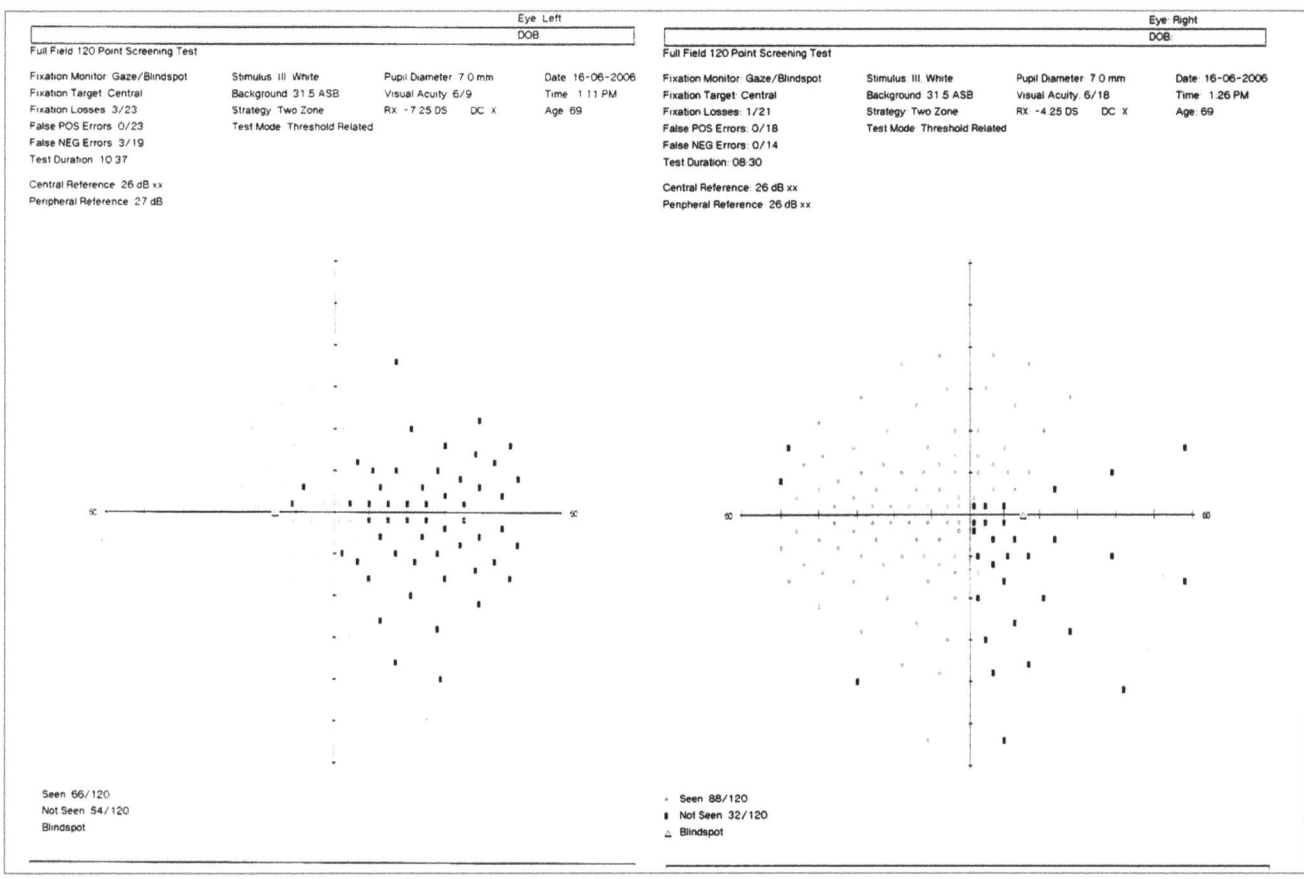

Fig. 4: This elderly patient could identify compromise in the right side of his visual field but could not cooperate well for threshold perimetry. However, the 120-point screening test picked up right incongruous hemianopia.
Courtesy: Sankara Nethralaya

disc or visual pathway lesions that are behind the lateral geniculate body.

Perimetry can also pick up early optic nerve decompensation in conditions such as pseudotumor cerebri or Graves' disease.

Visual Fields to Localize Site of Lesion in the Visual Pathway

Often there is a significant variability in perimetry when testing a diseased optic nerve. This variability, or fluctuation may either obscure typical defects **(Figs. 8A and B)** or may produce localizing visual field characteristics when in fact they are not. It is therefore a good rule to repeat visual field testing if there is any question of the validity of the test. Most optic neuropathies produce a generalized reduction in optic nerve function with characteristic focal damage superimposed to it **(Figs. 9A and B)**.[1] Papilledema in the early stage leads to enlargement of the blind spots. An altitudinal visual field defect is typically seen in anterior ischemic optic neuropathy **(Fig. 10)**. Central or cecocentral defects are typically macular or optic nerve, respectively in origin.

Central scotoma is the most common visual field defect seen in Ethambutol toxicity.[6] If the fellow eye is normal, most of the uniocular visual field defects are caused by the lesions which are anterior to the optic chiasm.

The hallmark visual field defect of chiasmal disease is bitemporal hemianopia.[7] The presence of this defect is a reliable indication of a problem localized to the chiasmal region that can be found out by doing neuroimaging (*see* **Fig. 2**). Unfortunately, many a time chiasmal disease is not sufficiently picked up early by ophthalmologists because of failure to perform visual fields. A high level of suspicion for chiasmal disease must accompany evaluation of patients with unexplained visual loss, optic disc pallor, or obscure visual complaints.[5] Partial bitemporal hemianopia demands more attention. This visual field defect can progress from superior to inferior bitemporal region if the optic chiasm is compressed from below, e.g., by a pituitary adenoma or vice-a-versa if the chiasm is pressed from above, e.g., by a craniopharyngioma, if the compression is not relieved sufficiently early.

Lesions of the visual pathway posterior to the chiasm produce defects in both eyes on the same side of the vertical

SECTION 3: Special Situations

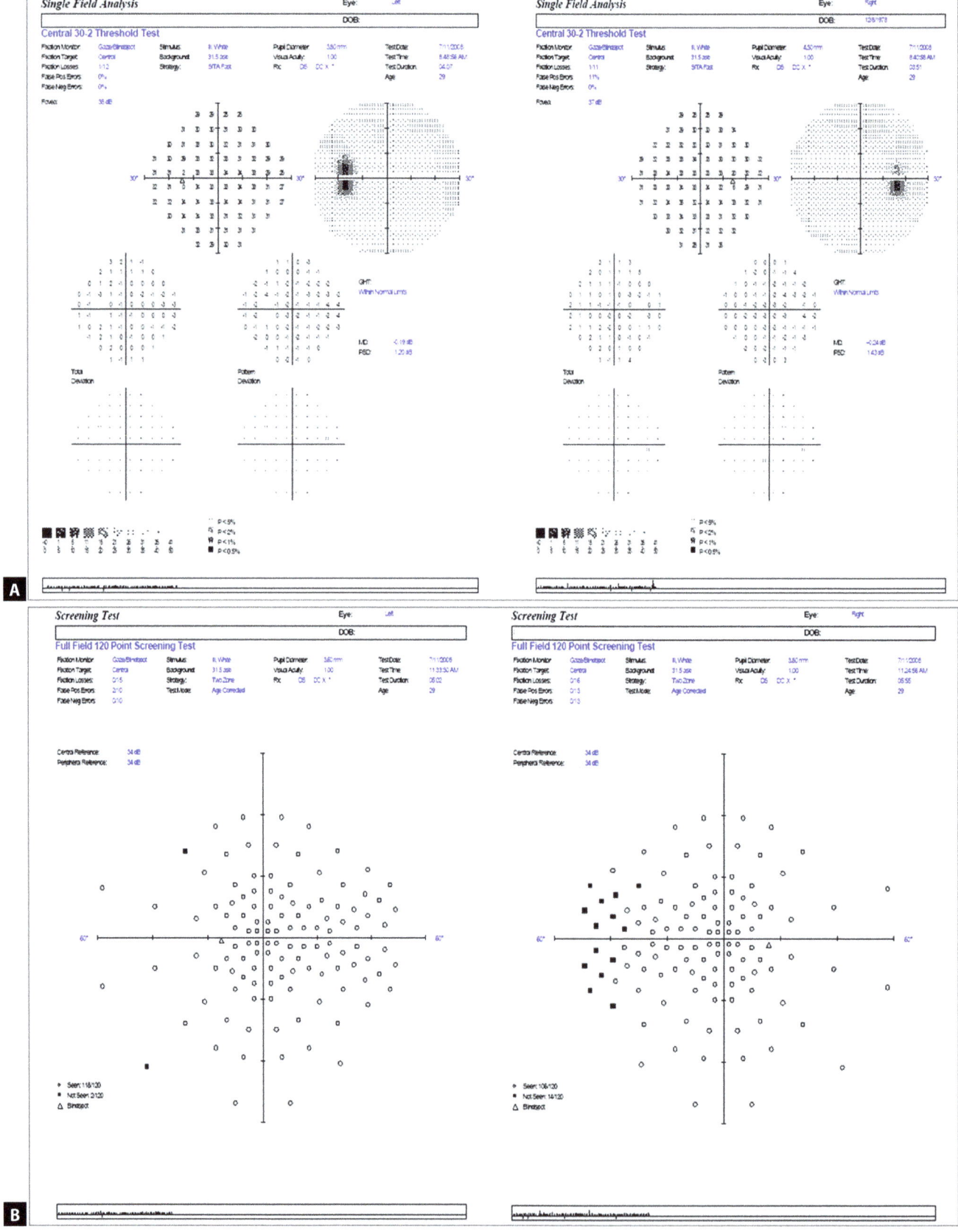

Figs. 5A and B

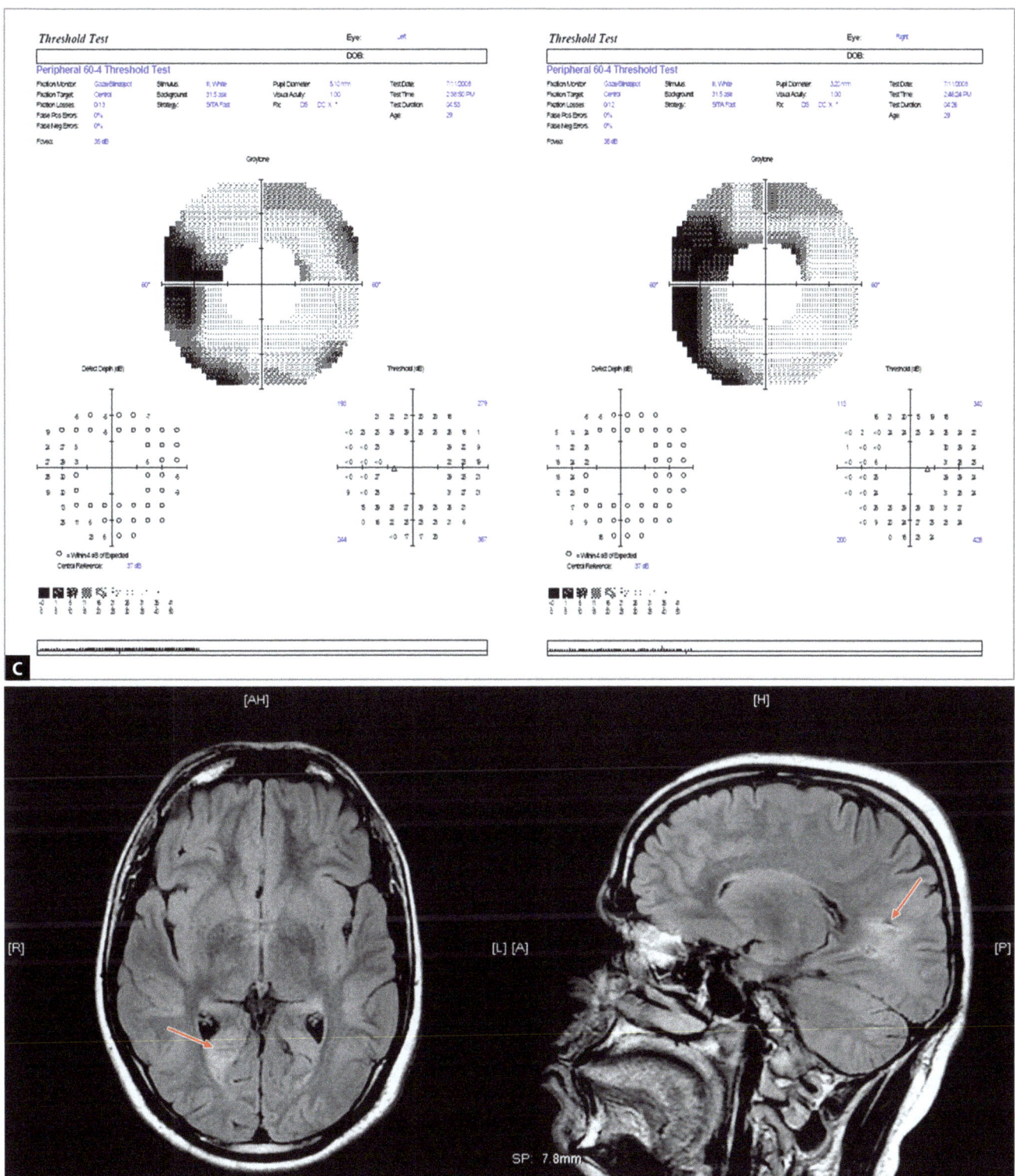

Figs. 5C and D

Figs. 5A to D: (A) This was a 29-year-old male patient who complained of difficulty in left-sided vision following a sun stroke 2 months ago. His ocular examination was normal so were the 30-2 visual fields; (B) Because of his consistent and well defined complain, a 120-point field was ordered. The latter did reveal defect in the nasal peripheral field of the right eye. Note presence of very few testing locations in the peripheral temporal field of the left eye in this program of the perimeter; (C) The 60-4 threshold confirmed left homonymous ring scotoma; (D) His MRI brain showed infarct in right intermediate visual cortex that explains the scotoma.
Case courtesy: Sankara Nethralaya

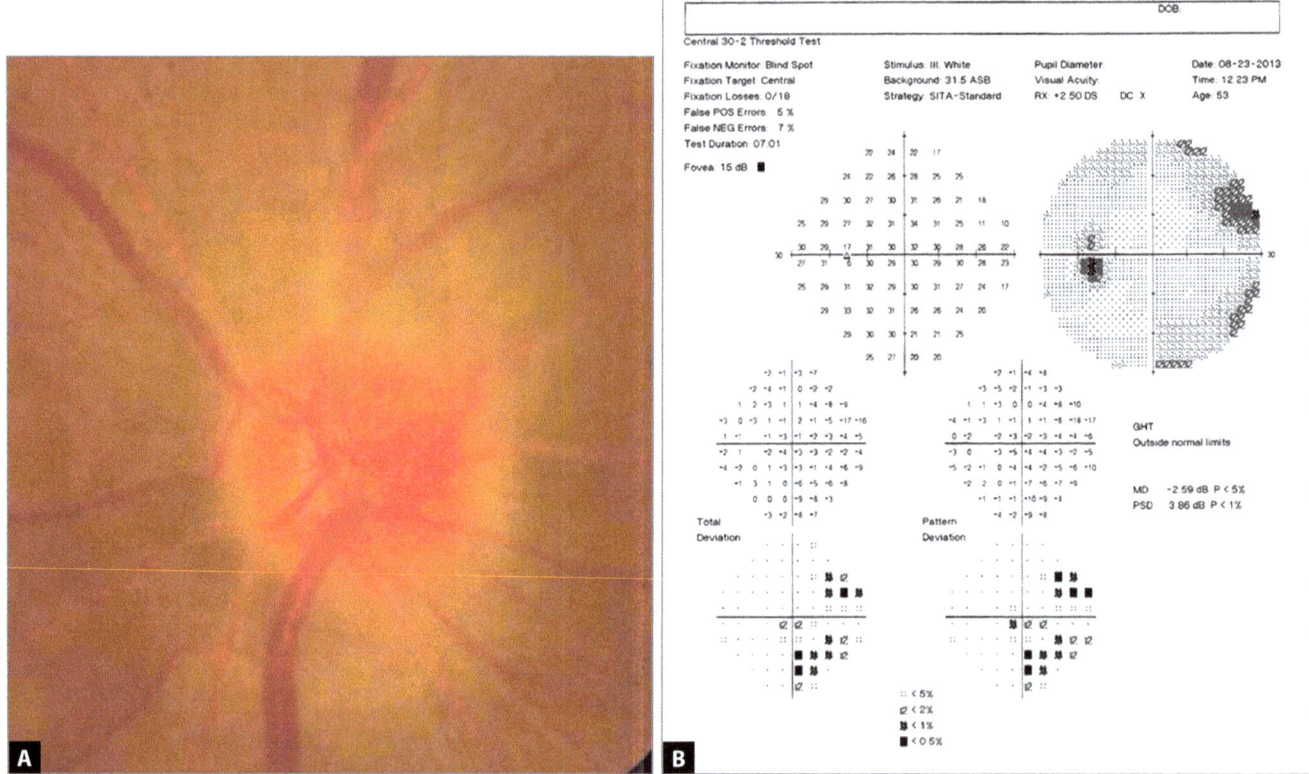

Figs. 6A and B: This diabetic patient gave history of recent history of fluctuating blood sugar levels following a leg injury. The optic disc photograph indicates diabetic papillopathy; (A) Note mild, pallid optic disc edema, and superficial telangiectatic vessels; (B) The visual field defect doesn't correlate with the appearance of the optic disc.

meridian, i.e., a homonymous hemianopia. It is possible to have 6/6 vision using the macular fibers from only one hemifield, therefore hemianopic visual fields may not have defective visual acuity.[8] Lesions just posterior to the chiasm in the optic tracts tend to be quite non congruous (i.e., even though the visual field defects lie on the same side of the vertical meridian in both eyes, the defects are quite dissimilar between the eyes, **Figs. 1 and 4**). On the other hand, lesions in the posterior visual pathway are congruous.

Visual Fields in the Follow Up of a Neuro-ophthalmic Condition

Follow-up visual fields can indicate resolution, progression (**Fig. 11**) or recurrence of disease processes affecting the visual pathway. There are several statistical analytical packages available to monitor changes in serial visual fields. However, as stated above, the available packages are designed to detect progression of glaucomatous visual field defects and do not yet have neuro-ophthalmic application.

Several important factors should be kept in mind while evaluating serial visual fields. The test strategies, target sizes, and other test conditions should be similar to compare the results, e.g., visual fields done with either 24-2 or 30-2 program on Humphrey perimeter can be compared keeping the difference in the number of test locations in mind. On the other hand, visual fields done with stimulus sizes 3 and 5, for example, cannot be compared with each other. The patient conditions from one visual field to the other should also be comparable, e.g., visual fields done with upper lid taped on one occasion and not taped on other occasion cannot be compared with each other. Most importantly, it is difficult to differentiate short- or long-term variability in the visual fields from true progression. Other factors such as perimetrist-patient interaction, patient fatigue, and experience add to the complexity of the decision. Therefore, unless the visual field change is dramatic and collaborates with the patient's clinical presentation, it is best to repeat the testing on a separate visit to confirm the suspected change. The important decisions about visual field stability or progression are best taken on the basis of the entire series of the visual fields, whenever available.[2]

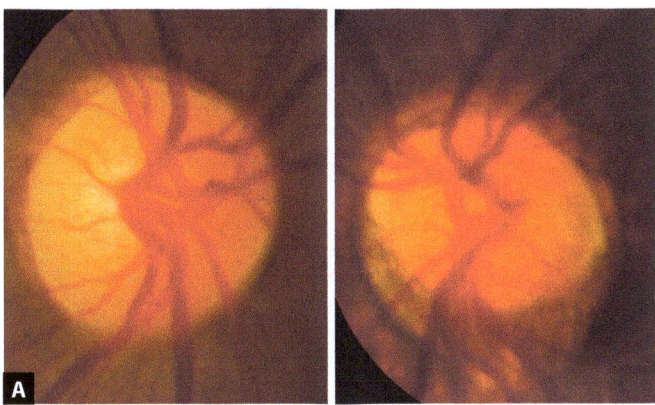

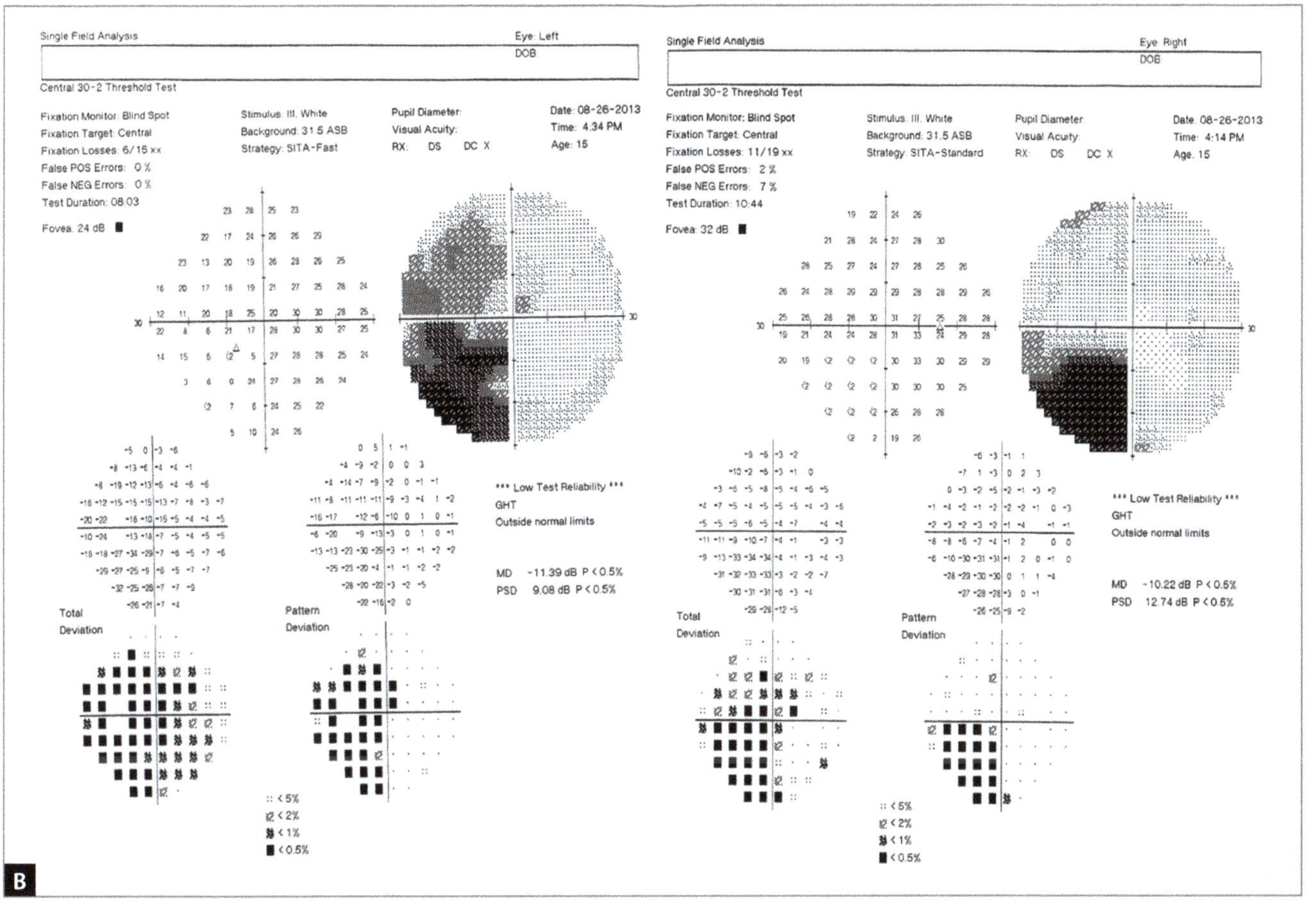

Figs. 7A and B: This 15-year-old girl came with 6-month history of decreased vision in her left eye; (A) Her right optic disc had temporal pallor while the left had band shaped pallor; (B) Her visual fields showed left incongruous homonymous hemianopia that was denser in the inferior half (see the gray scales). This is another example of poor correlation between the appearance of the optic disc and the pattern of visual field defects as often seen in neuro-ophthalmic diseases. Her MRI brain revealed focal atrophy in right parietal lobe and periventricular demyelinated lesions typical of multiple sclerosis.

■ STEPPING INTO THE FUTURE

Automated perimetry is not an easy test to take. It requires the patient to remain attentive on the visual target for several minutes at a time. The test is not entertaining in any way. Moreover, the test demands a fair amount of perimetrist's time and energy. Given these realities, attempts are being made to develop portable perimeters that use tablets, personal computers, or head-mounted displays. The approach is potentially inexpensive, might allow home-based and frequent testing, and thereby reduce traveling of elderly and remotely located individuals. The test output can also be electronic medical record system friendly. This

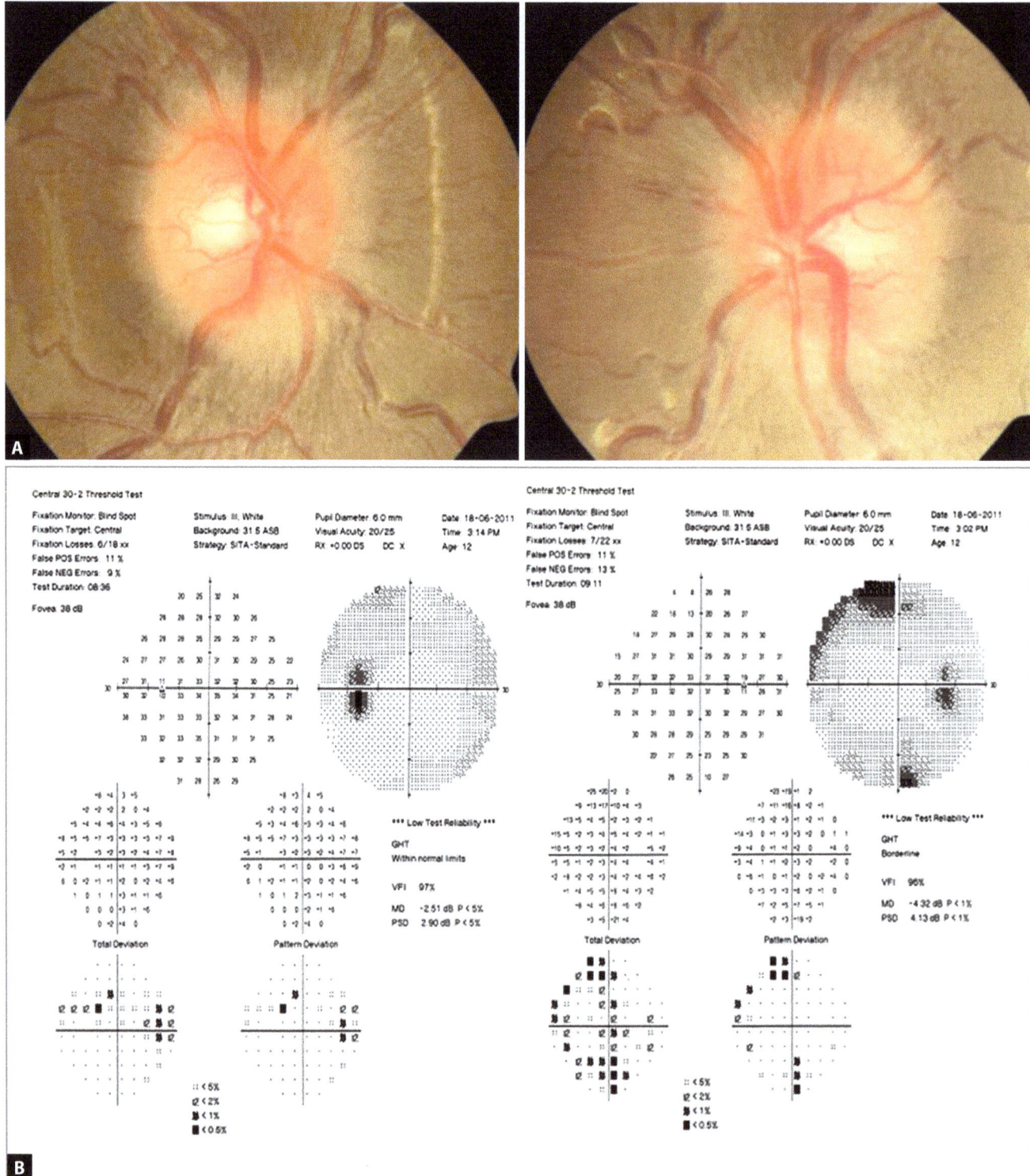

Figs. 8A and B: (A) This was a 12-year-old girl with left 6th cranial nerve palsy and optic disc edema due to idiopathic intracranial hypertension; (B) Note enlarged blind spot only in the visual field of the left eye and bizarre peripheral defect in the visual field of the right eye. She also had significant fixation losses.

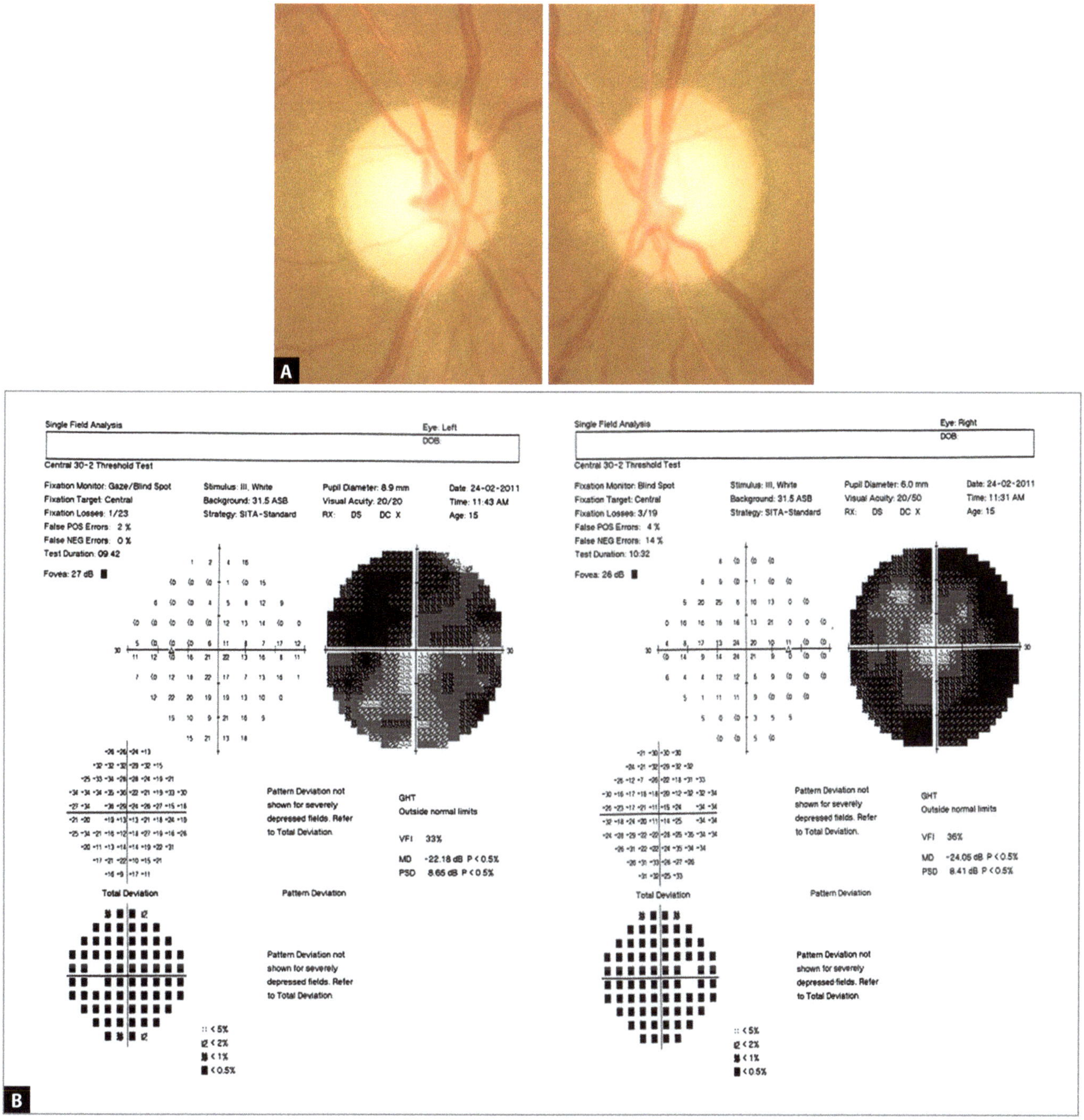

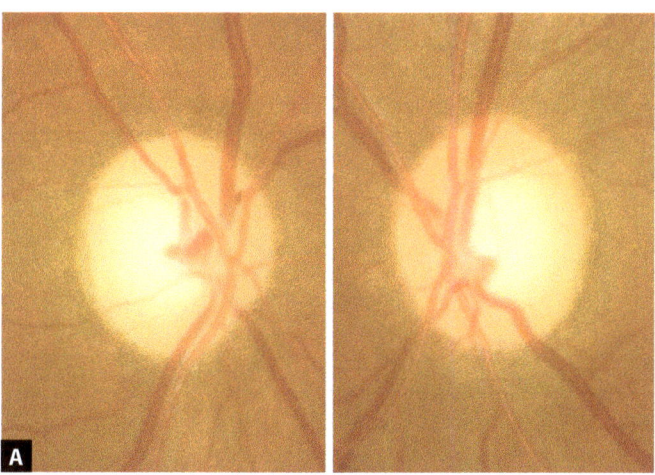

Figs. 9A and B: This was a 15-year-old boy who had multiple episodes of postinfectious optic neuritis. (A) Note gross optic disc pallor and (B) severe constriction of visual fields.

approach may suit neuro-ophthalmology because of the lesser dependence on quantitative visual field assessment. However, currently the devices are under development and there is uncertainty about their performance.[9,10]

automated visual fields in neuro-ophthalmic disorders **(Table 1)**. An intelligent choice of automated test programs and paying attention to the vertical meridian will result in optimal use of perimetry in neuro-ophthalmic conditions.

■ CONCLUSION

The ophthalmologist should understand and follow the not so difficult but different interpretation strategy for evaluating

■ ACKNOWLEDGMENTS

We thank G Chandra Sekhar, Vice Chair and Director of Hyderabad Campus, LV Prasad Eye Institute and Ronnie

TABLE 1: Interpretation of automated visual fields in glaucoma vis-a-vis in neuro-ophthalmology.

Parameter	Glaucomatous visual field defect	Neuro-ophthalmic visual field defect
Purpose of testing	To find earliest pathological field defect or detect progression	• Diagnosis, narrowing differential diagnosis of neuro-ophthalmic condition • To find nature of visual field defect to localize site of visual pathway involvement
Preferred type of perimetry	Static	Kinetic
Preferred program on automated perimetry	24-2, 10-2	30-2
Technique of evaluating reports of automated perimetry	Can evaluate reports of individual eye	Reports from both eyes must be evaluated simultaneously by keeping left eye report on left side and right eye report on right side
Preferred analysis in automated perimetry	Pattern deviation plot and other statistical analytical packages	Grayscale plot, Overview printout (Humphrey perimeter)
Nature of visual field defects	Respect horizontal meridian	Respect vertical meridian (except few exceptions)
Typical visual field defects	Nasal step, arcuate defect, tubular field	Enlarged blind spot, cecocentral defect, altitudinal defect, hemianopia, bitemporal defect
Correlation between clinical signs and visual field defect(s)	Often good	Often fair to poor

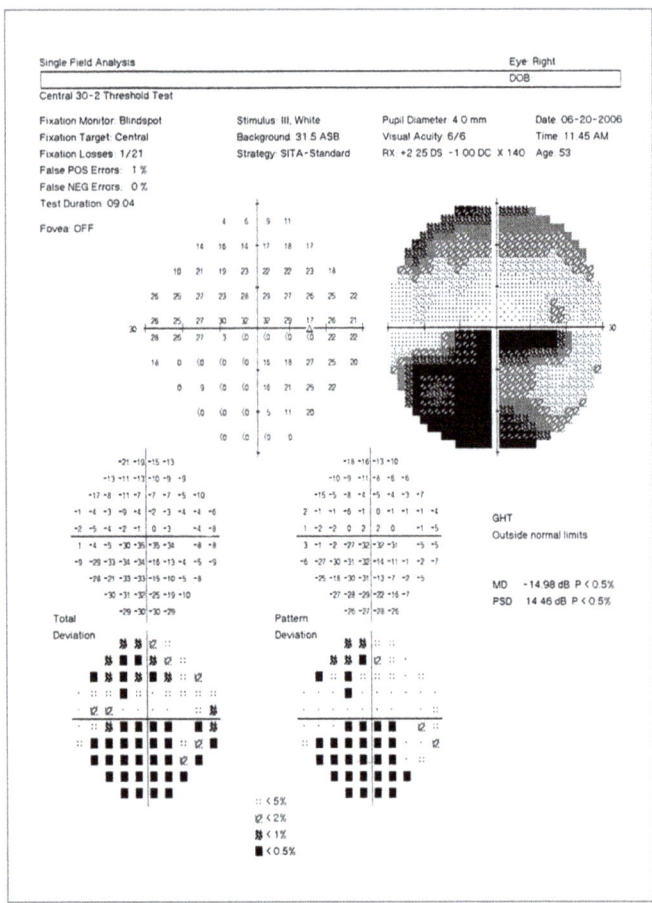

Fig. 10: The first impression of this visual field defect is an incomplete inferior arcuate scotoma. But majority of the depressed points have sensitivity dropped to 0 dB (see the numeric plot). Moreover, look at the drop off of light sensitivity across the horizontal meridian; from 30s to 0 dB. This is atypical of glaucoma. The patient had ischemic optic neuropathy.
Courtesy: Sankara Nethralaya

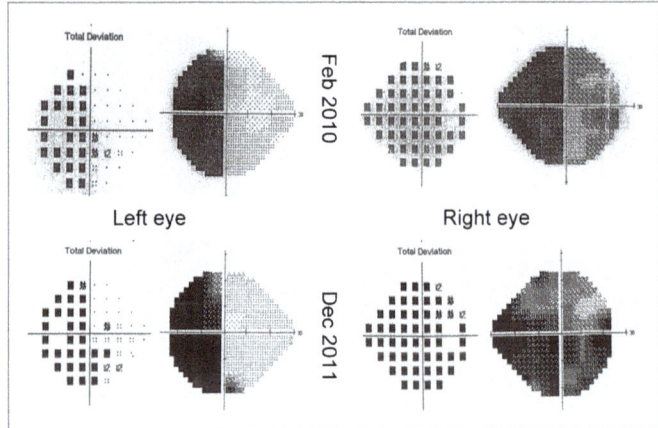

Fig. 11: These fields are of a 50-year-old man who had chiasmal compression by a craniopharyngioma. The tumor was not picked up sufficiently early. The visual fields show progression in both eyes (this is same patient as in **Figure 3**).

George, Senior Consultant, Department of Glaucoma, Sankara Nethralaya, Chennai for reviewing this chapter.

REFERENCES

1. Mills RP. Automated perimetry in neuro-ophthalmology. Int Ophthalmol Clin. 1991;31:51-70.
2. Wall M, Johnson CA. Principles and techniques of the examination of the visual sensory system. In: Miller NR, Newman NJ, Biousse V, Kerrison JB (Eds). Walsh and Hoyt's Clinical Neuro-ophthalmology. Philadelphia: Lippincott Williams & Wilkins, 2005. pp. 96-128.
3. Thomas R, George R. Interpreting automated perimetry. Indian J Ophthalmol. 2001;49:125-40.
4. Carl Zeiss Meditec Inc., Dublin, CA, USA. (2023). Perimetry brochure. [online] Available from: https://www.zeiss.com/content/dam/Meditec/us/download/

certified-pre-owned-systems/Perimetry_Brochure_US_PER4622_REVB_2014.pdf [Last accessed April, 2023].
5. Choudhari NS, Neog A, Fudnawala V, George R. Cupped disc with normal intraocular pressure: the long road to avoid misdiagnosis. Indian J Ophthalmol. 2011;59:491-7.
6. Sharma P, Sharma R. Toxic optic neuropathy. Indian J Ophthalmol. 2011;59(2):137-41.
7. Chiu EK, Nichols JW. Sellar lesions and visual loss: Key concepts in neuro-ophthalmology. Expert Rev Anticancer Ther. 2006;6 Suppl 9:S23-8.
8. Purvin VA, Kawasaki A. Misinterpretation of visual fields. In: Common neuro-ophthalmic pitfalls. New Delhi: Cambridge university press, 2009. Pp.117-35.
9. Odayappan A, Sivakumar P, Kotawala S, Raman R, Nachiappan S, Pachiyappan A, et al. Comparison of a New Head Mount Virtual Reality Perimeter (C3 Field Analyzer) With Automated Field Analyzer in Neuro-Ophthalmic Disorders. J Neuroophthalmol. 2023;43(2):232-6.
10. Daka Q, Mustafa R, Neziri B, Virgili G, Azuara-Blanco A. Home-based perimetry for glaucoma: Where are we now? J Glaucoma. 2022;31(6):361-74.

CHAPTER 11

Role of Perimetry in Diagnosis and Management of Retinal or Macular Disorders

Sathidevi AV, Gowri J Murthy, Rajani S Battu, Vinaya Kumar Konana, Supriya Dabir, Padmamalini Mahendradas, Chitralekha De, Priyanka Sudhakar

■ INTRODUCTION

Retinal disorders are predominantly diagnosed and assessed by structural examination, either by ophthalmoscopy or by imaging. Functional evaluation, like perimetry, is done only in a few specific circumstances. However, it is desirable to be aware of the functional correlates, for retinal disorders, as this can complement the assessment. Perimetry can also document and quantify improvement in visual function.

Often, a patient with long-standing glaucoma could develop retinal disease. In this situation, one needs to differentiate field loss due to one or the other disease and avoid misdiagnosing glaucomatous progression. Occasionally, field defects found accidentally, on routine testing for other indications, can lead to diagnosis of retinal disease. Arcuate defects caused by retinal diseases such as branch vein occlusion or retinochoroiditis may be mistaken for glaucomatous field defects. In a patient with cataract and multiple pathologies involving the retina and optic nerve, performing perimetry and foveal thresholding as a measure of foveal function could help in predicting postoperative vision and aid appropriate counseling of the patient about expectations of visual recovery.

A meticulous assessment of the disc and retina and correlating it with the visual field defects is very important, and perimetry results should not be viewed in isolation, in any circumstance.

Field defects caused by retinal lesions are generally deep with sharp borders, with lesser test–retest variability than glaucomatous lesions.

■ TYPES OF PERIMETRY

Qualitative techniques such as confrontation testing are useful in eyes with poor vision and extensive areas of retinal involvement and as quick bedside tests.

Tangent screen and Amsler grid are also useful as qualitative techniques, especially for testing the central field.

Quantitative techniques of perimetry have proven to be extremely useful, providing understanding of the nature of visual disturbance that the patient with retinal pathology experiences. The Goldmann perimeter and kinetic perimetry may be used for monitoring peripheral visual field loss, in disorders such as retinitis pigmentosa (RP) and large scotomata. However, with the advent of static automated threshold perimetry such as the Octopus and the Humphrey visual field (HVF) analyzers, quantitative evaluation of retinal disease received a tremendous boost. The role of frequency doubling technology and other newer visual field-testing strategies, like high pass resolution perimetry, have been researched, but are not used widely clinically.[1,2] Short-wavelength automated perimetry (SWAP) has also been studied in retinal disorders, but has not gained widespread acceptance.[3,4]

Microperimetry (MP) is a newer method of visual field testing that is particularly useful in the diagnosis and follow-up of macular pathology. It features a confocal line scanning laser ophthalmoscope (SLO), real-time eye-tracker, and 4-2 threshold fundus perimetry (microperimetry). Perimetry can be performed at specific locations in the fundus, while simultaneously observing the retina, as seen by fundus imaging (fundus-related perimetry). Thus, the anatomic pathology is correlated with loss of visual function. This technique can also be used in patients with unstable/noncentral fixation. It helps in assessing the peripheral point of fixation called the preferred retinal locus (PRL), seen in people with macular disease.[5,6] Macular Integrity Assessment (MAIA) is a third-generation-automated macular perimeter that allows quantitative evaluation of macular function based on threshold sensitivity and fixation analysis.[7]

■ CHOOSING THE TEST

The choice of testing strategy (30-2/24-2/10-2/peripheral testing) used varies depending on the extent and location of retinal disease. Full-field suprathreshold testing may be used in patients where information about the peripheral field is essential, as in RP. In patients with macular disease and poor central vision, testing must be carried out using the large/small diamond fixation target, as the patient will be unable to see the central fixation target.

PERIMETRY IN SPECIFIC RETINAL DISEASES

Retinal Dystrophies

Retinitis Pigmentosa (Cases 1 and 2)

Visual fields help in assessing the extent of visual field loss. Follow-up fields aid in monitoring disease progression. A standard threshold 30-2 or a suprathreshold test that includes the peripheral field would be preferable. In early stages of the disease, isolated scotomata may be seen in the midperipheral fields. These eventually coalesce to form the classical ring scotoma, involving the midperiphery of the visual field. With progression of the peripheral field loss, the patient is left with a small, central island of vision. In advanced disease, this also may be lost. Documenting the remaining field by perimetry is also required to decide eligibility for driving license, in patients with RP, in some countries. MP has been advocated as a potential outcome measure of macular function for clinical trials involving patients with RP.[8]

Cone Dystrophy

The pigmentary disturbance at the macula produces progressive central visual loss. Visual field testing demonstrates central scotomata with relative sparing of the fovea. A central 10-2/10° testing would be preferable in such eyes, and larger target size can be used in case of decreased visual acuity.

Stargardt Disease (Cases 3 and 4)

Central or paracentral scotoma may be seen. With MP, fixation can be assessed to be central or shifted. In Stargardt disease, there is relative sparing of the peripapillary area, and it has been suggested that this is a region of interest for monitoring the efficacy of treatment in this disease. Spectral domain optical coherence tomography (SDOCT) and MP studies show that there is a greater photoreceptor sensitivity loss in temporal than nasal area of extramacular region as compared to relative sparing noticed in the peripapillary region in these patients.[9]

The ProgStar Study Group reported on MP a mean baseline macular sensitivity of 10.73 dB in patients with a mean age of 33.7 years at the time of the assessment, and a mean decrease in the macular sensitivity of 0.87 dB/year.[10,11]

Diabetic Retinopathy (Cases 5 and 6)

Roth et al.[12] found central field defects in about 40% of eyes without visible retinopathy and in all diabetic patients with retinopathy. SWAP and MP are more sensitive than standard white-on-white perimetry in detecting scotoma in patients with clinically significant macular edema. Mild background retinopathy usually shows no field loss at all on standard white-on-white perimetry. Bell and Feldon[13] used Octopus static perimetry to show that visual sensitivity is quantitatively correlated with retinal perfusion in preproliferative diabetic retinopathy.

It is important to remember that laser photocoagulation for the treatment of diabetic retinopathy in itself may produce visual field defects. Panretinal photocoagulation often produces a marked concentric contraction of the visual field. Studies have also reported reduced retinal sensitivity in eyes with diabetic macular ischemia (DMI). This reduction in sensitivity could be noted despite visual acuity being normal, highlighting superiority of MP over visual acuity in eyes with DMI. Eyes with DMI may have normal visual acuity despite reduced retinal sensitivity, suggesting that MP is more sensitive than the visual acuity, or the changes in the sensitivities may precede the reduction of the visual acuity in DMI.[14-17] Santos et al. reported that the eyes with better retinal sensitivities before intravitreal antivascular endothelial growth factor (anti-VEGF) treatment were associated with better best-corrected visual acuity (BCVA) outcomes after therapy, suggesting that better sensitivity on MP preoperatively is associated with good prognosis. MP, therefore, can help predict response to anti-VEGF treatment.[18]

Other Vascular Diseases and Nondiabetic Macular Edema

Vascular Occlusions (Cases 7–9)

Arterial occlusions typically produce absolute field defects, while venous occlusions produce highly variable field loss. These involve the hemifield opposite the occlusion, with defects often respecting the horizontal meridian, and corresponding exactly to the distribution of the occluded vessel. Recovery of visual field loss has been noted using HVF and MP after central and branch artery occlusions.[19,20] Visual fields assessment by kinetic perimetry can be useful in documenting preserved visual fields in patients with nonarteritic central retinal artery occlusion (CRAO).[21]

Central Serous Retinopathy (Case 10)

A mild central depression of retinal sensitivity may be seen. Even after resolution of edema, these patients demonstrate residual Amsler and perimetric defects.[22,23] Presence of fluid in the macula in Irvine–Gass syndrome, trauma (Berlin's edema), or retinal vasculitis produces similar field changes.

Age-related Macular Degeneration and Other Maculopathies (Cases 11 and 12)

Macular drusen may show some reduction of retinal sensitivity using SWAP and MP, but not with standard techniques. MP has been used to quantify the loss in visual sensitivity over time even in individuals with progressive atrophic macular disease with stable visual acuity.

Shintaro et al. noted the ability of MP to plan placement of the stimuli on the retinal regions of interest. This helps in studying the functional impact of specific anatomic biomarkers of interest, which are associated with a higher risk of progression to late age-related macular degeneration (AMD).[24]

Central scotomata with sloping margins and variable density are seen in pigmentary type of AMD. Dense central scotomata are seen in disciform scarring due to exudative AMD.[25]

Monitoring the functional impact of enlargement of atrophy, especially at the margin, is an important application of MP, especially in therapeutic trials.[24]

Myopic Traction Maculopathy

Baptista et al. reported that the MP sensitivity was significantly reduced in eyes with atrophic areas compared with those eyes with only schisis. They concluded that MP helps in precise functional assessment in patients with myopic maculopathy.[26]

Macular Holes and Epiretinal Membrane (Case 13)

Macular holes result in dense scotomata with steep margins. However, cysts in the macula may not produce appreciable scotomata. MP can be a useful tool in assessing postoperative functional outcome in eyes with focal vitreomacular pathologies, where BCVA would underestimate the surgical benefits.

Microperimetry allows for more reliable and objective examination of functional retinal sensitivity in patients with macular holes. Wang et al. studied the predictive value of preoperative macular sensitivity testing in predicting visual prognosis in a study of 44 eyes using microperimeter. They noted positive linear correlation between preoperative macular sensitivity and postoperative BCVA at 4 months.[27]

To peel or not to peel internal limiting membrane (ILM) in eyes with epiretinal membrane (ERM) is controversial. Even MP studies on ERM peeling with or without ILM peeling remains inconclusive.[28-30]

Toxic Retinopathies (Cases 14 and 15)

Chloroquine maculopathy causes a ring-like central scotoma, with a small island of slightly less visual loss in its center, commonly referred to as a "bull's eye." Screening for chloroquine and hydroxychloroquine (HCQ) toxicity is performed using a 10-2 white-on-white perimetry.[31]

Classic bull's eye appearance in HCQ toxicity is infrequently seen in the Asian population, who often show an extramacular pattern of damage. Hence, American Academy of Ophthalmology Recommendations on Screening for Chloroquine and Hydroxychloroquine Retinopathy recommends 30-2 fields in the Asian patients.[32,33]

Infectious and Inflammatory Retinopathies (Cases 16 and 17)

Visual field defects in infectious and inflammatory retinopathies correspond to the area of retinal involvement. Toxoplasmosis produces focal chorioretinal scars with corresponding dense, isolated scotomata with steep margins.[34] In conditions causing more disseminated inflammation, a diffuse depression of visual field function is seen. Using MP, areas of decreased sensitivity were shown to correlate with affected areas of the retina in multiple evanescent white-dot syndrome, acute posterior multifocal placoid pigment epitheliopathy, serpiginous choroiditis, and birdshot chorioretinopathy.

Autoimmune Retinopathy (Case 18)

Autoimmune retinopathy is a group of rare inflammatory autoimmune retinal degenerative diseases presumably caused by cross-reactivity of serum autoantibodies against retinal antigens. It is characterized by vision loss, scotomas, visual field deficits, photoreceptor dysfunction, and the presence of circulating antiretinal antibodies. Visual field testing shows constriction and central or paracentral scotomas.[35]

Ferreyra et al. studied 24 nonparaneoplastic autoimmune retinopathy patients who received therapy with various combinations of systemic and local immunosuppressants such as prednisone, cyclosporine, azathioprine, mycophenolate mofetil, periocular, or intravitreal steroid injections. 15 of the 24 (62.5%) showed varying degrees of improvement in visual acuity or visual field.[36]

Retinal Detachment (Case 19)

Typically, rhegmatogenous retinal detachments have sloping isopters on kinetic perimetry and relative defects. Occasionally, this feature helps in differentiating a retinal detachment from a retinoschisis, which is characterized by dense, absolute defects with steep margins. However, long-standing retinal detachments may develop steep isopters and in this situation, recovery of visual field sensitivity is incomplete. Since these conditions usually involve the peripheral retina, conventional fields involving the central

30° field may not be useful except in detecting the inner border of a defect in the midperiphery.[37-39]

Tumors

Anterior melanomas produce localized constriction of the visual field, whereas posterior melanomas produce dense scotomata with steep borders. On the other hand, only a subtle field defect may be produced by a choroidal nevus. Long-term visual field defects that correspond to tumor size, location, and treatment modality have been documented in eyes with retinoblastoma.[40]

■ CASES

Case 1: A 46-year-old female patient presented with bilateral, severe RP. 10-2 fields (performed with stimulus size V) show severe constriction of fields with central sparing. With progression of the disease, fixation may be affected.

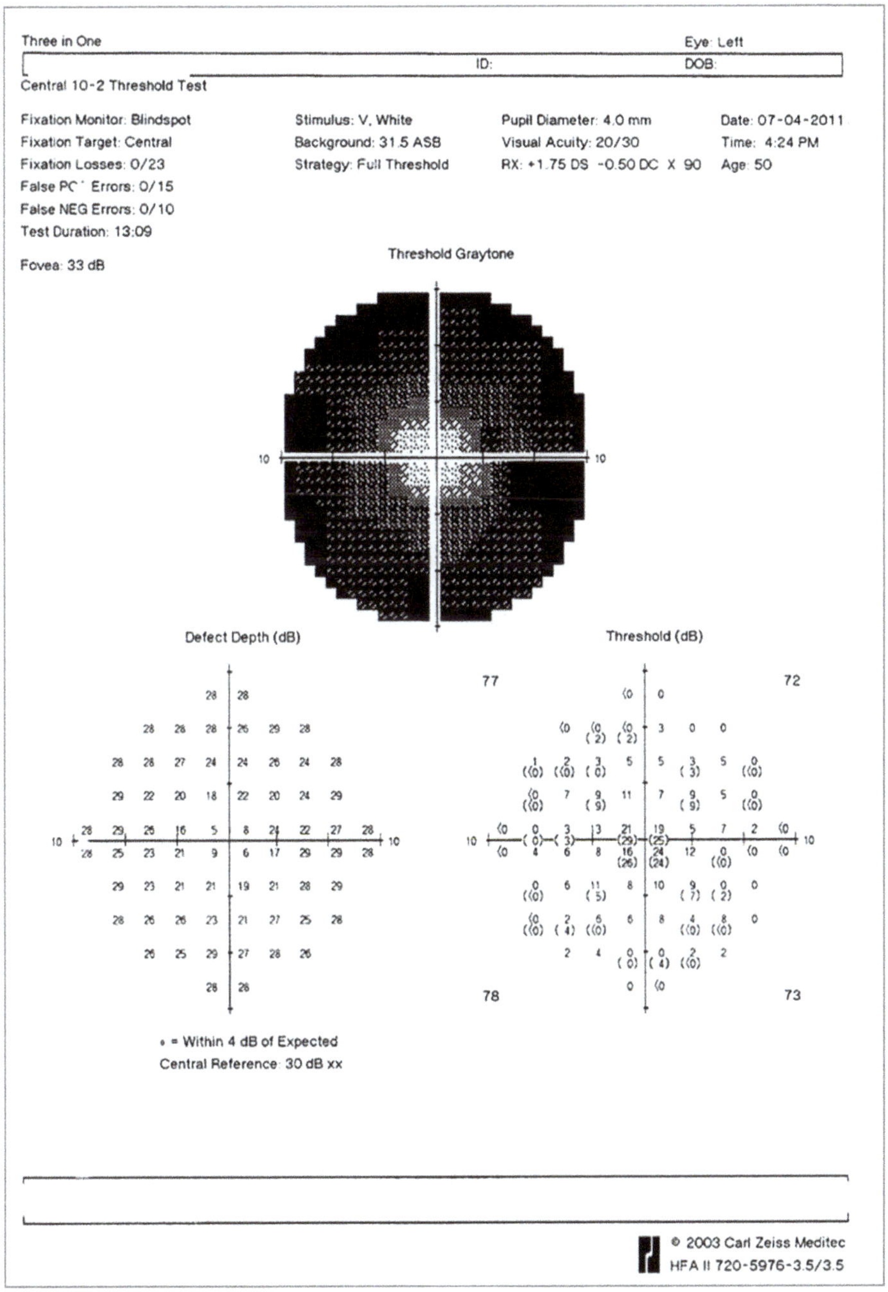

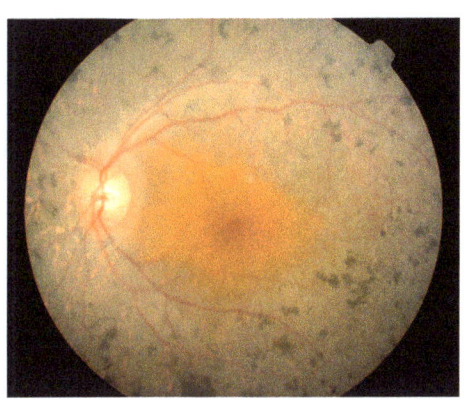

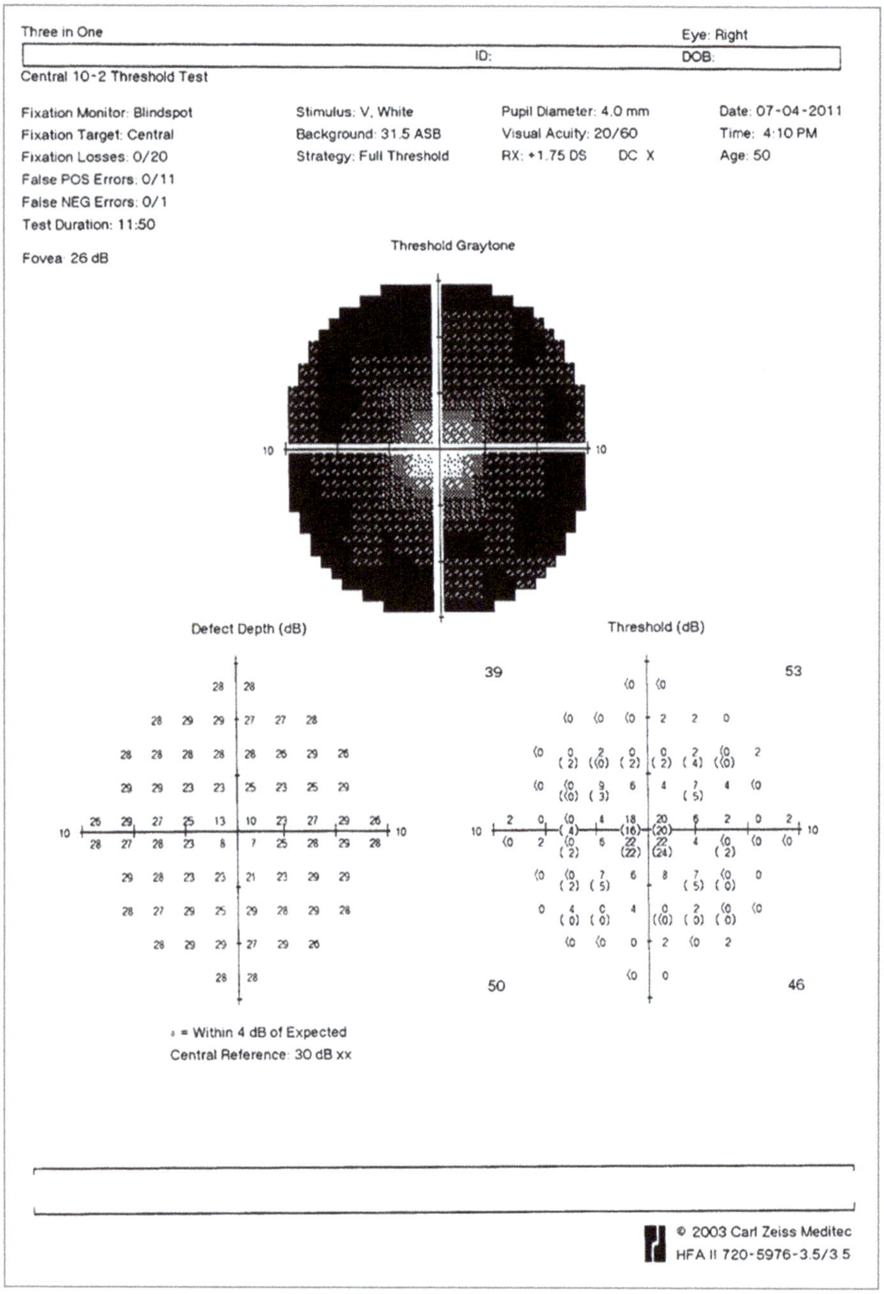

SECTION 3: Special Situations

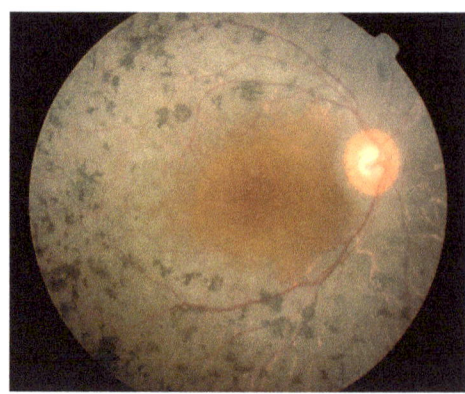

Case 2: A 19-year-old female patient presented with night blindness and atypical retinitis pigmentosa (RP). Visual field testing shows typical ring scotoma in the paracentral region. These lesions are more typical of late onset, slowly progressive RP, and are less likely to affect fixation.

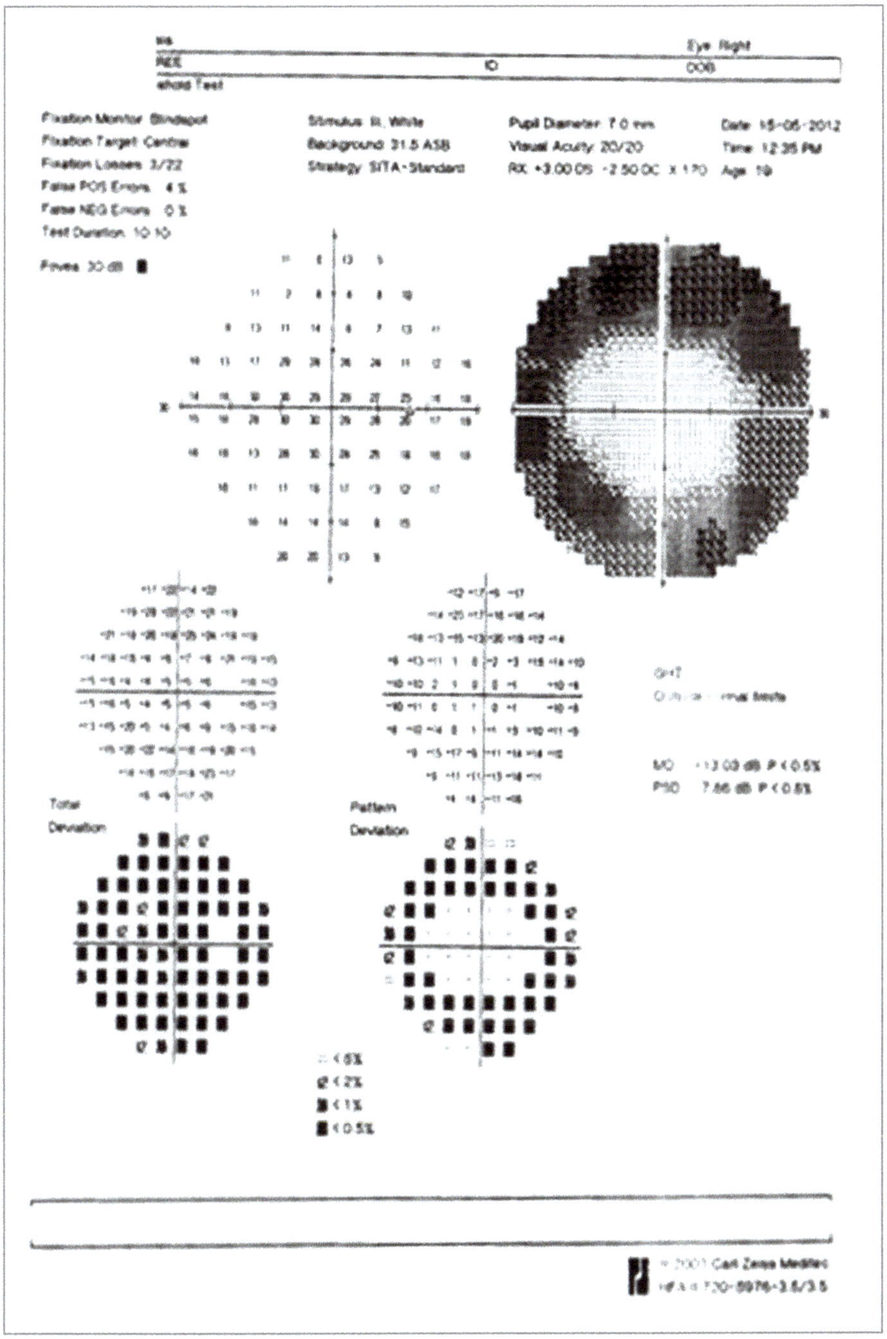

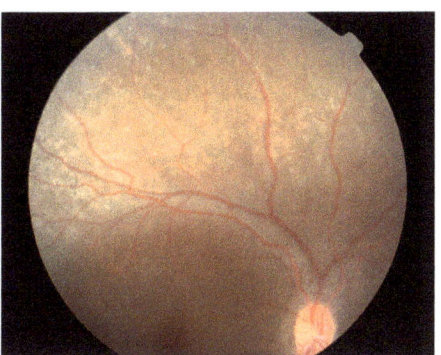

Case 3: Macular Integrity Assessment in this 50-year-old patient with Stargardt's and progressive loss of vision shows reduced macular sensitivity inferiorly in both the eyes, (seen on sensitivity and threshold maps), corresponding to the location of the lesion. It is important to remember that MP is fundus-correlated perimetry. Unlike conventional perimetry where an inferior lesion causes a superior field defect, in MP, the exact correlation of retinal pathology and functional vision is possible. Also note that the bivariate contour ellipse area (BCEA), a quantification of fixation stability, is smaller in the right eye, corresponding to more stable fixation. The advantage of using MAIA or the MP-3 is that these devices can provide a broader tracking system with a clear and detailed retinal image. Due to the quality of these images, this results in a higher reliability.

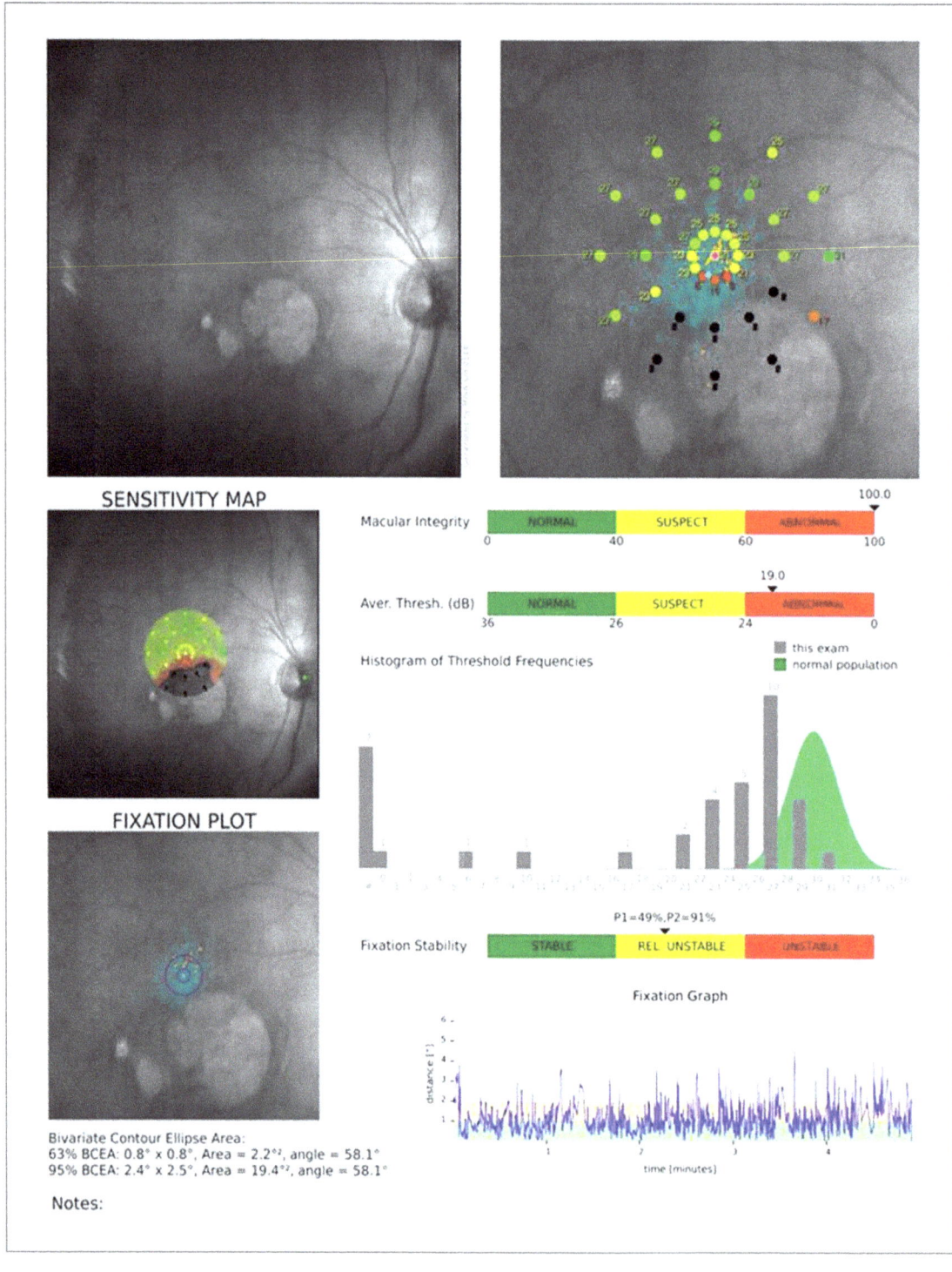

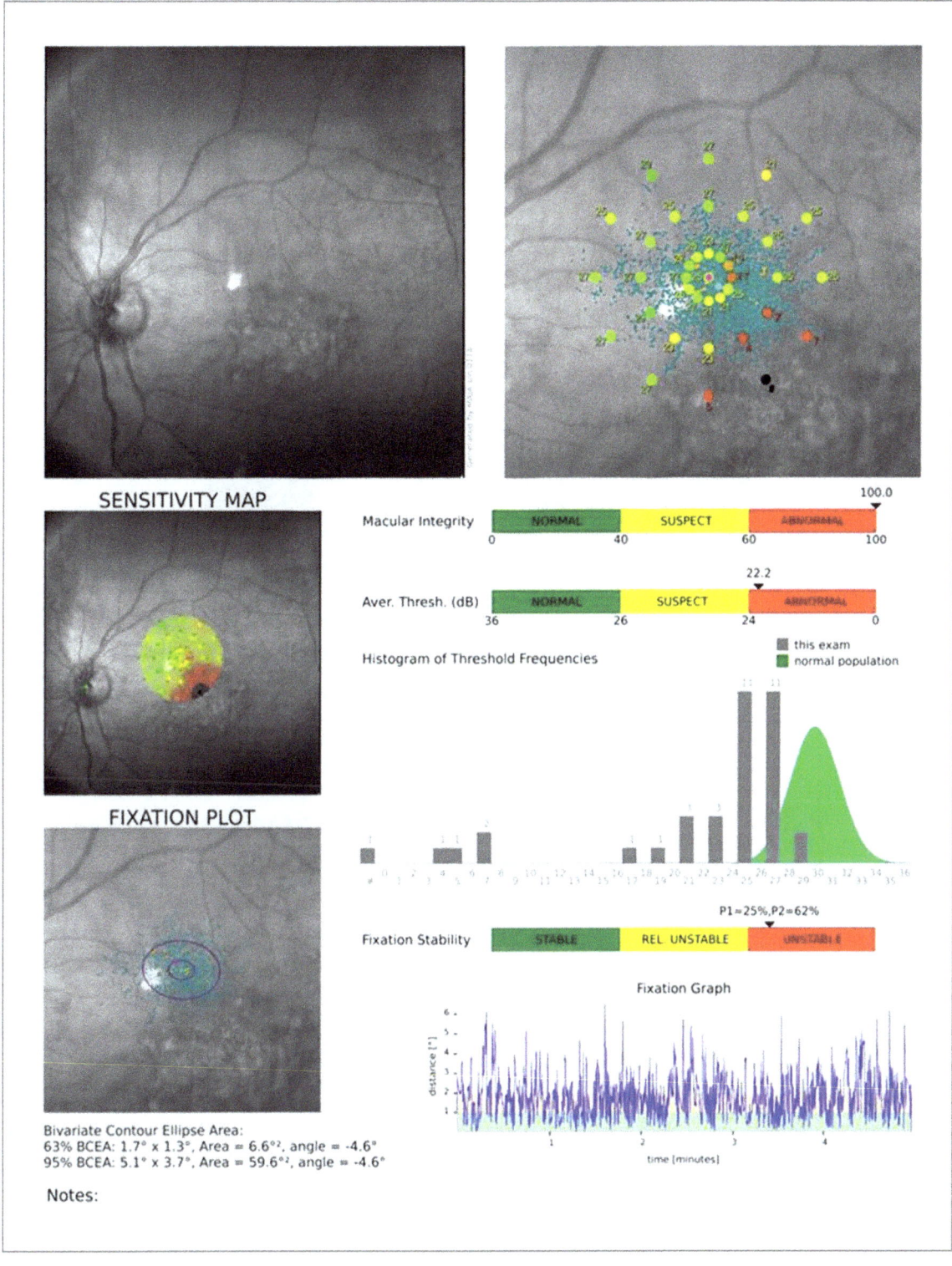

Case 4: A 21-year-old male with Stargardt's dystrophy shows a dense centrocecal scotoma. The 10-2 field report provides more details about the scotoma.

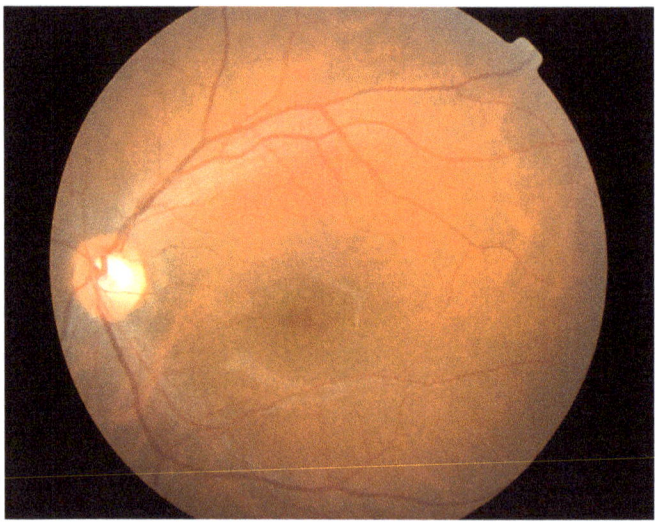

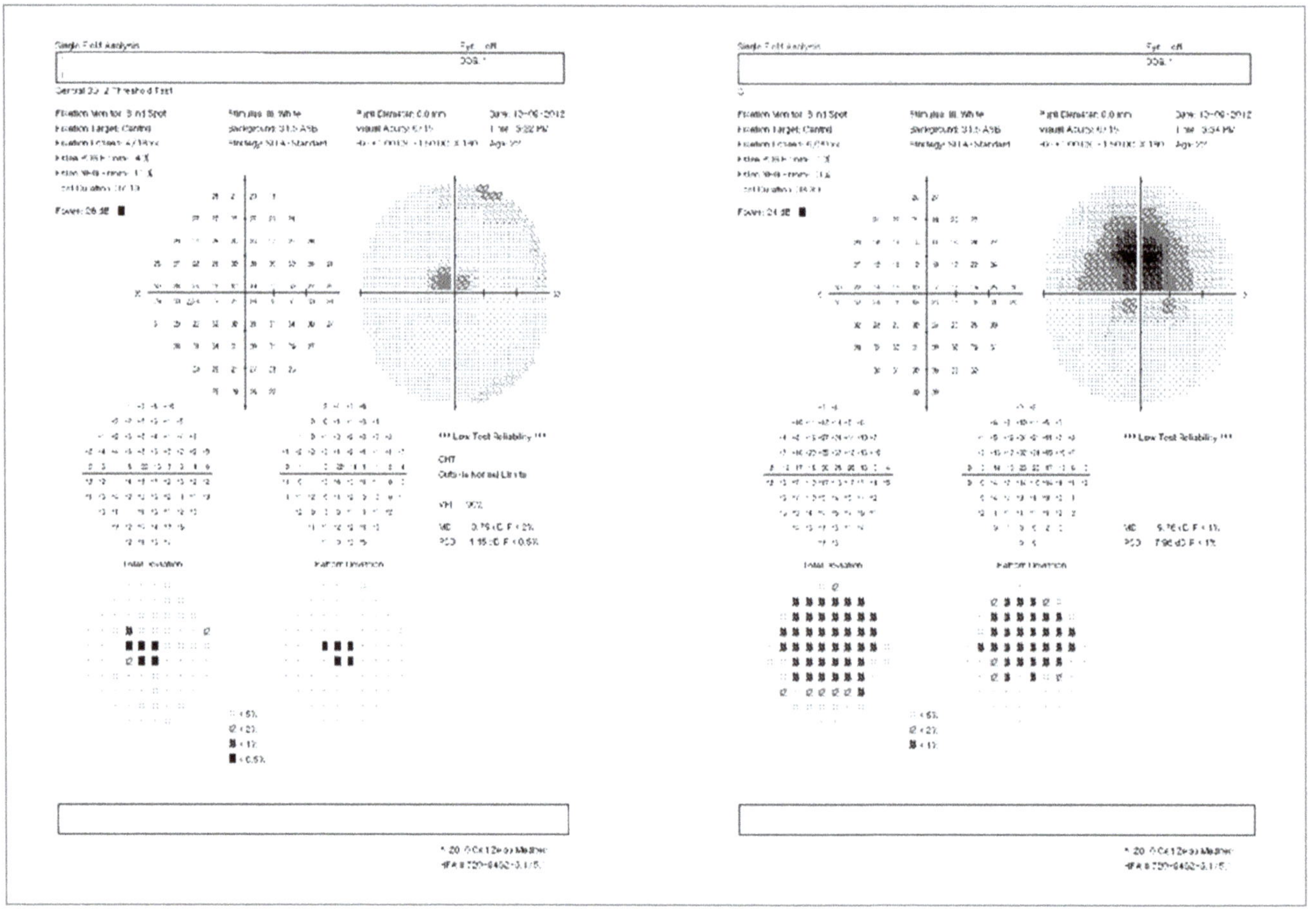

Case 5: A 53-year-old gentleman, with nonproliferative diabetic retinopathy, was started on antituberculosis therapy (ATT) for pulmonary tuberculosis. He complained of decreased vision in both eyes and was found to have ethambutol toxicity. The fundus photo shows retinal pigment epithelium (RPE) alterations in the fovea, and fields show a cecocentral scotoma, and decreased foveal threshold.

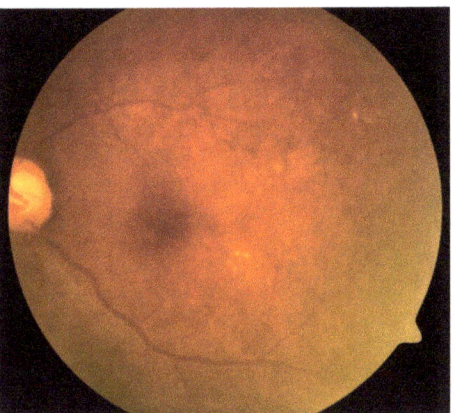
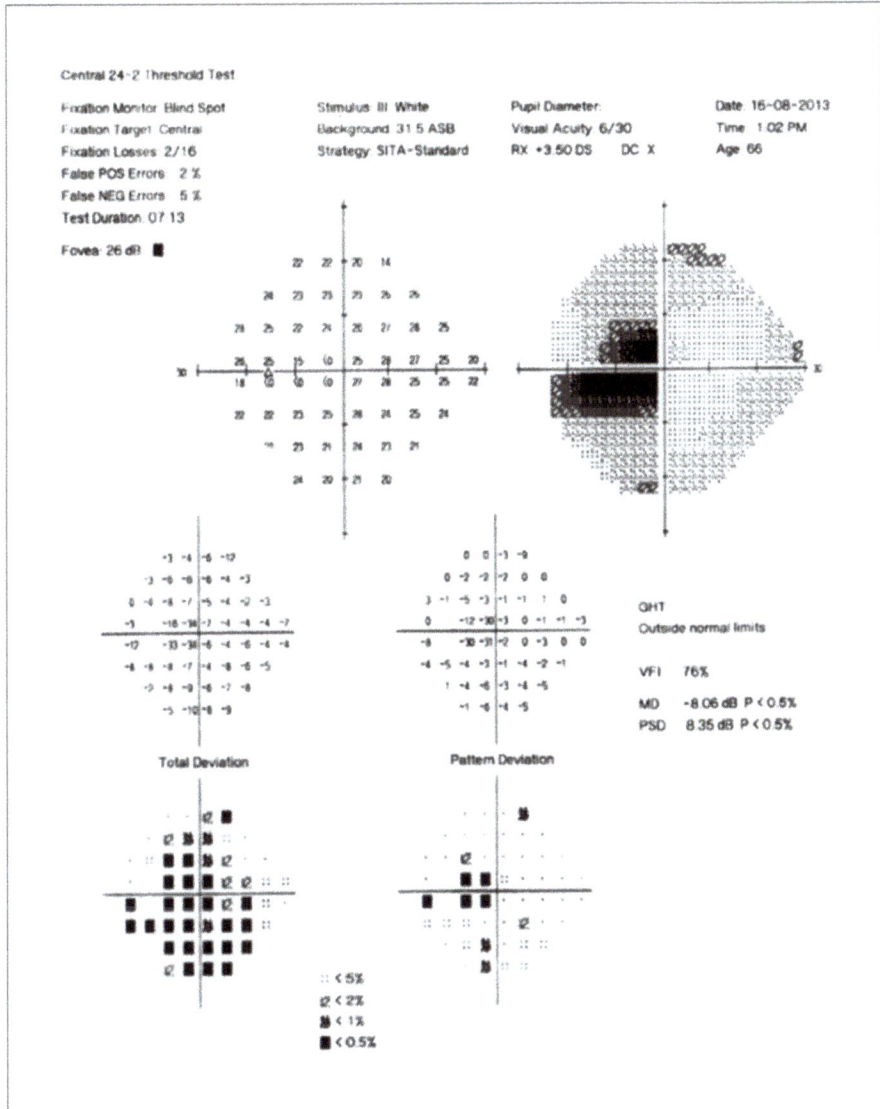

SECTION 3: Special Situations

Case 6: A 63-year-old male patient with proliferative diabetic retinopathy, status postpanretinal photocoagulation (PRP), shows localized scotomas seen on the gray scale and deviation plots corresponding to the laser scars. PRP can cause dense constriction of the peripheral visual field.

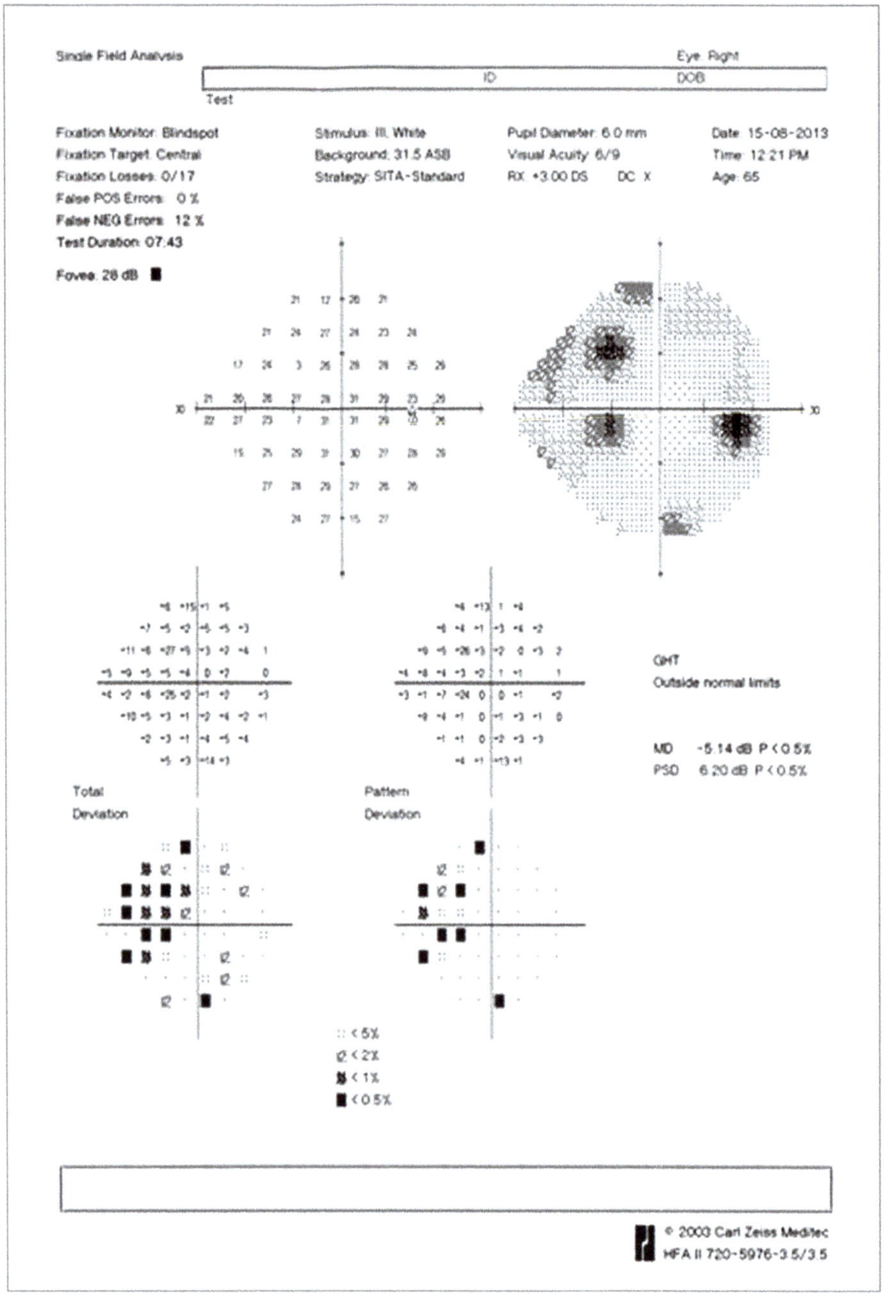

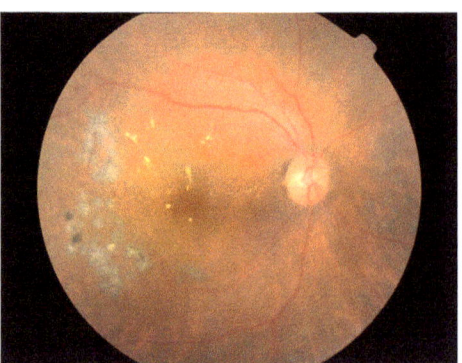

CHAPTER 11: Role of Perimetry in Diagnosis and Management of Retinal or Macular Disorders

Case 7: A 64-year-old female, with ocular hypertension, has an old branch retinal vein occlusion (BRVO) in the left eye. The field defect corresponds to the area of vein occlusion.

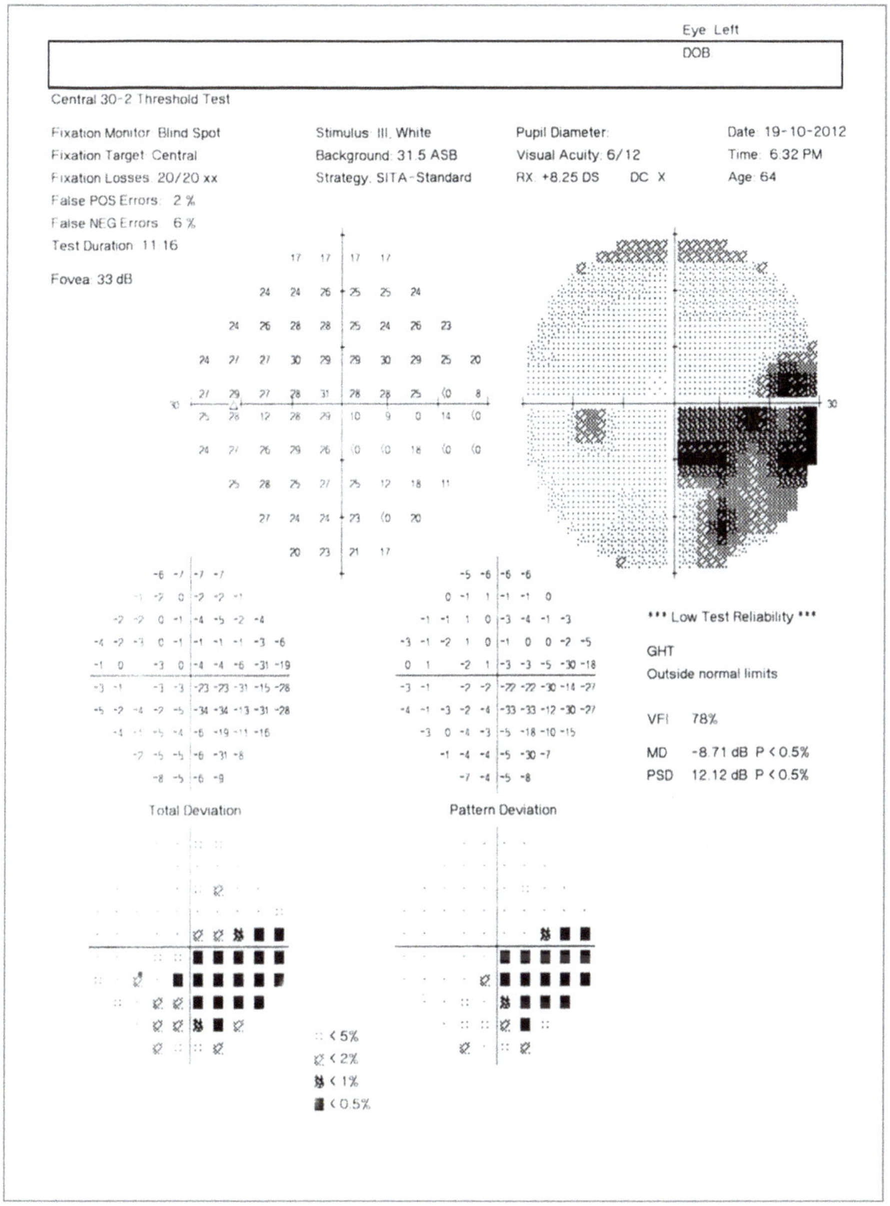

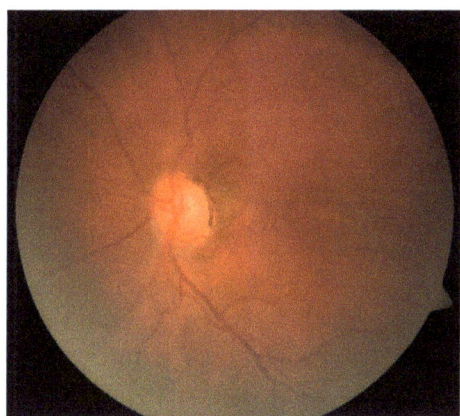

SECTION 3: Special Situations

Case 8: A 44-year-old female patient, known to be diabetic and hypertensive, has an old superotemporal BRVO in the left eye (LE), for which she has undergone grid laser 8 months back. HVF reveals an inferior arcuate scotoma corresponding to the retinal pathology. Macular edema has resolved following intravitreal injection of anti-VEGF agent. The patient's vision improved to 6/6, N6. Foveal threshold value is 32 dB.

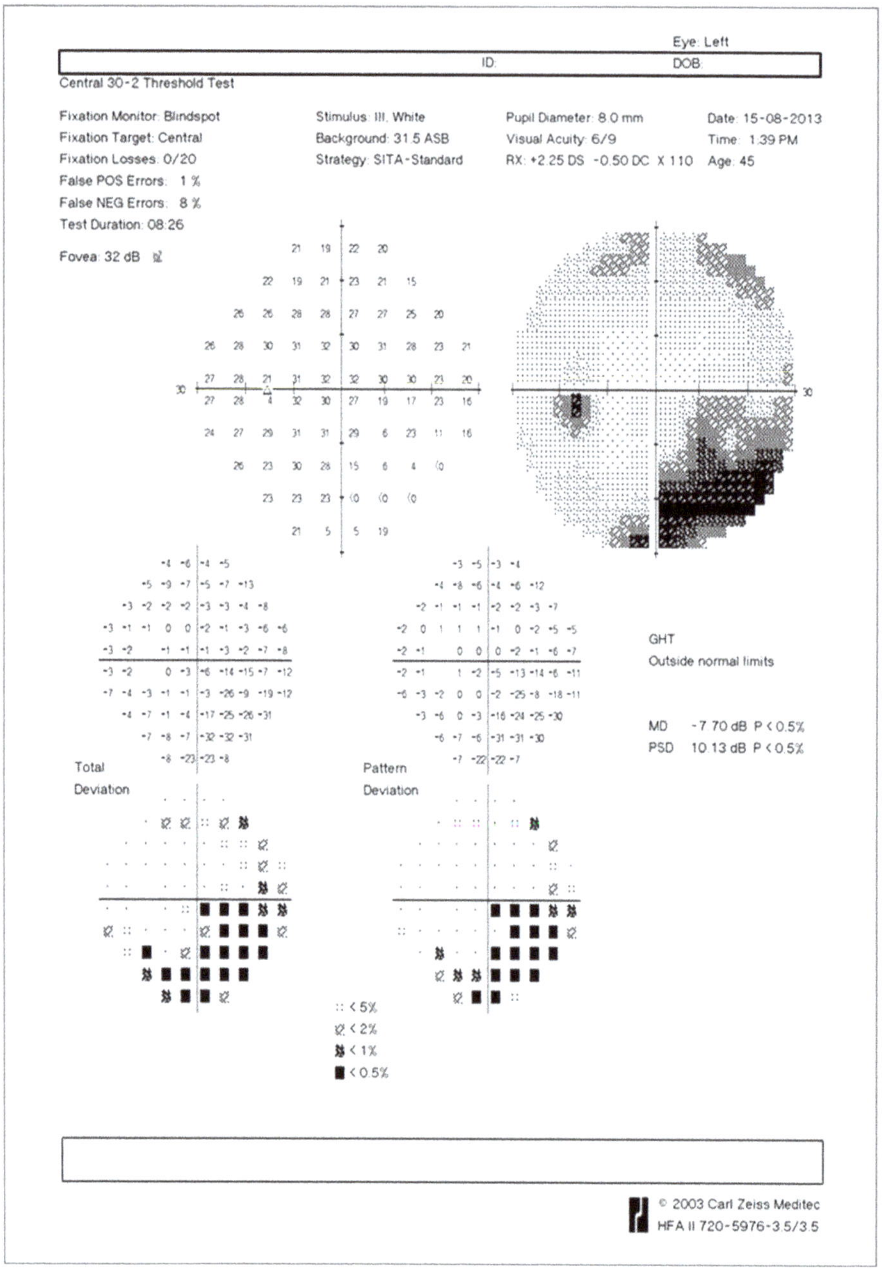

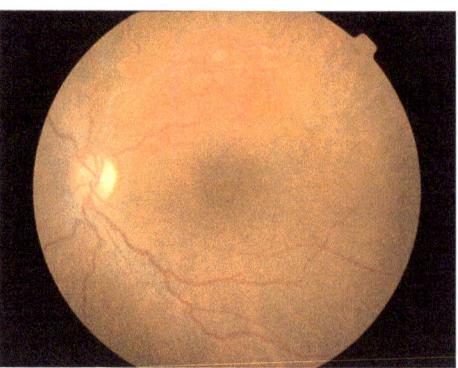

Case 9: An 80-year-old gentleman, who presented with sudden onset of blurring of vision in the right eye (RE), was noted to have multiple branch retinal artery occlusion and cilioretinal artery occlusion in the RE. Fundus picture shows multiple emboli. HVF shows absolute scotoma below fixation, corresponding to the area of retinal involvement just above the fovea. The superior scotoma in the arcuate area corresponds to the occlusion involving the inferior retina.

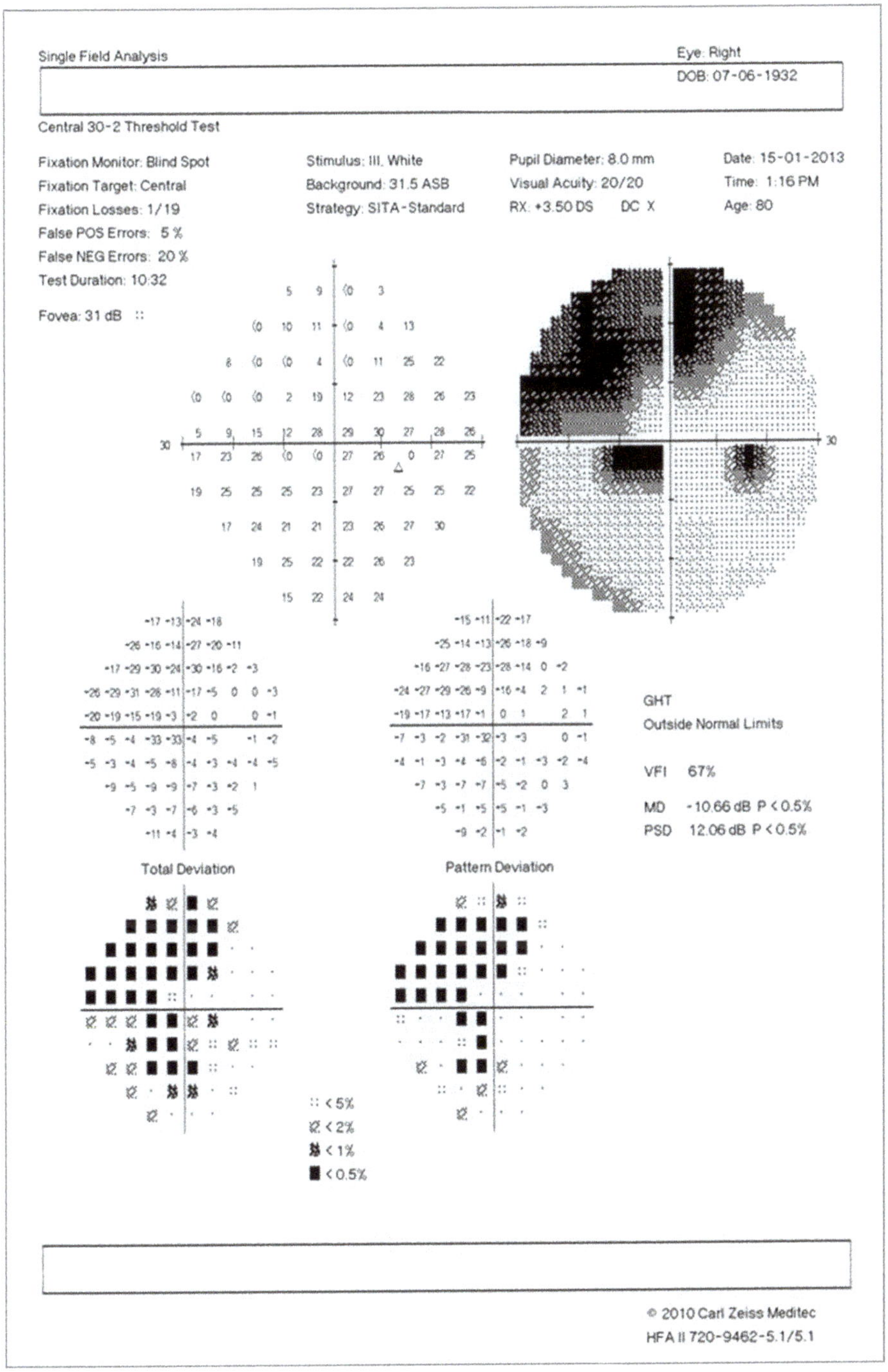

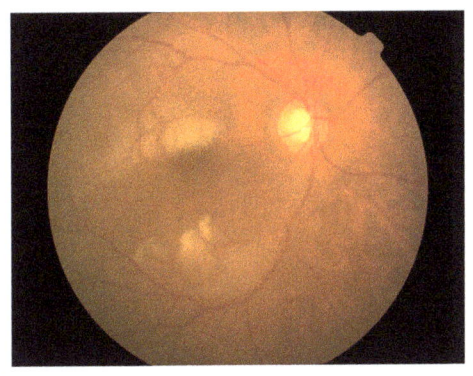

SECTION 3: Special Situations

Case 10: A 49-year-old male patient who presented with a drop in vision in his left eye. Fundus examination revealed the presence of central serous retinopathy. Humphrey visual fields 10-2 reveal mild depression of central values best seen on the deviation plots. MAIA reveals threshold values superimposed on the fundus image of the lesion. Lower threshold values are seen close to fovea as well as in the area of retina superior to the fovea. These correspond to the areas of RPE changes in the same area.

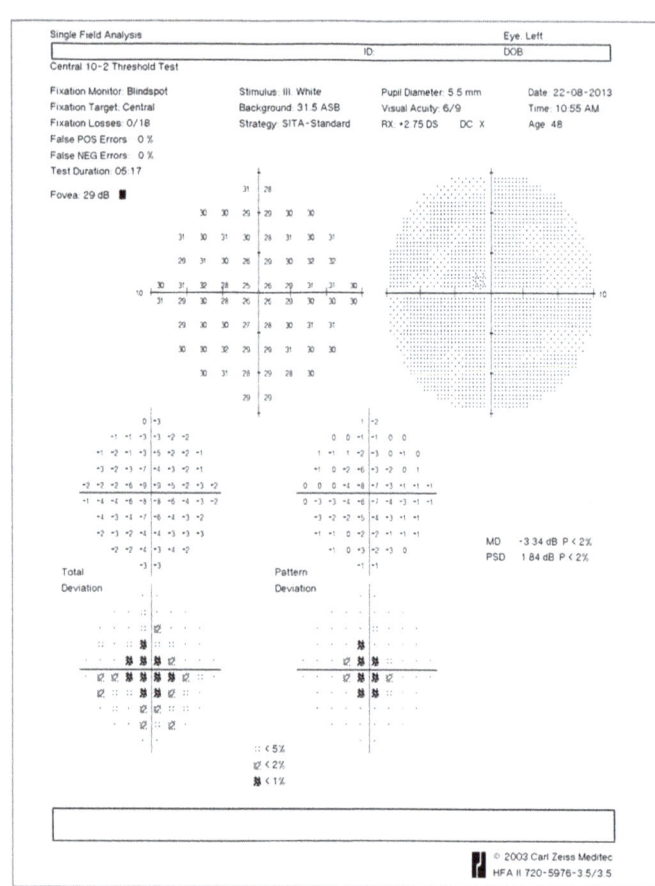

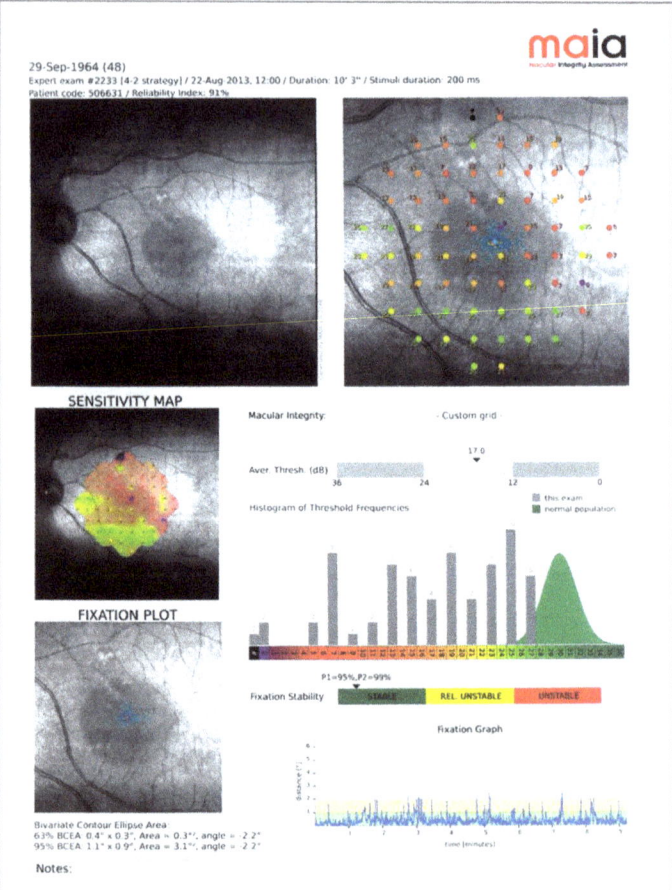

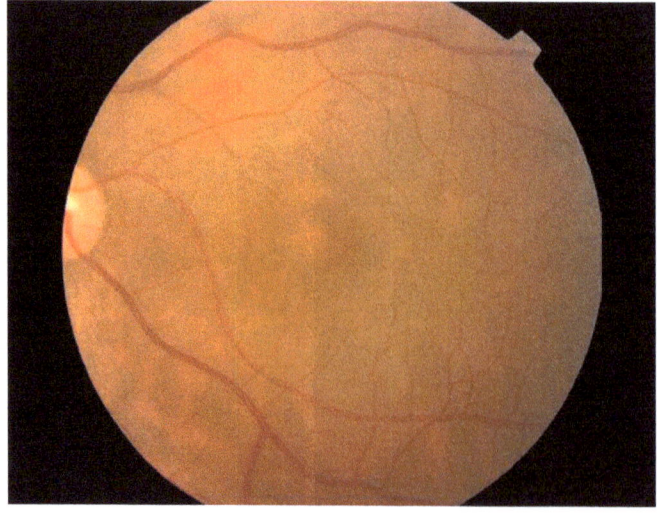

Case 11: A 71-year-old male patient, disc suspect [cup-to-disc (CD) ratio 0.7], has atrophic changes at the macula. Visual fields do not show glaucomatous field defects (correlating with the healthy neuroretinal rim). Generalized reduction of sensitivity and paracentral scotoma (seen on the gray scale) correspond to the macular pathology.

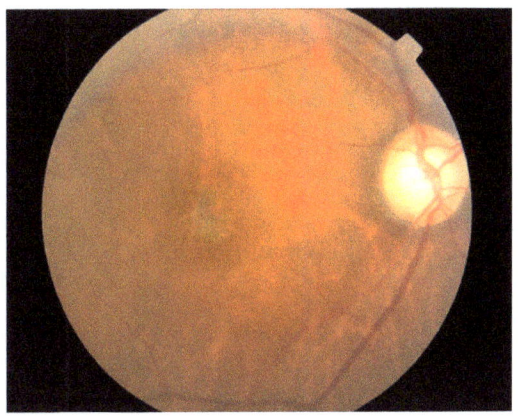

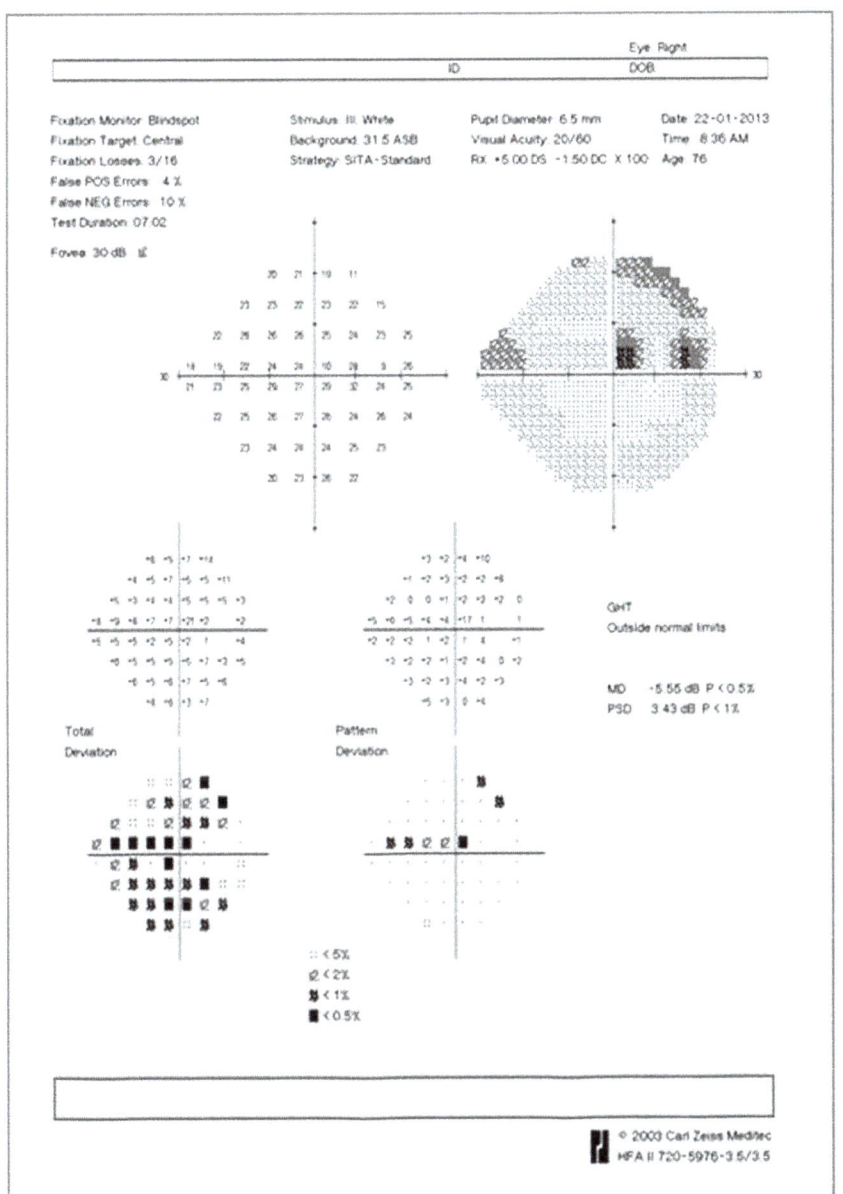

SECTION 3: Special Situations

Case 12: A 57-year-old lady presented with parafoveal telangiectasia and choroidal neovascular membranes (CNVM). The CNVM in the left eye has scarred following intravitreal anti-VEGF injections, whereas the CNVM in the right eye is still active. Fields show predominantly central scotoma, corresponding to the retinal lesions, with decreased foveal threshold.

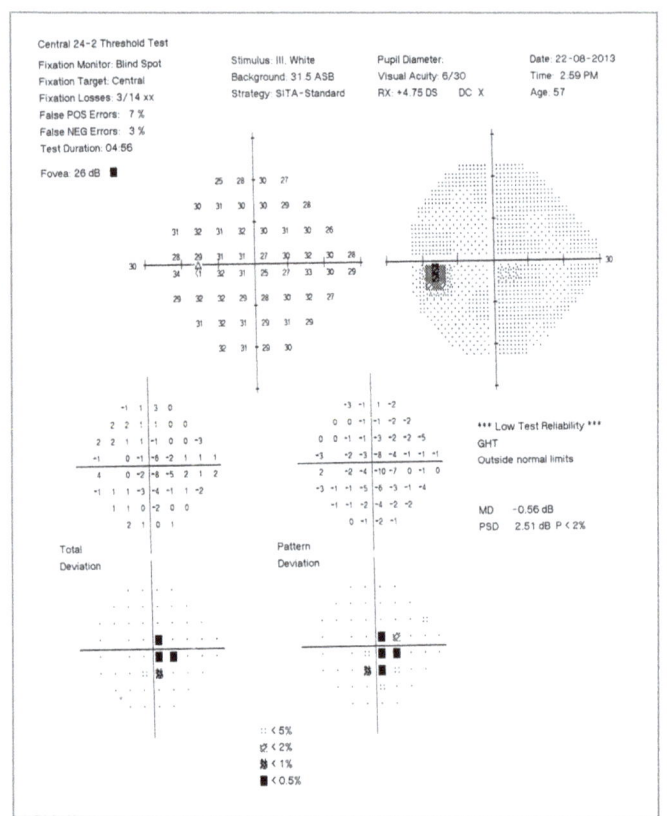
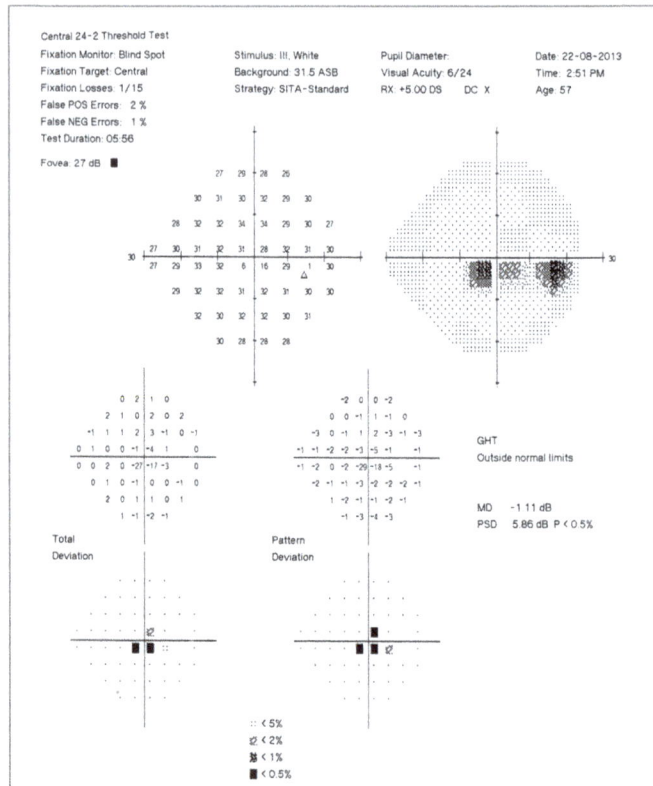
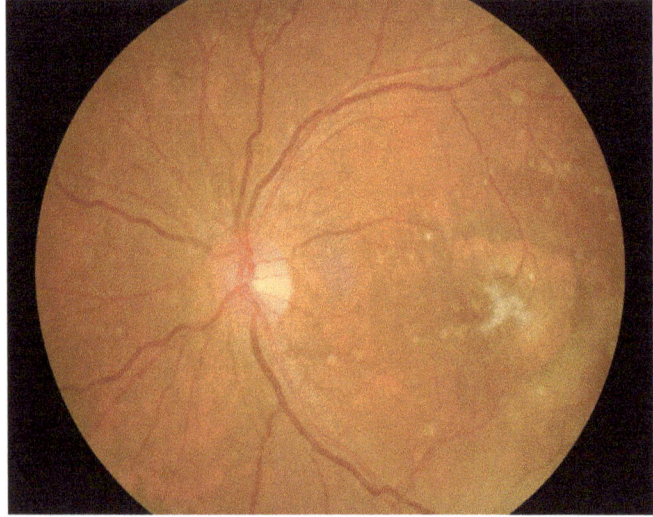
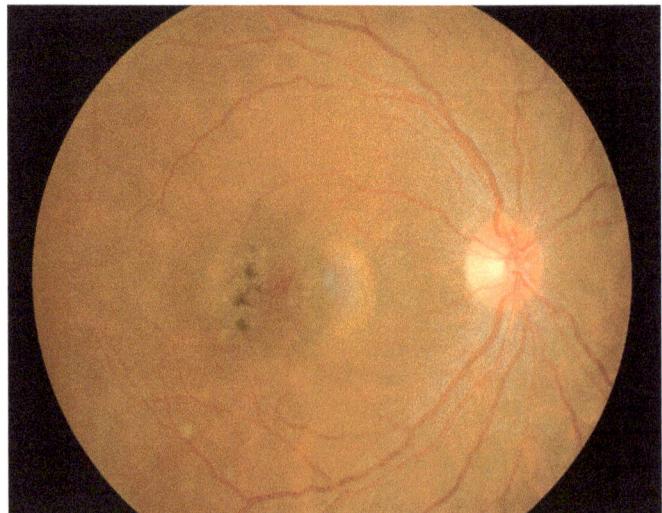

Case 13: A 74-year-old lady presented with macular hole in the left eye. MAIA done preoperatively (left) and postsurgery for hole (right) shows definite improvement in visual function at the macula (seen on actual threshold and sensitivity maps). Vision improved from counting finger (Cf) 3 meters to 6/12, N6 postoperative.

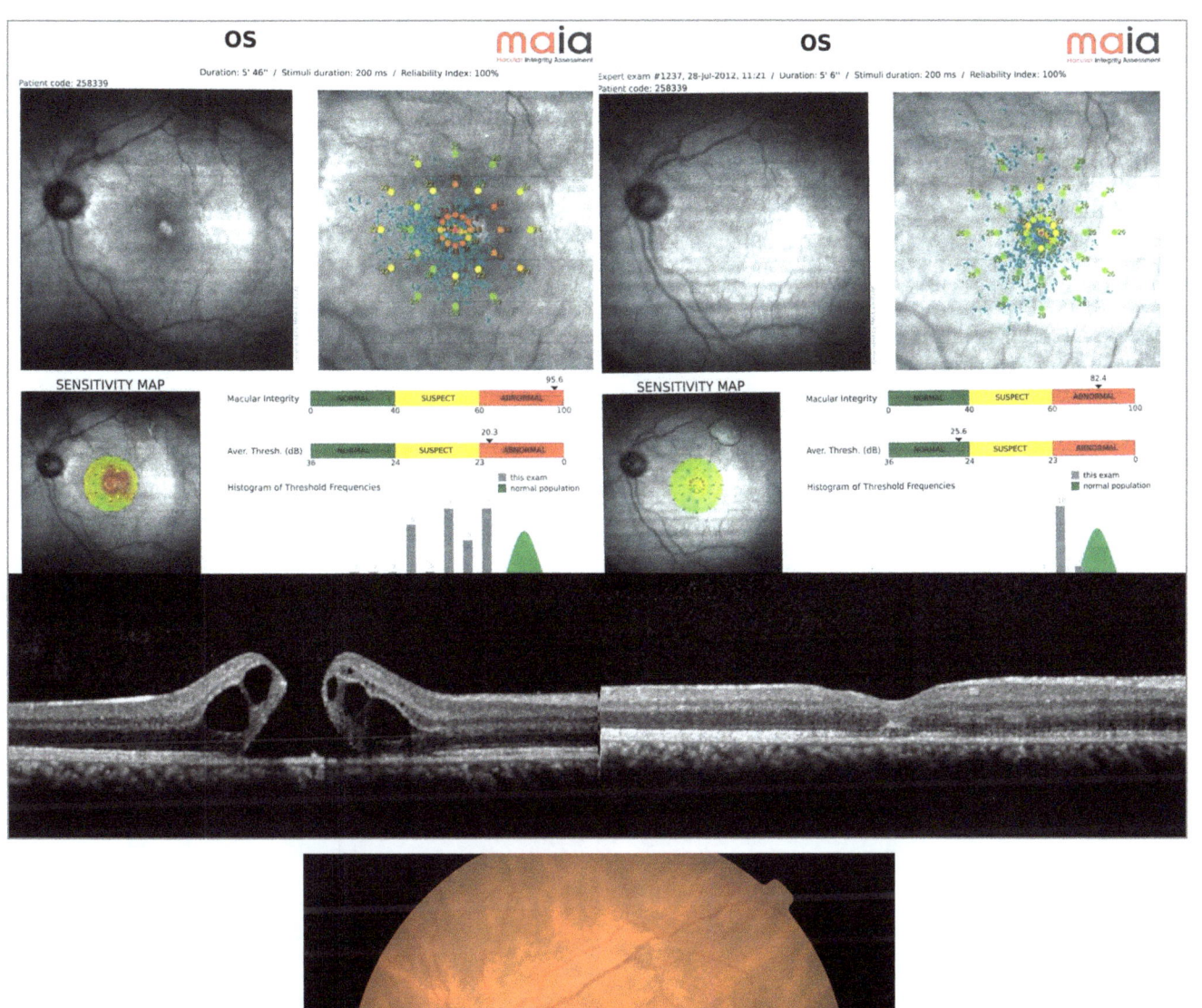

Case 14: Hydroxychloroquine (HCQ) toxicity shows bilateral central ring scotomas on central 10-2 visual field testing. MAIA performed in both eyes shows areas of decreased macular sensitivity. Following discontinuation of HCQ, improved macular function (macular integrity index and average threshold values now in normal range) documented on MAIA.

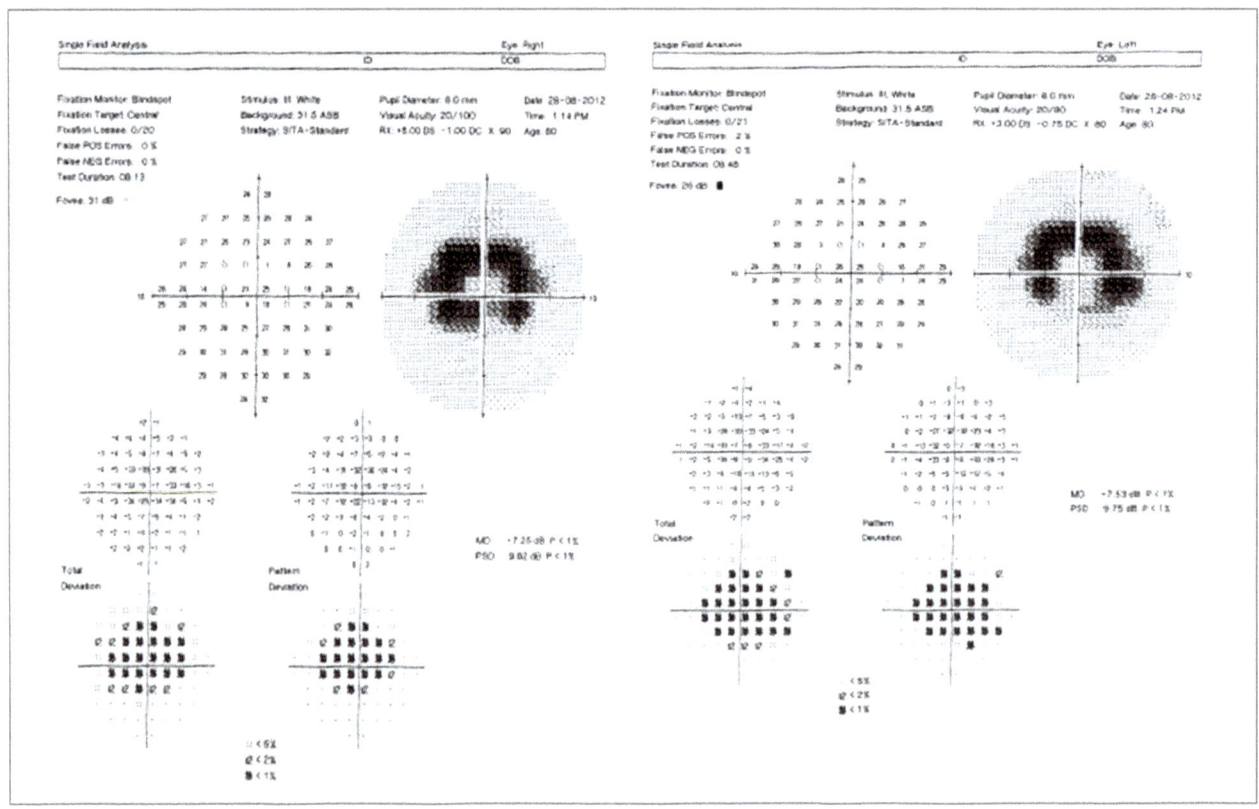

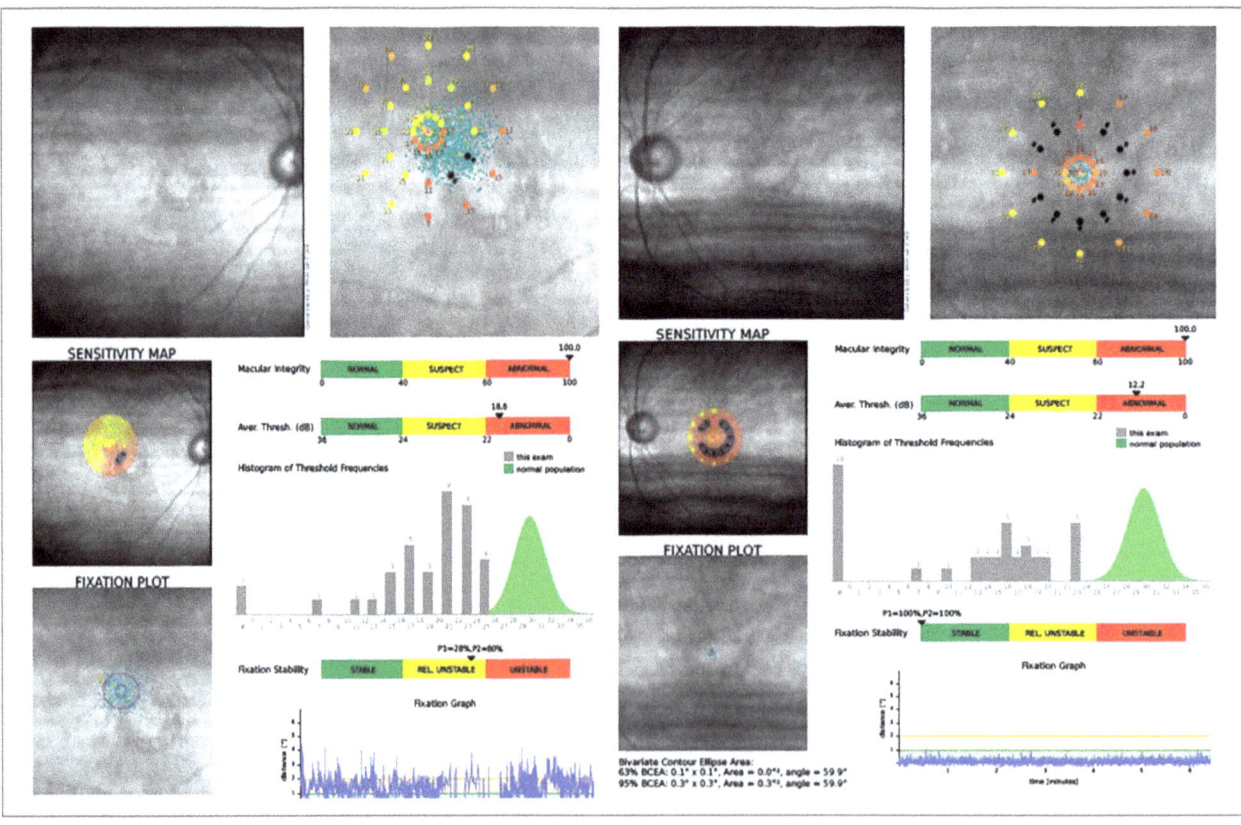

CHAPTER 11: Role of Perimetry in Diagnosis and Management of Retinal or Macular Disorders

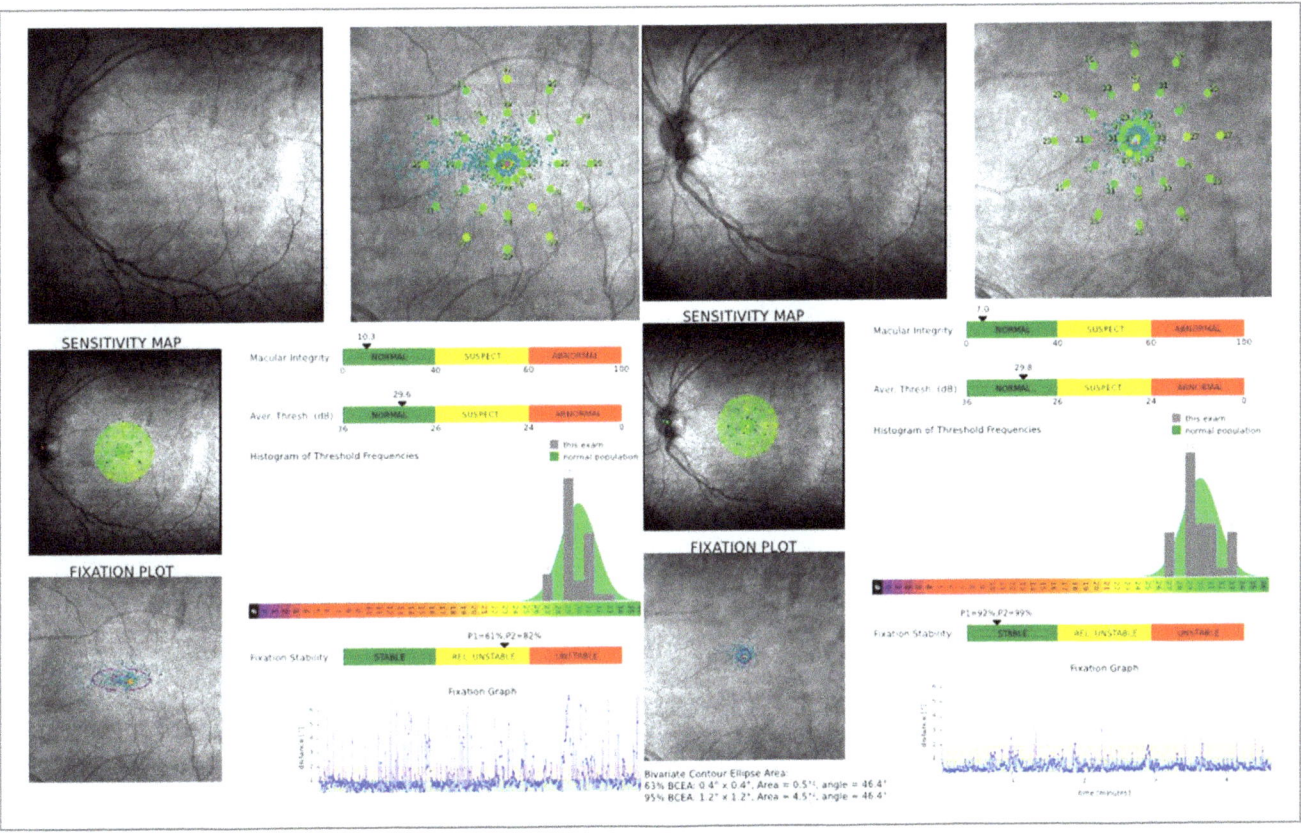

Case 15: A 65-year-old female, who was on hydroxychloroquine for 6 years, was noted to have peripheral field defects on 30-2 (right eye more than left eye). Both eyes fundus photos show few drusen at macula. Both eyes optical coherence tomography (OCT) images show ellipsoid zone disruption in extramacular region (yellow arrow).

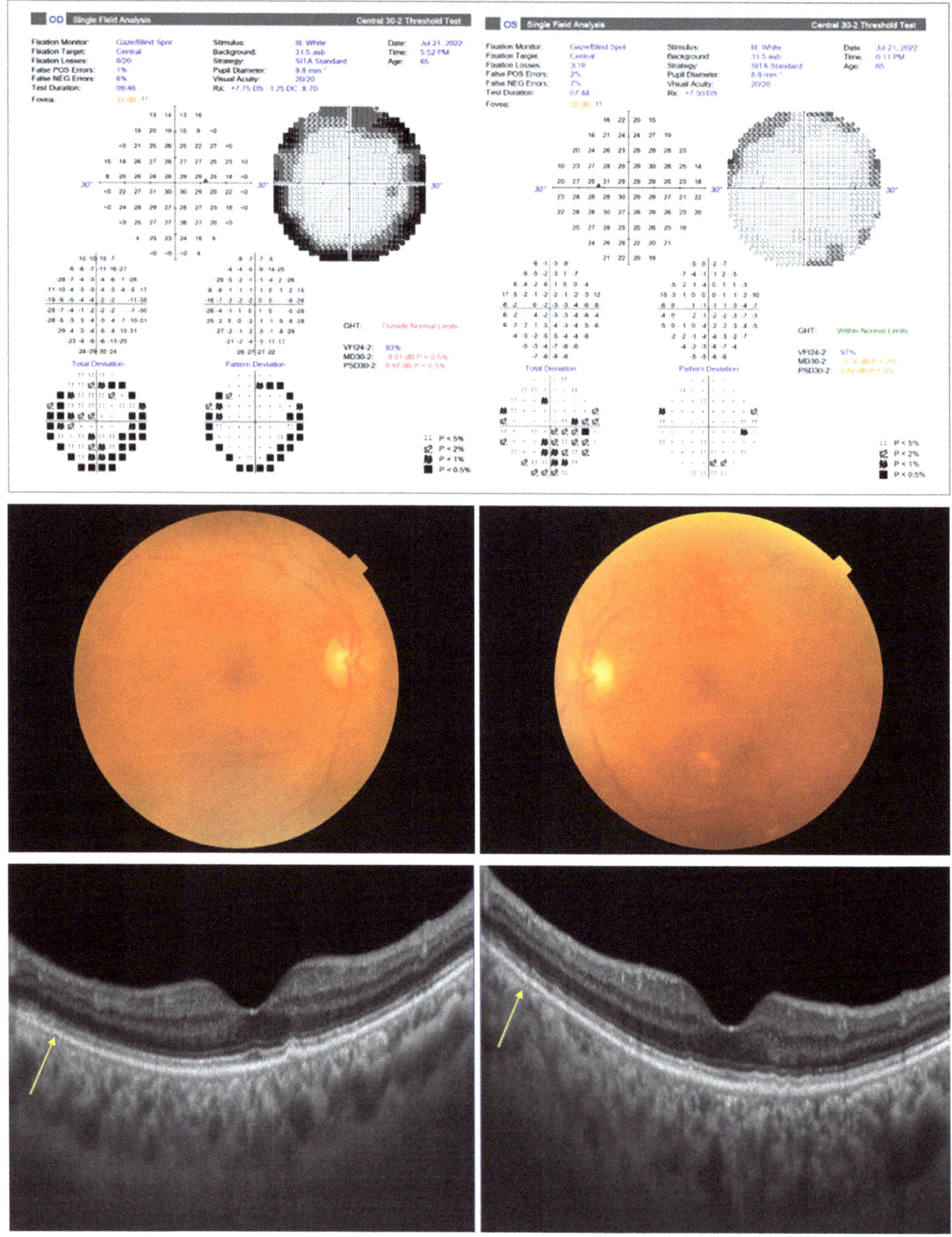

Case 16: A 23-year-old male presented with blurring of vision and loss of lower visual fields in both eyes. He was diagnosed to have acute zonal occult outer retinopathy (AZOOR). Fundus examination revealed vitritis with multiple hypopigmented lesions in the midperiphery. Fundus fluorescein angiography showed multiple hypofluorescent spots in both eyes in the early phase that turned hyperfluorescent in the late phases. Visual field testing on a Humphrey field analyzer (HFA) showed bilateral inferior arcuate defects, more dense in the left eye.

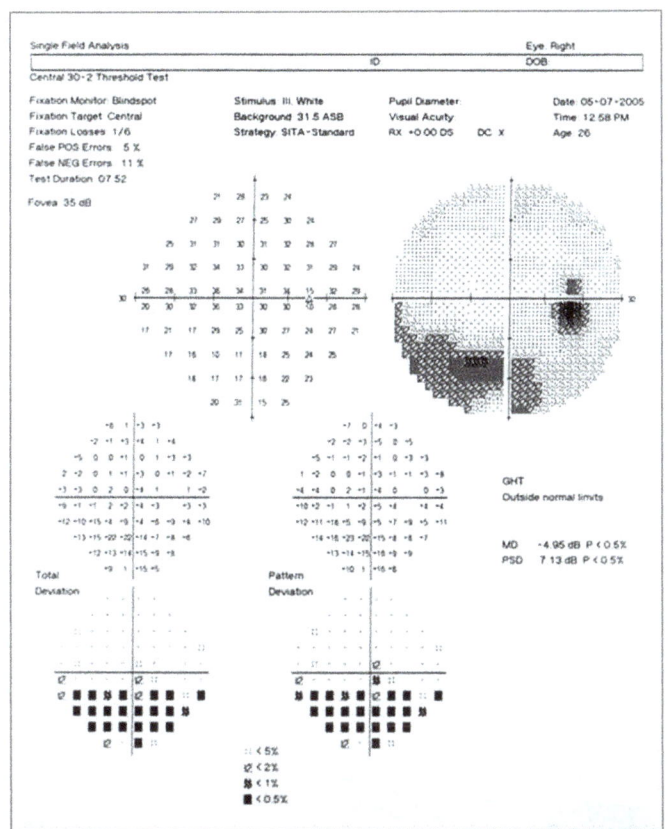
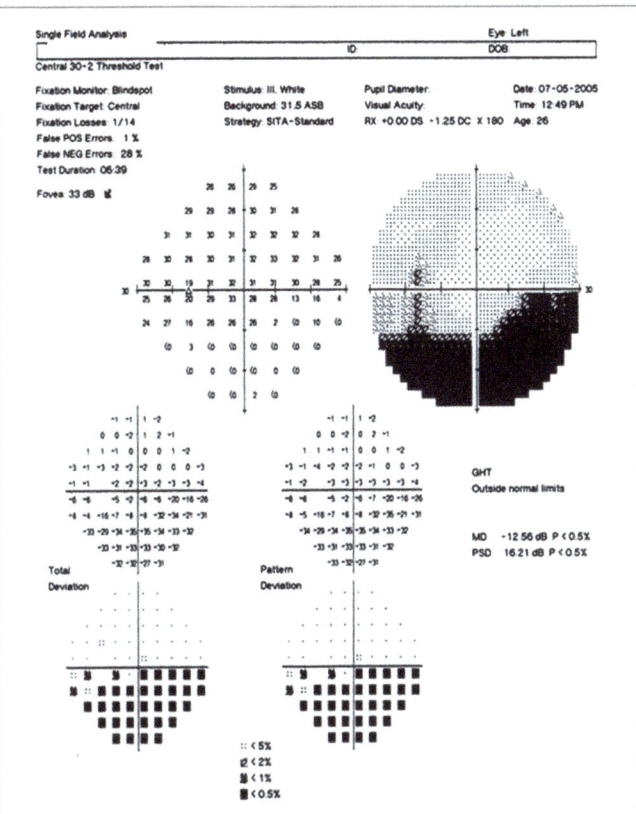
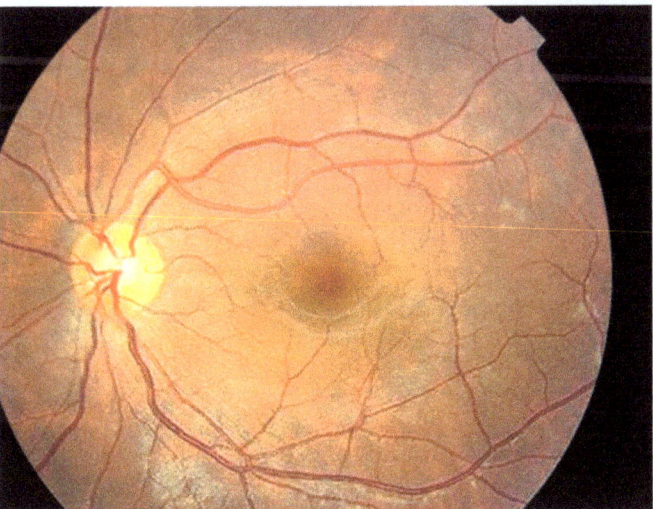
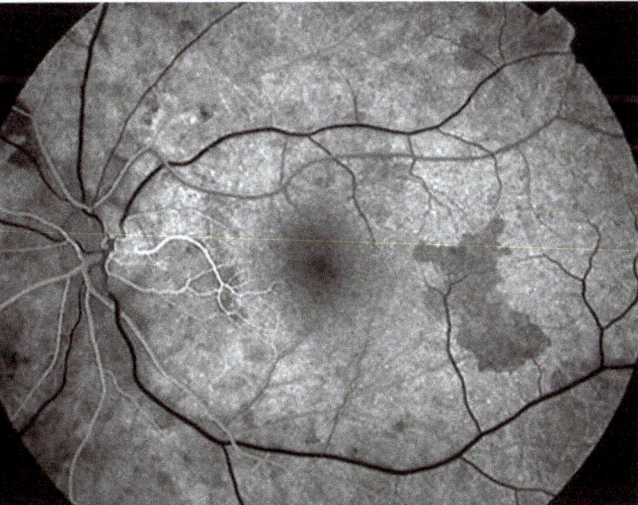

Case 17: A 42-year-old female patient presented with complaints of sudden, painless, blurring of vision associated with flashes in her left eye. Fundus examination revealed multiple, discrete, yellowish-white dots in the retina, suggestive of multiple evanescent white dot syndrome (MEWDS). Visual field of the left eye showed diffuse depression on the total deviation plot and an enlarged blind spot.

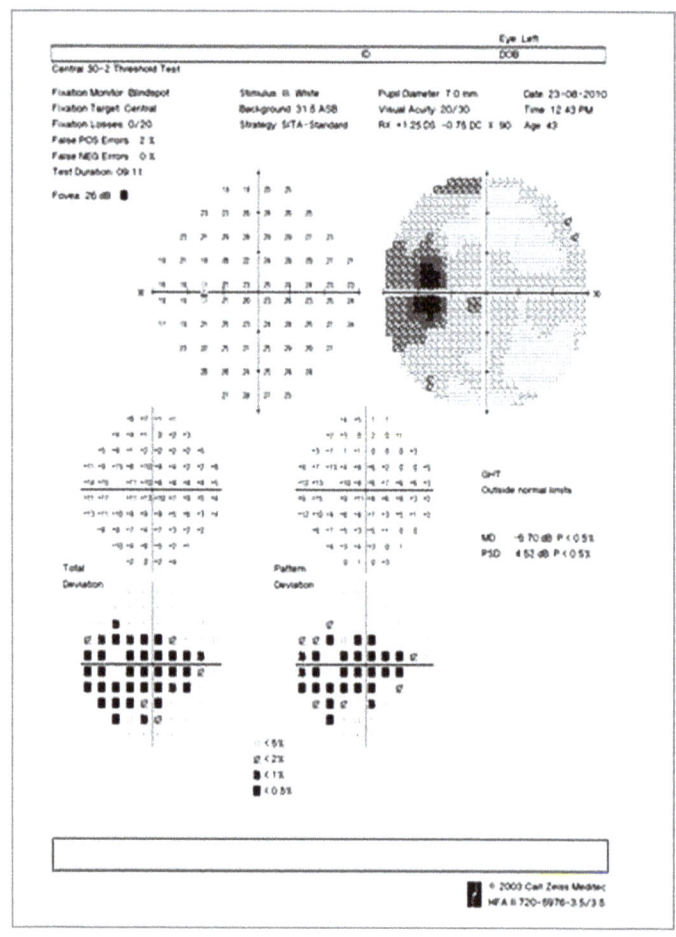
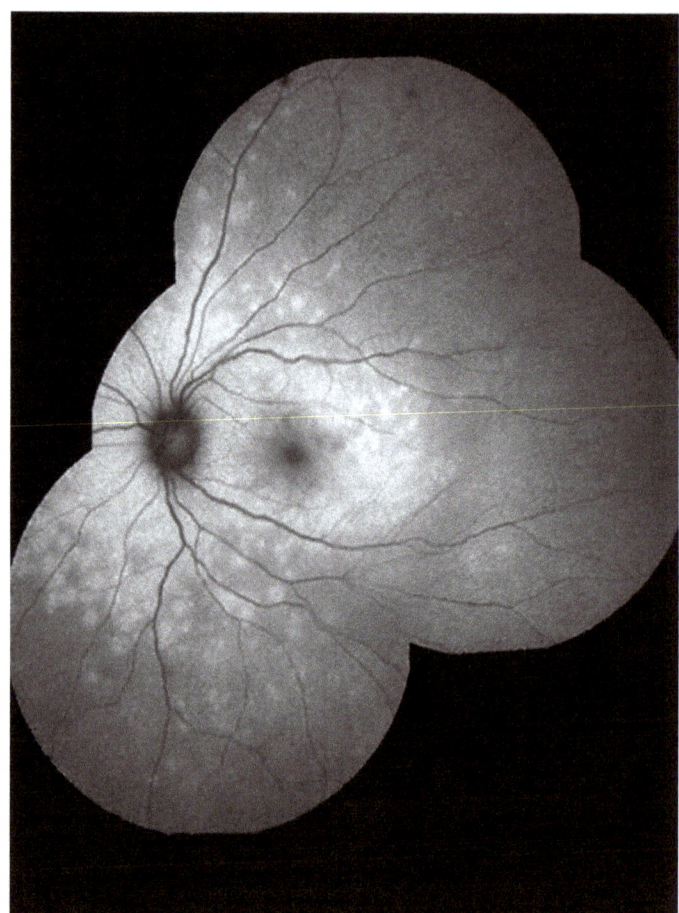

Case 18: A 62-year-old female was diagnosed with autoimmune retinopathy with significant constriction of visual fields on 30-2 in both eyes. Both eyes fundus photos show arteriolar narrowing with retinal pigment epithelial alterations in both eyes.

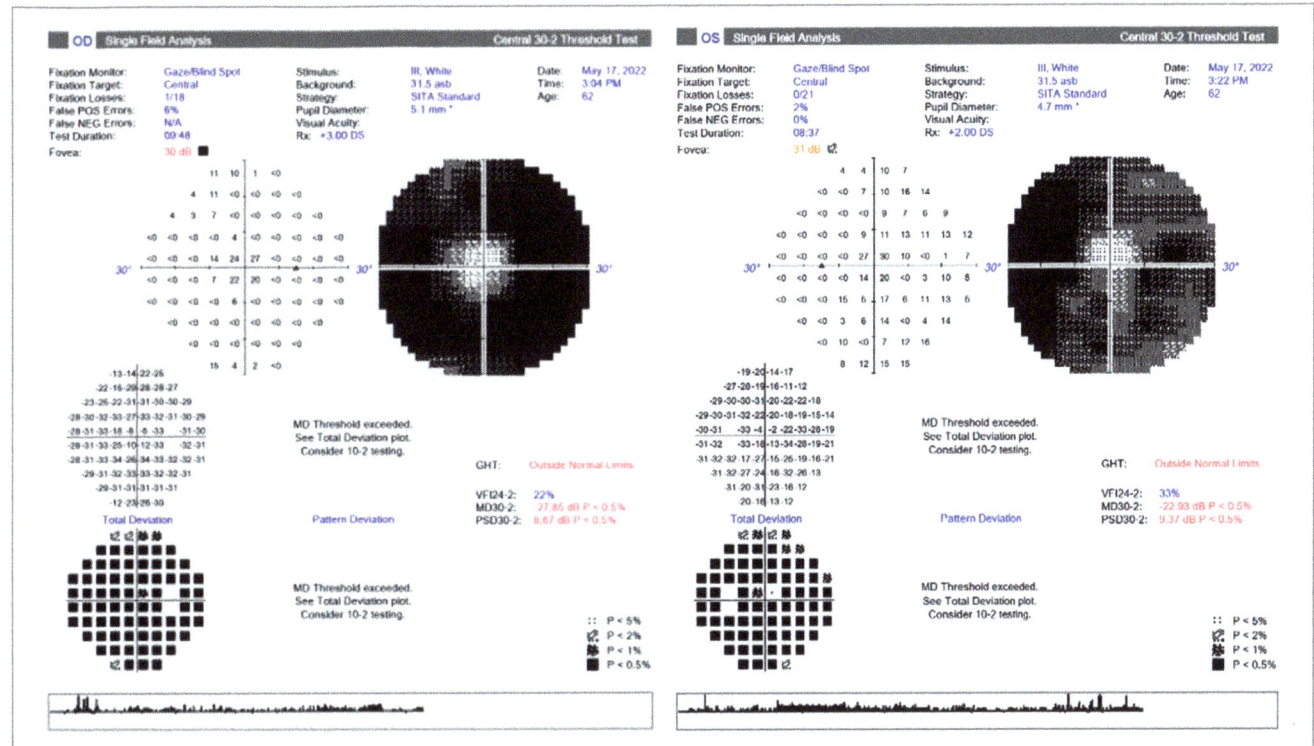

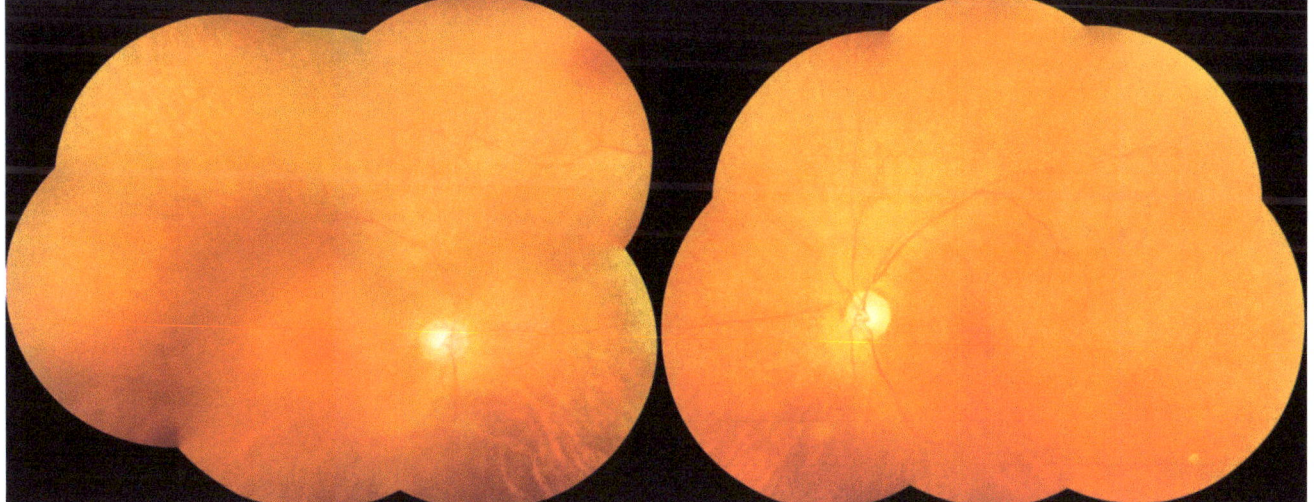

Case 19: Fundus photos show inferior rhegmatogenous retinal detachment in this 17-year-old myope. As the detachment involves the posterior pole, even a central 24-2 fields reveal the corresponding superior scotoma. The defect has sloping margins (relative defect at the borders of the scotoma). In long-standing detachments, the defect has sharp borders. Also note the generalized reduction in sensitivity seen on total deviation plot and high fixation losses.

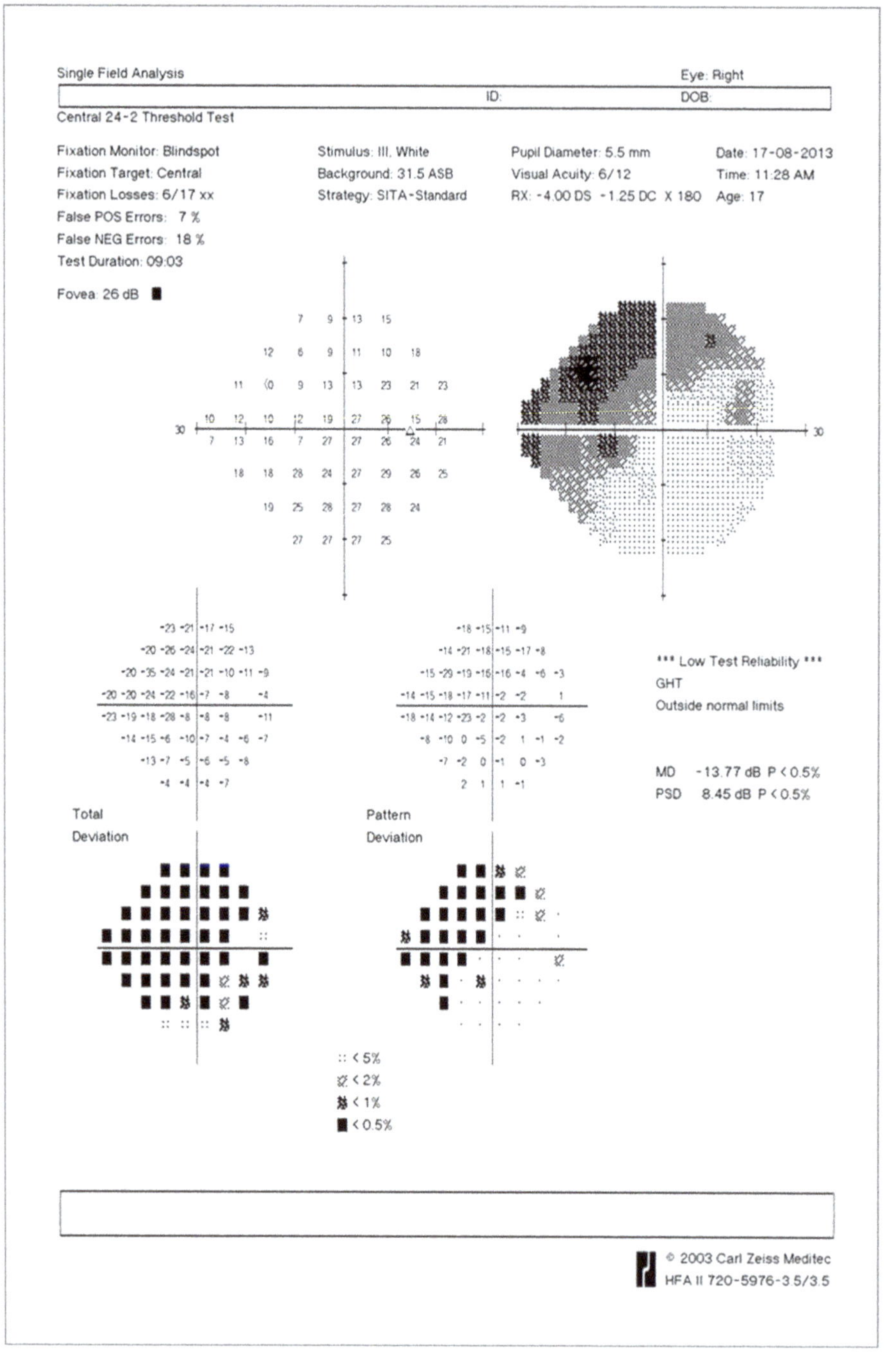

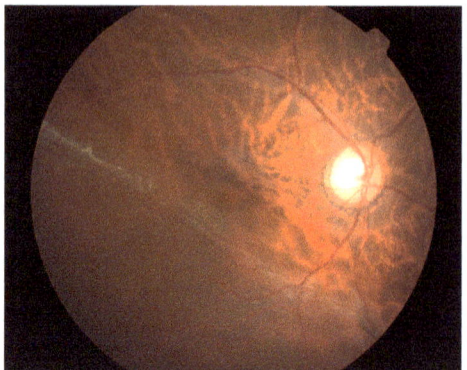

CONCLUSION

Perimetry provides a standardized, reliable, and reproducible method for evaluation and follow-up of retinal disease. MP helps in quantifying visual function of the macula in a variety of retinal diseases. Understanding the pathology and its impact on function may help in developing screening algorithms and treatment modalities for management of retinal diseases.

REFERENCES

1. Sheu SJ, Chen YY, Lin HC, Chen HL, Lee IY, Wu TT. Frequency doubling technology perimetry in retinal diseases—preliminary report. Kaohsiung J Med Sci. 2001;17(1):25-8.
2. Jackson GR, Scott IU, Quillen DA, Walter LE, Gardner TW. Inner retinal visual dysfunction is a sensitive marker of nonproliferative diabetic retinopathy. Br J Ophthalmol. 2012;96(5):699-703.
3. Remky A, Weber A, Hendricks S, Lichtenberg K, Arend O. Short-wavelength automated perimetry in patients with diabetes mellitus without macular edema. Graefes Arch Clin Exp Ophthalmol. 2003;241(6):468-71.
4. Bengtsson B, Heijl A, Agardh E. Visual fields correlate better than visual acuity to severity of diabetic retinopathy. Diabetologia. 2005;48(12):2494-500.
5. Varano M, Scassa C. Scanning laser ophthalmoscope microperimetry. Semin Ophthalmol. 1998;13:203-9.
6. Plummer DJ, Azen SP, Freeman WR. Scanning laser entoptic perimetry for the screening of macular and peripheral retinal disease. Arch Ophthalmol. 2000;118(9):1205-10.
7. Alexander P, Mushtaq F, Osmond C, Amoaku W. Microperimetric changes in neovascular age-related macular degeneration treated with ranibizumab. Eye (Lond). 2012;26(5):678-83.
8. Cideciyan AV, Swider M, Aleman TS, Feuer WJ, Schwartz SB, Russell RC, et al. Macular function in macular degenerations: Repeatability of microperimetry as a potential outcome measure for ABCA4-associated retinopathy trials. Invest Ophthalmol Vis Sci. 2012;53(2):841-52.
9. Acton JH, Greenstein VC. Fundus-driven perimetry (microperimetry) compared to conventional static automated perimetry: Similarities, differences, and clinical applications. Can J Ophthalmol. 2013;48(5):358-63.
10. Schönbach EM, Janeschitz-Kriegl L, Strauss RW, Cattaneo MEGV, Fujinami K, Birch DG, et al. The progression of Stargardt disease using volumetric hill of vision analyses over 24 months: ProgStar Report No.15. Am J Ophthalmol. 2021;230:123-33.
11. Schönbach EM, Wolfson Y, Strauss RW, Ibrahim MA, Kong X, Muñoz B, et al. Macular sensitivity measured with microperimetry in Stargardt disease in the progression of atrophy secondary to Stargardt disease (ProgStar) Study: Report No. 7. JAMA Ophthalmol. 2017;135(7):696-703.
12. Roth JA. Central visual field in diabetes. Br J Ophthalmol. 1969;53:16-25.
13. Bell JA, Feldon SE. Retinal microangiopathy: Correlation of Octopus perimetry with fluorescein angiography. Arch Ophthalmol. 1984;102:1294-8.
14. Tsai ASH, Gan ATL, Ting DSW, Wong CW, Teo KYC, Tan ACS, et al. Diabetic macular ischemia: Correlation of retinal vasculature changes by optical coherence tomography angiography and functional deficit. Retina. 2019;40:2184-90.
15. Tsai ASH, Jordan-Yu JM, Gan ATL, Teo KYC, Tan GSW, Lee SY, et al. Diabetic macular ischemia: Influence of optical coherence tomography angiography parameters on changes in functional outcomes over one year. Invest Ophthalmol Vis Sci. 2021;62:9.
16. Alonso-Plasencia M, Abreu-Gonzalez R, Gomez-Culebras MA. Structure-function correlation using OCT angiography and microperimetry in diabetic retinopathy. Clin Ophthalmol. 2019;13:2181-8
17. Mokrane A, Zureik A, Bonin S, Erginay A, Lavia C, Gaudric A, et al. Retinal sensitivity correlates with the superficial vessel density and inner layer thickness in diabetic retinopathy. Invest Ophthalmol Vis Sci. 2021;62:28.
18. Santos AR, Raimundo M, Alves D, Lopes M, Pestana S, Figueira J, et al. Microperimetry and mfERG as functional measurements in diabetic macular oedema undergoing intravitreal ranibizumab treatment. Eye (Lond). 2021;35: 1384-92.
19. Imasawa M, Tsumura T, Kikuchi T, Sekine A, Iijima H. Humphrey perimetry as a predictor of visual improvement after photodynamic therapy. Jpn J Ophthalmol. 2009;53:281-2.
20. Chalam KV, Agarwal S, Gupta SK, Shah GY. Recovery of retinal sensitivity after transient branch retinal artery occlusion. Ophthalm Surg Lasers Imaging. 2007;38:328-9.
21. Hayreh SS, Zimmerman MB. Central retinal artery occlusion: Visual outcome. Am J Ophthalmol. 2005;140:376-91.
22. Baran NV, Gurlu VP, Esgin H. Long-term macular function in eyes with central serous chorioretinopathy. Clin Experiment Ophthalmol. 2005;33:369-72.
23. Ozdemir H, Karacorlu SA, Senturk F, Karacorlu M, Uysal O. Assessment of macular function by microperimetry in unilateral resolved central serous chorioretinopathy. Eye (Lond). 2008;22:204-8.
24. Horie S, Giulia C, Esmaeilkhanian H, Sadda SR. Cheung CMG, Ham Y. Microperimetry in Retinal Diseases. Asia Pac J Ophthalmol (Phila). 2023;12(2):211-27.
25. Acton JH, Gibson JM, Cubbidge RP. Quantification of visual field loss in age-related macular degeneration. PLoS One. 2012;7(6):e39944.
26. Baptista PM, Silva N, Coelho J, José D, Almeida D, Meireles A. Microperimetry as part of multimodal assessment to evaluate and monitor myopic traction maculopathy. Clin Ophthalmol. 2021;15:235-42.
27. Chen WC, Wang Y, Li XX. Morphologic and functional evaluation before and after successful macular hole surgery using spectral-domain optical coherence tomography combined with microperimetry. Retina. 2012;32:1733-42.
28. Ripandelli G, Scarinci F, Piaggi P, Guidi G, Pileri M, Cupo G, et al. Macular pucker: To peel or not to peel the internal limiting membrane? A microperimetric response. Retina. 2015;35:498-507.

29. Russo A, Morescalchi F, Gambicorti E, Cancarini A, Costagliola C, Semeraro F. Epiretinal membrane removal with foveal-sparing internal limiting membrane peeling: A pilot study. Retina. 2019;39:2116-24.
30. Blautain B, Glacet-Bernard A, Blanco-Garavito R, Toutée A, Jung C, Ortoli M, et al. Long-term follow-up of retinal sensitivity assessed by microperimetry in patients with internal limiting membrane peeling. Eur J Ophthalmol. 2022;32(1):539-45.
31. Marmor MF, Kellner U, Lai TY, Melles RB, Mieler WF; American Academy of Ophthalmology. Recommendations on Screening for Chloroquine and Hydroxychloroquine Retinopathy (2016 Revision). Ophthalmology. 2016;123(6):1386-94.
32. Melles RB, Marmor MF. Pericentral retinopathy and racial differences in hydroxychloroquine toxicity. Ophthalmology. 2015;122:110-6.
33. Lee DH, Melles RB, Joe SG, Lee JY, Kim JG, Lee CK, et al. Pericentral hydroxychloroquine retinopathy in Korean patients. Ophthalmology. 2015;122:1252-6.
34. Stanford MR, Tomlin EA, Comyn O, Holland K, Pavesio C. The visual field in toxoplasmic retinochoroiditis. Br J Ophthalmol. 2005;89:812-4.
35. Grange L, Dalal M, Nussenblatt RB, Sen HN. Autoimmune retinopathy. Am J Ophthalmol. 2014;157(2):266-72.e1.
36. Ferreyra HA, Jayasundera T, Khan NW, He S, Lu Y, Heckenlively JR. Management of autoimmune retinopathies with immunosuppression. Arch Ophthalmol. 2009;127(4):390-7.
37. Budenz DL. Atlas of Visual Fields. Michigan: Lippincott–Raven; 1997.
38. Anders H, Vincent PM. Essential Perimetry: The Field Analyzer Primer, 3rd edition. Germany: Carl Zeiss Meditec, Inc.; 2002.
39. Ryan SJ, Sadda SR (Eds). Retina. Visual Fields in Retinal Disease, 5th edition. London: Saunders; 2013.
40. Abramson DH, Melson MR, Servodidio C. Visual fields in retinoblastoma survivors. Arch Ophthalmol. 2004;122:1324-30.

CHAPTER 12

Frequency Doubling Perimetry

Parul Ichhpujani, Shibal Bhartiya, Dewang Angmo, Tanuj Dada

■ INTRODUCTION

Perimetry is required to detect visual field loss, and to determine the specific patterns of the field defects. This is essential for both the differential diagnosis, as well as monitoring progression of the disease process and the consequent visual field loss. Standard achromatic or automated perimetry (SAP) is the gold standard to accomplish these management goals, but the procedure has certain inherent drawbacks. Frequency doubling perimetry (FDP) addresses the need for a faster diagnostic technique for screening, diagnosis, as well as serial monitoring of the disease process. In this alone, it does have a slight advantage over SAP. It also examines motion attributes of vision which may be affected in early glaucoma which may be missed by conventional perimetry.[1-9]

■ CONCERNS WITH STANDARD AUTOMATED PERIMETRY

The SAP, despite being the "gold standard" to assess visual function, has certain limitations and disadvantages. The most important of these include:

- *SAP is nonselective:* SAP evaluates differential light sensitivity using a small (0.47°) white flash (200 ms) on a dim (31.5 asb) white background. All the primary retinal ganglion cell (RGC) types responsible for vision respond to this stimulus, hence it becomes nonselective.
- *SAP may miss early glaucomatous ganglion cell loss:* SAP may not provide adequate sensitivity to detect early glaucomatous changes due to the inherent redundancy of the visual system. It is able to detect functional deficits only after a significant amount of ganglion cell loss has already occurred (25-50%).[10,11]
- *SAP protocol has an inherent high test-retest variability and progression is therefore difficult to ascertain:* There is a high test-retest variability, particularly in regions of visual field deficits, making it difficult to assess whether the visual field is worsening on serial examination.[12]

■ FREQUENCY DOUBLING PRINCIPLE

The optic nerve is made up of the axons of approximately 1.2-1.5 million RGC. The irreversible loss of these RGC fibers results in glaucoma and certain other ocular conditions, which affect the field of vision. There is evidence in literature that a considerable loss of RGC fibers can go undetected, and for any notable visual field loss/symptoms to occur, up to 40% of RGCs may be lost. An average of 3-5 years of gradual nerve fiber loss may pass, before an apparent visual field loss is detected.

To understand the pathophysiology of this complex interaction, it is essential to understand the basic retinal anatomy and physiology.

Retinal nerve fibers transmit signals from the retinal receptor cells by way of the optic nerve to the lateral geniculate body and ultimately to the visual cortex. These are broadly classified into the magnocellular (or M) cells, and the parvocellular (or P) cells.

- *P Cells:* The P-cell pathway is responsible for high contrast, low temporal frequency (or static) stimulus detection.
- *M Cells:* The M-cell pathway detects low contrast; high temporal frequency (or motion) stimuli,[13] and constitutes approximately 10% of the total retinal nerve fibers.

Nonlinear M cells are a subset of the large diameter M cells, and are affected before any other cell type in glaucoma. Therefore, detection of this cell loss helps to identify RGC loss before it can be detected by traditional automated perimetry.[14]

■ FREQUENCY DOUBLING ILLUSION

When a low spatial frequency sinusoidal grating with alternating wide light and dark bars undergoes high temporal-frequency counter phase flicker, (i.e., the black and white bands reverse to become white and black, respectively in a rapid sequence) the spatial frequency of the grating appears doubled. This is known as frequency doubling illusion.

Selective testing of the magnocellular pathway by presenting alternate grating stimuli therefore may help in early detection of glaucomatous cell loss.[14]

The reduced redundancy theory, on the other hand, works on the presumption that visual field loss may be detected earlier if only a subset of the visual system is tested, i.e., the sensitivity of the test may be is higher if only one of the two major transmission pathways are tested.[15]

The frequency doubling technology (FDT) perimeter (Humphrey FDT perimeter using the Welch Allyn Frequency Doubling Technology) was developed keeping in mind both these physiological attributes of the RGC layer. FDT perimetry is thought to be mediated by a subset of the RGCs with large axonal diameter, called the M6y ganglion cells that project to the magnocellular (M) pathway. Recent research has, however, suggested that the origins of the response are most likely cortical.[16]

Frequency Doubling Technology versus Standard Automated Perimetry

Target: In FDP, rather than using a small spot of light as in SAP, a large low spatial frequency sinusoidal grating (<1 cycle/degree) that consists of black and white bars undergoes a rapid counter phase flicker (>15 Hz) so that the black bars become white, and the white bars become black (**Figs. 1A and B**).

The rapid flickering of the target results in the frequency doubling illusion, that is, at a particular contrast level, the visible lines become double in number. The person observing the stimulus, therefore, sees double the number of bars than actual present in the grating.

Area stimulated: FDP uses a target that stimulates a significantly larger retinal area. The standard FDP target is a square 10° in diameter. The size III Goldmann target equivalent subtends a spot of light 0.43° in diameter onto the retina, while the size V Goldmann target, is 1.72° in diameter. Even the largest size available (size V Goldmann target) for SAP in patients with significantly reduced visual fields, thus, is significantly smaller than the FDP target. FDP therefore tests larger areas, and is capable of detecting certain subtle diffuse changes that may not be elicited with other perimetry protocols. The corollary to this is the fact that FDP can miss shallow localized defects, since the area stimulated is much larger than in conventional perimetry.[17]

FREQUENCY DOUBLING PERIMETRY DEVICES

First Generation (Frequency Doubling Perimetry 1)

- It is a portable device which comprises a compact video display unit and a moveable binocular cowling piece to shield ambient room light. A video display unit presents 10° square target and a central 5° radius target.
- A view finder slides from side to side to allow monocular viewing without the need of patching.
- Fixation is monitored by a video camera focused on the observer's eye.

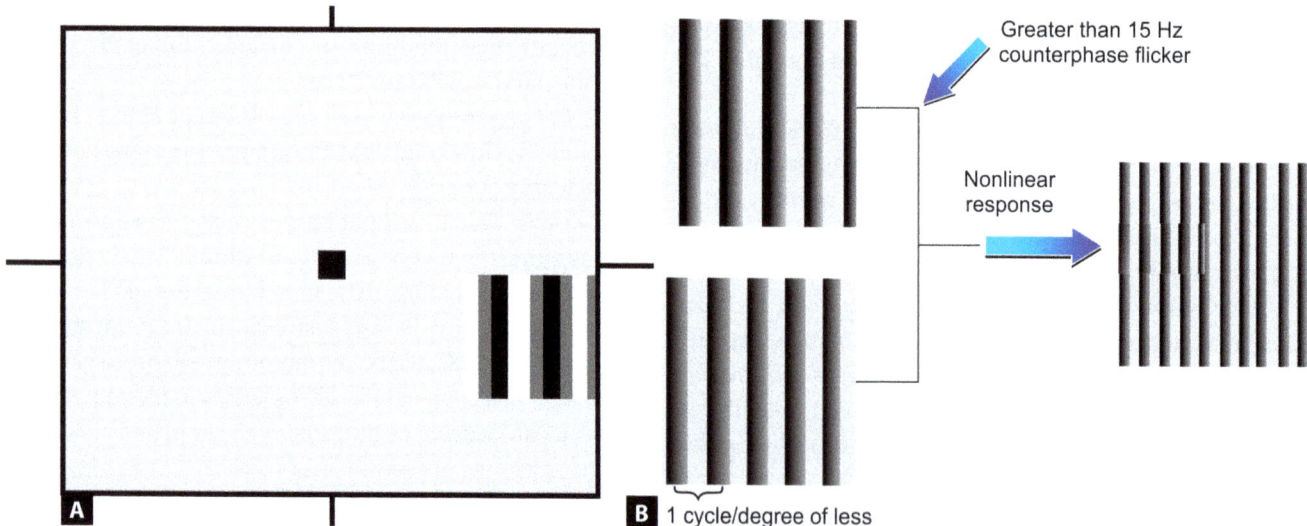

Figs. 1A and B: Frequency doubling perimetry (FDP) target: Sinusoidal gratings consisting of alternate black and white bars; and rapid counterphase flicker.

- The stimulus is a monochrome sine-wave sinusoidal pattern of vertical gray stripes with a spatial frequency of 0.25 cycles per degree and temporal frequency of 25 Hz.
- The contrast of the stimulus is modified for each of the locations (17 or 19) in the visual field. 10° × 10° targets are used, 4 per quadrant within the central 20°, along with one smaller central target (5° diameter circle) projected on the macular region to measure contrast sensitivity.
- The stimulus is presented for no >720 ms, in order to avoid temporal transients. In this time, the contrast is gradually ramped up to the level of contrast selected initially, remains at that level for some time, before gradually decreasing to zero.
- The time interval between presentation of stimuli varies by up to 500 ms. This ensures that there are no "rhythmic or as-expected responses" by the patient.
- If the patient presses the response button between 100 ms and 1 s after its presentation, the stimulus is recorded as *"seen"* at that specific contrast level for the specified location. Otherwise, it is recorded as *"not seen"*.
- Since targets are seen to be at optical infinity, it is imperative that the patients be corrected for distance with appropriate lenses (both bifocals and progressive ones may be used). Near correction is not required since the large targets with the lower spatial frequency are not impacted by refractive errors of <6 diopters.

Testing Modes for Frequency Doubling Perimetry 1

Suprathreshold Strategy

The suprathreshold strategy is basically employed as a screening protocol, with a test duration that ranges from 45 to 90 seconds, depending on the severity of the field defect. The two types of screening methods are denoted by the suffixes –1 and –5. Each specific location is tested at different contrast levels. This testing may vary from once, to four times, depending on the subject reporting the target to be seen or not.[18]

- *1 screening test*: Stimuli are presented at a contrast level that can be detected by 99% of healthy age-matched subjects. Only those targets that remain unseen are tested again. In case the target is still not seen, it is presented for the third time. However, the contrast level presented is such that 99.5% of healthy, age-matched subjects of can see it.

  If the target is seen, the location is labeled as $p < 1\%$. If not, the target is presented again at maximum contrast (about 100%), and marked as $p < 0.5\%$, if seen. If not, the location is labeled as "not seen at maximum".
- *5 screening test*: In this protocol, targets are presented at a contrast level that may be detected by 95% of healthy age-matched subjects. If the target is seen, the location is labeled as normal at $p \geq 5$. If unseen, the target is presented again without changing contrast. If this is also not seen, the target is then presented at contrast level that may be seen by 98% of healthy normals.

The location is labeled as $p < 5$ if seen, and if not seen, the location is tested again. This time, a higher contrast level at p of 1% is used, which should be seen by 99% of healthy normals. If seen, the location is marked as $p < 2\%$, and if missed, the location is marked as $p < 1\%$.

The –1 protocol thus has higher specificity (which implies low false positives), while the –5 procedure has a higher sensitivity (which implies low false negatives). This means early defects at picked up with greater sensitivity, with a consequent lower specificity.

Test options include a screening field (screening C-20-1) in which gratings with three contrast levels are shown at 17 locations in the central 20° field and it takes about 45 seconds. Other is suprathreshold screening C-30 program.

Interpretation

The FDT screening mode perimetry is considered abnormal in case the following criteria are met:
- Any defect in the central five locations
- Two mild or moderate defects in the outer 12 squares
- One severe defect in the outer 12 squares
- Screening test time > 90 seconds per eye

Full Threshold Strategy

There are two variants in the full threshold (FT) strategy—(1) C-20 and (2) N-30.

C-20 versus N-30

- C-20 strategy examines the central 20° at 17 locations, while
- N-30 evaluates two additional points nasally (total 19 locations).
- C-20 is a rapid strategy, taking about three and a half minutes. On the other hand, N-30 takes significantly longer, about 6 minutes.
- Nasal targets of N-30 are beyond the width of the FDT screen. To test the nasal loci, the fixation point is moved temporally. The redirection of the fixation point 10° temporally is done once the other points have been mapped.

Threshold sensitivity is measured by one of the two protocols—(1) method of adjustment (MOA) or (2) modified binary search (MOBS).[19]

1. *Method of adjustment:* For each stimulus pattern, the geometric mean of three contrast threshold adjustments is determined as the final contrast threshold value.

2. *Modified binary search:* MOBS is a staircase test strategy. Testing continues until the specified number of response reversals are documented and the difference between the upper and lower stack values is equal or less than a specified interval. The final threshold is therefore marked as the mid-point between the upper and lower limits, when both of the aforementioned specifications are satisfied.

■ NEWER STRATEGIES

- *Rapid efficiency binary search technique (REBS):* The REBS strategy is based on MOBS. The termination criteria for REBS, however, are more stringent—two response reversals are required(with the upper to lower limit interval within 3 dB).
- *Zippy estimation of sequential testing (ZEST):* In ZEST, a probability density function (PDF). The test depicts the relative likelihood of threshold values within the population, and is assumed for threshold before the test starts. Both ZEST and REBS are 40%, 50%, faster than MOBS.[20]

All protocols (including screening and threshold) such as SAP, compare each test results to specific age-matched contrast sensitivity values. The normative database has >700 eyes of 450 "normal" subjects between the ages of 18 and 85. They also correct for decrease in the sensitivity due to increasing age; as well as the first versus second eye.

Frequency Doubling Perimetry Printout (Figs. 2 to 4)

When evaluating FDP printouts, the following areas are evaluated:
- Number of points depressed
- Location of involved points
- Pattern of involved points
- Depth of depression
- Comparison between the two eyes
- Correlate any field loss with ocular examination (lens, optic nerve, and retina)

Reliability indices (fixation errors, false-positive errors, and false-negative errors) are provided, as well as mean deviation (MD) and pattern standard deviation (PSD) indices for the threshold tests, similar to the indices provided with traditional automated threshold perimetry statistical analyses.

Correlation of FDP1 with SAP

Percent correlation to Humphrey 30-2 threshold visual field is reported to be approximately 100% sensitivity and specificity [area under the curve (AUC) 1.0] for detecting advanced glaucomatous visual field loss. The same is about 96% sensitivity and 96% specificity (AUC, 0.9751) for detection of moderate glaucomatous field loss, decreasing to 85% sensitivity and 90% specificity (AUC, 0.9261) for early glaucomatous damage. Overall sensitivity of FDT for glaucoma diagnosis varies from 80 to 93%, while specificity is from 93 to 100%.[1-3,6]

Custom 24-2 Frequency Doubling Perimetry

Some commercially available FDT perimeters use bigger targets and fewer visual locations during testing. Johnson et al.[15] reported that a custom designed FDT perimeter (Quadravision) with 4° target using 24-2 stimulus presentation pattern, working under the presumption that smaller targets and multiple visual field locations would increase sensitivity and specificity of the testing protocols. 54 stimuli of 4° targets with 6° grid spacing were used in a 24-2 stimulus presentation pattern, and the authors found that the 24-2 stimulus pattern appears to have a slightly better sensitivity for detecting early glaucomatous field loss. It also provided a better description and characterization of the field loss pattern. The increased sensitivity, however, came at a significant cost, viz., time taken for the screening—the protocol took approximately twice as much time as conventional FDP.[21,22]

Second Generation: Matrix Frequency Doubling Technology

- The Humphrey matrix (FDT2)[23,24] uses a similar, but smaller FDT stimuli.
- It provides up to 69 stimuli, 5° × 5° each. Except foveal stimulus, the stimuli are 5° square windows of a vertical grating with spatial frequency of 0.5 cyc/deg, counterphase flickered at 18 Hz.
- Matrix FDT can fully delineate visual field loss patterns. It also performs a progression analysis of serial examinations.
- ZEST is Bayesian strategy with a fixed number of presentations at each test location and a flat previous PDF. This reduces the test time for FT perimetry to almost 50%, with no compromise on accuracy and reliability.
- Five threshold testing methods are available at present, and these provide quantitative measurements of the visual field at each location. The results are thereafter compared to the normative database (which includes >270 individuals between 18 and 85 years of age).
  - *N-30-F test*: It is analogous to the 19-point threshold test found on the original FDT. Matrix uses a two-reversal MOBS strategy (instead of four reversals in the original machine) for determining threshold. This

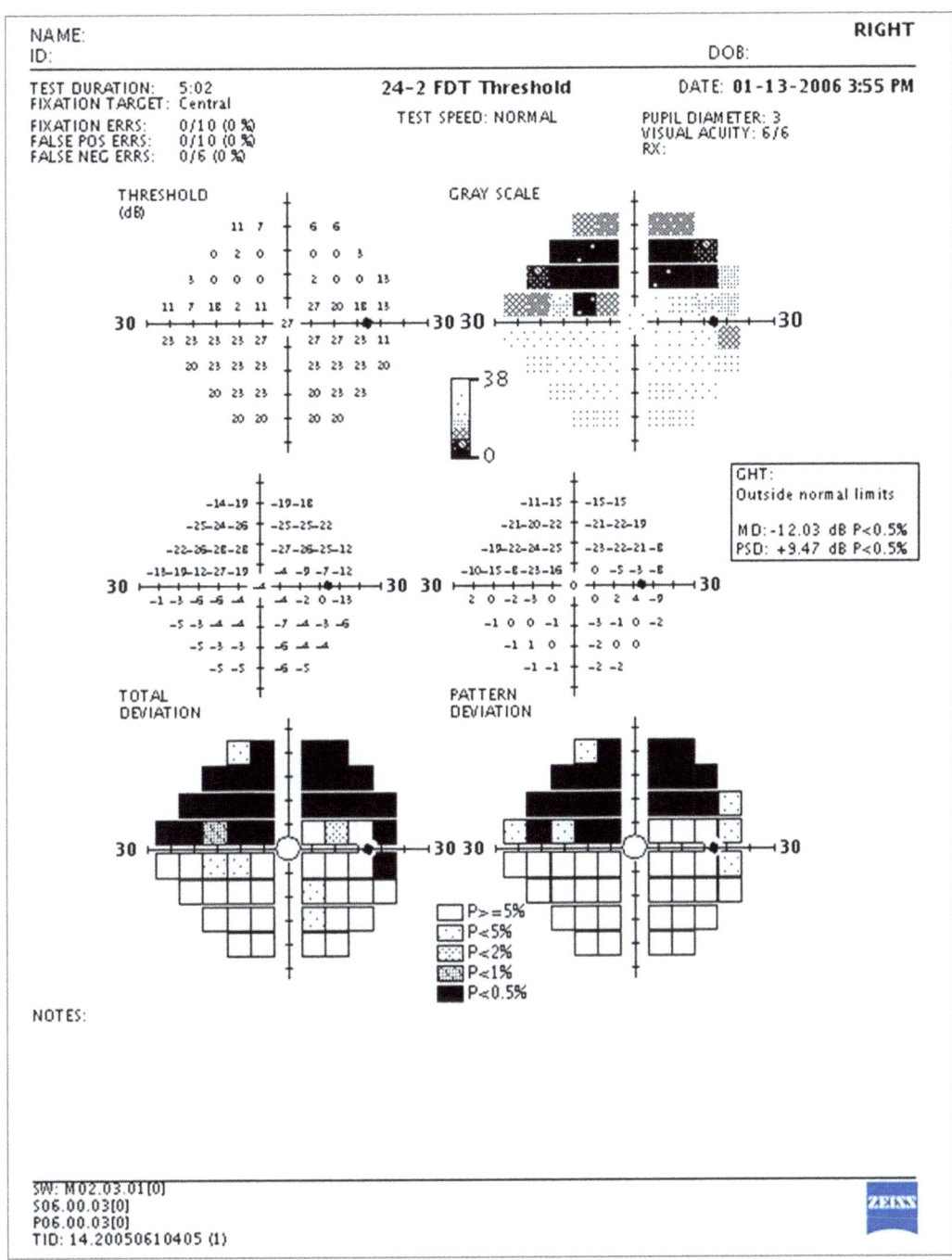

Fig. 2: Humphrey matrix frequency doubling perimetry using 24-2 threshold test procedure shows right eye of a patient with superior arcuate field defect.

is therefore a more efficient algorithm, with a lesser testing duration. Also, moving fixation is not needed for the test.

- *24-2 and 30-2 tests*: The 24-2 and 30-2 tests use 5° targets to test and characterize 55 and 69 locations, respectively. The temporal counterphase flickering rate is 18 Hz. The pattern of stimulus presentation is analogous to that in HFA II, with most points being similar except for the 14 most peripheral locations within the central 30° tested with the 30-2 test.
- *10-2 and Macula test*: The 10-2 and Macula tests use 2° targets with a temporal flickering rate of 12 Hz. This enables the flicker sensitivity instead of FD response. The 10-2 evaluates a total of 42 locations, while the Macula protocol evaluates 16 points.

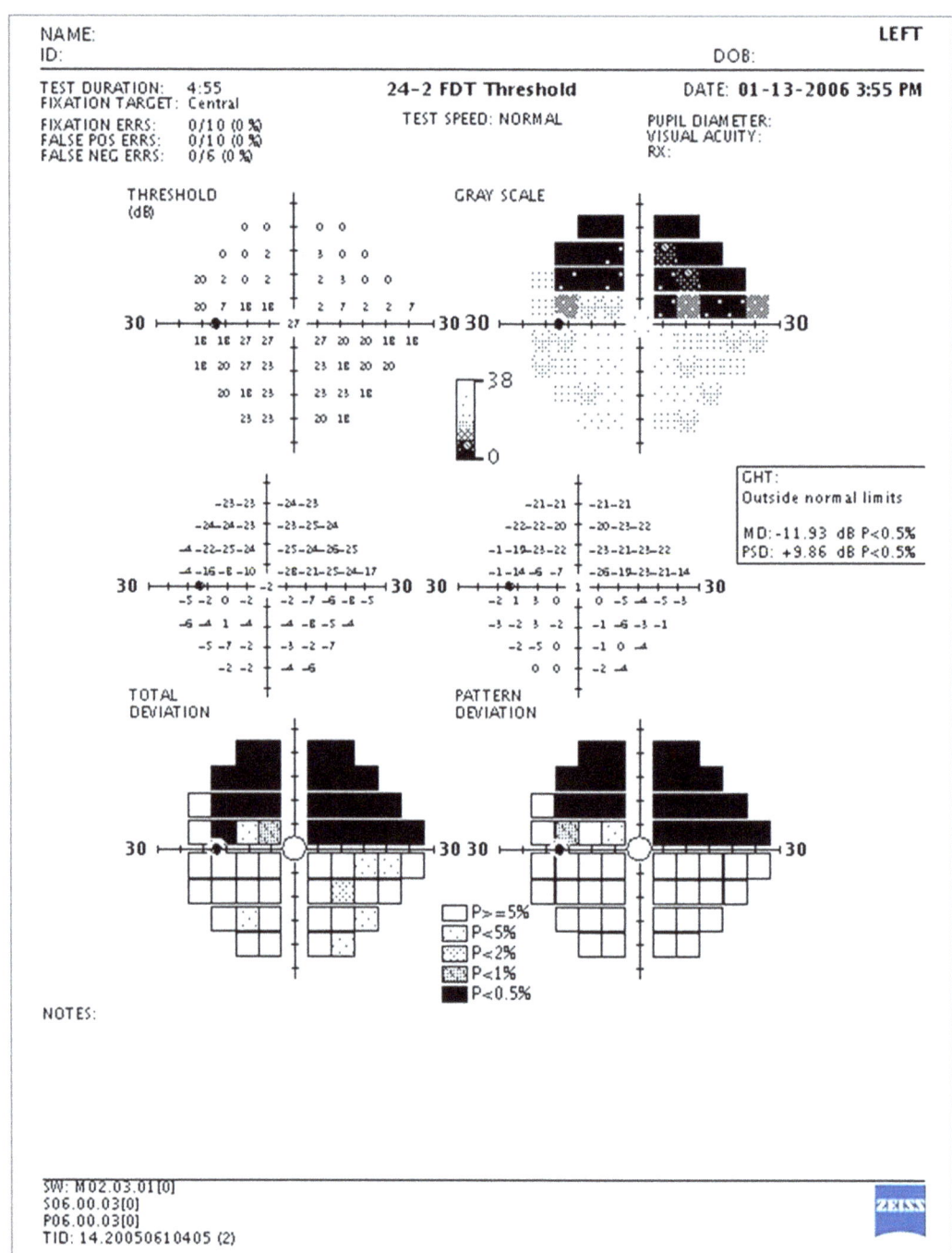

Fig. 3: Humphrey Matrix Frequency Doubling Perimeter using 24-2 threshold test procedure shows left eye of a patient with superior arcuate field defect.

Spry et al., compared threshold testing using the FDT Matrix and SAP and found the two to be comparable when the 24-2 test pattern is used.[23] Global visual field indices including the MD and PSD of FDT and SAP were found to correlate highly. The test–retest variability of FDT2 was found to be uniform over the measurement range of the machine, as reported by Artes et al.[24]

Advantages of Frequency Doubling Perimetry

- Short test duration (4–5 minutes for FT), portability, and lower cost makes it useful for glaucoma screening.
- Its ease of use by both patient and examiner, as also the flat learning curve means it may be used in children as well.[25]
- Very tolerant to defocus and blur (+ 6 D sphere),[14] not affected by pupil size.

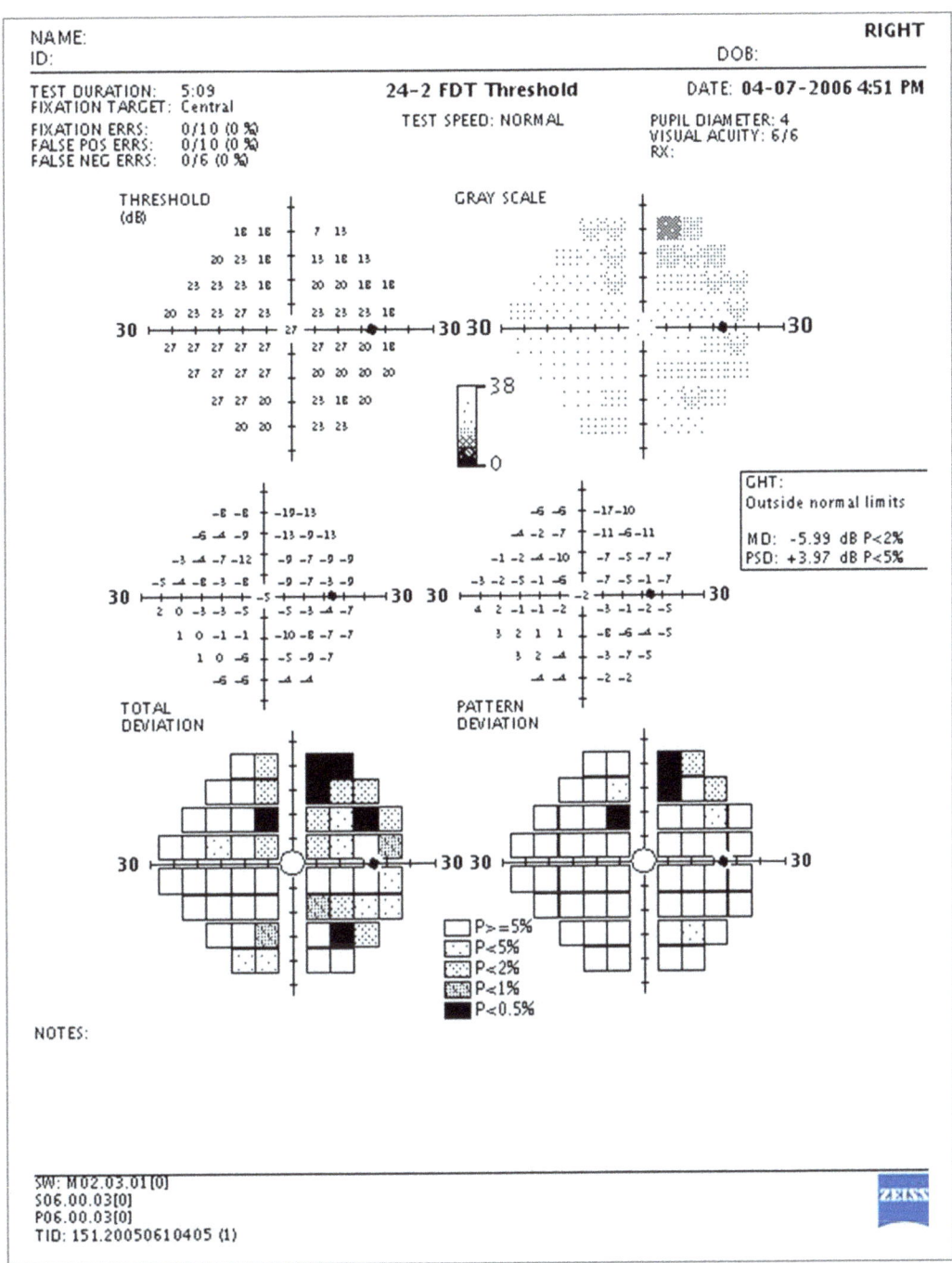

Fig. 4: Humphrey Matrix Frequency Doubling Perimeter using 24-2 threshold test procedure shows right eye of a patient with early superior arcuate field defect, correlating clinically with an inferotemporal notching.

- Patient can wear spectacles with bifocals.
- Test-retest reliability of the FDP is good and can thus be used to follow glaucoma progression over time with the computed MD and PSD values.

Disadvantages of Frequency Doubling Perimetry

- May miss focal defects, and especially nasal steps in the central 20° field

- Lack of longitudinal data for comparison over time
- Follow-up in cases with early progression is difficult.

SCIENTIFIC EVIDENCE

Frequency doubling perimetry has been evaluated for both sensitivity and specificity for various stages of glaucoma. Johnson et al. reported a sensitivity of 82% with a specificity of 95% for early glaucomas, 96% sensitivity and 99% specificity for moderate glaucomas and 100% sensitivity and 100% specificity for advanced glaucoma.[1]

Allen et al.[26] reported a low false positive rate and a good positive predictive value comparing the FDT screening algorithm (C 20-1) to the HFA 24-2 Swedish Interactive Threshold Algorithm (SITA) Fast for screening.

Frequency doubling perimetry has been evaluated for its sensitivity and specificity for detecting visual field defects associated with neuro-ophthalmic conditions such as anterior ischemic optic neuropathy (AION) compressive optic neuropathies and pseudotumor cerebri.[27] The sensitivity of FDT was reported by Wlland et al. to be 81.3%, with a specificity of 76.2%. When compared with sensitivity and specificity of Humphrey perimetry 87.5% and 81.0%, respectively, the difference was not statistically significant.

The agreement between the predictive powers of FDT, and clinical examination of optic disc, nerve fiber layer, and FDP, was evaluated by Quigley et al. and the authors concluded that FDP may be used as a screening tool for detecting glaucomatous optic nerve damage.[3]

Sponsel's clinical scoring algorithm for FDP modeled after the Hodapp-Parrish-Anderson (HAP) criteria for scoring Humphrey visual field defect severe visual field loss proposes the following criteria for classifying glaucomatous field loss—>1 FDP sector at probability 0.5%; moderate visual field loss, not severe, with either 1.

Frequency doubling perimetry sector at probability 0.5% or >13 sectors at 1–5%; early visual field loss, not moderate, with >4 sectors at 1–5%.[4] FDT has been shown to have a lower intra- and intertest variability than SAP. The test-retest variability in glaucoma patients tested using the FDT does not increase as much with the severity of field defect, as compared to conventional perimetry.[7,8]

Boden et al.[28] found that FDT detects abnormal fields in more eyes than SAP-FT (SITA), especially in eyes with early field loss. Correlations of the global indices of both perimetry techniques were found to be similar, irrespective of the threshold strategy used in SAP.

The serial analysis of FDT examinations in glaucoma suspects by Medeiros et al.[29] during follow-up revealed that in 59% of those who developed glaucoma, the FDT detected visual field abnormalities 4 years before the visual field damage was detected by SAP. This loss detected by the SAP was noted in the in loci that had been labeled as abnormal earlier on FDP. Landers et al.[30] also concluded that FDP predicts future visual field loss with SAP, just like short-wavelength automated perimetry (SWAP).

Kogure and colleagues found that the best agreement of the results of FDT and HFA was seen in normal tension glaucoma (NTG) using threshold of HFA.[31] The eyes with higher intraocular pressure (IOP) showed lower agreement with more abnormal points reported with FDT. This implies that the sensitivity of FDT in eyes with NTG is better, and while the sensitivity of FDT is higher in primary open angle glaucoma (POAG).

Lamparter et al. reported a good correlation between SAP and Matrix-FDT in both ocular hypertensive and healthy subjects. In ocular hypertensives, poor agreement was found in the temporal, inferotemporal, and inferonasal disc sectors. The authors attributed this to possible early retinal nerve fiber layer damage in these regions of the disc, recognized by one of the visual field instruments.[32]

Kim et al. evaluated difference between FDT and SAP with respect to detected visual field damage, and the associated factors for this difference in early glaucoma. They reported that a higher SAP-FDT difference was seen with structural parameters such as lamina cribrosa depth (LCD) and lamina cribrosa curvature index (LCCI). A lower SAP-FDT difference, on the other hand, was in patients with disc hemorrhage and lower deep layer peripapillary vessel density. The authors concluded that the difference of SAP and FDT may be useful in the identification of the associated risk factors in early glaucoma.[33]

Bradvica et al. evaluated both FDT and SAP and reported that both tests were highly specific and sensitive in distinguishing diabetics from healthy subjects, but neither was better than the other. Bot tests, on the other hand, were unable to distinguish diabetics with retinopathy from those without.[34]

Richardson et al. reported that both FDT and Moorfields motion displacement test are both portable perimeters with fair diagnostic accuracy for glaucoma detection. They, however, cautioned that these tests cannot be used in isolation for glaucoma screening test but may be useful ancillary tests.[35]

CLINICAL RELEVANCE IN CURRENT GLAUCOMA PRACTICE

- Frequency doubling technology is an inexpensive, efficient, and relatively nonoperator dependent. The testing of one eye takes an average of 1.8 ± 0.7 minutes, making it extremely efficient.
- Patients can wear their own spectacles during the test, and the results are unaffected by a refractive blur of 7D.
- FDT shows a sensitivity and specificity levels of over 97% in detection of moderate to advanced glaucoma damage. These levels are 85% and 90%, respectively in detection of early glaucoma.
- The FDT machine is >30% lighter than the Humphreys (19 vs. 30 pounds) making it more portable, and

consequently useful for community screenings. However, in comparison to the new smartphone and iPad-based algorithms, its portability may no longer be considered its USP.

- FDT shows an acceptable correlation with SAP in detecting visual field defects in neuro-ophthalmologic disorders, and diabetic retinopathy.
- The recent iPad and smartphone-based FDT are yet to be validated. This may potentially revolutionize community-based glaucoma screening, improving efficiency, accessibility, and affordability of the test.

CONCLUSION

Frequency doubling technology offers several advantages over conventional perimetry for screening, diagnosis, and monitoring of glaucoma, being more patient and operator friendly, as well as significantly faster. Its place in the glaucoma treatment algorithm, as a test more sensitive than others, however, is yet to be established. Because of its ease of use, speed, affordability, and portability, FDT was the first choice for both population-based screening and research in glaucoma and other ophthalmic disorders that require evaluation of the visual fields. However, with the advent of smartphone based and iPad-based algorithms for glaucoma screening, FDT may be considered as one of the efficient options for community-based screening programs.

REFERENCES

1. Johnson CA, Samuels SJ. Screening for glaucomatous visual filed loss with the frequency-doubling perimetry. Invest Ophthalmol Vis Sci. 1997;38:413-25.
2. Yamada N, Chen PP, Mills RP, Leen MM, Lieberman MF, Stamper RL, et al. Screening for glaucoma with frequency-doubling technology and damatocampimetry. Arch Ophthalmol. 1999;117(11):1479-84.
3. Quigley HA. Identification of glaucoma-related visual field abnormality with the screening protocol of frequency doubling technology. Am J Ophthalmol. 1998;125(6):819-29.
4. Sponsel WE, Arango S, Trigo Y, Mensah J. Clinical classification of glaucomatous visual field loss by frequency doubling perimetry. Am J Ophthal. 1998;125(6):830-6.
5. Turpin A, McKendrick AM, Jhonson, Vingrys AJ. Performance of efficient test procedure for frequency-doubling technology perimetry in normal and glaucomatous eyes. Invest Ophthalmol Vis Sci. 2002;43:709-15.
6. Wadood AC, Azuara-Blanco A, Aspinall P, Taguri A, King AJW. Sensitivity and specificity of frequency doubling perimetry, Tendency oriented perimetry, and Humphrey Swedish Interactive Threshold Algorithm-fast perimetry in a glaucoma practice. Am J Ophthal. 2002;133:327-32.
7. Chauhan BC, Jhonson CA. Test-retest variability of frequency doubling perimetry and conventional perimetry in glaucoma patients and normal subjects. Invest Ophthalmol Vis Sci. 1999;40:648-56.
8. Spry PGD, Johonson CA, McKendrick AM, Turpin A. Variability components of standard automated perimetry and frequency- doubling technology perimetry. Invest Ophthalmol Vis Sci. 2001;42:1404-10.
9. Casson R, James B, Rubinstein A, Ali H. Clinical comparison of frequency doubling technology perimetry and Humphrey-perimetry. Br J Ophthalmol. 2001;85:360-2.
10. Quigley HA, Dunkelberger GR, Green WR. Retinal ganglion cell atrophy correlated with automated perimetry in human eyes with glaucoma. Am J Ophthalmol. 1989;107:453-64.
11. Kerrigan-Baumrind LA, Quigley HA, Pease ME, Kerrigan DF, Mitchell RS. Number of ganglion cells in glaucoma eyes compared with threshold visual field tests in the same persons. Invest Ophthalmol Vis Sci. 2000;41:741-8.
12. Keltner JL, Johnson CA, Levine RA, Fan J, Cello KE, Kass MA, et al. Normal visual field test results following glaucomatous visual field end points in the Ocular Hypertension Treatment Study. Arch Ophthalmol. 2005;123:1201-6.
13. Maddess T, Henry GH. Performance of nonlinear visual units in ocular hypertension and glaucoma. Clin Vis Sci. 1992;7:371-83.
14. Maddess T, Goldberg I, Dobinson J, Wine S, James AC. Clinical trials of the frequency doubled illusion as an indicator of glaucoma. Invest Ophthalmol Vis Sci. 1995;38:413-25.
15. Johnson CA. Selective versus nonselective losses inglaucoma. J Glaucoma (suppl). 1994;3:S32-S44.
16. Wall M, Johnson CA, Kardon RH, Crabb DP. Use of a continuous probability scale to display visual field damage. Arch Ophthalmol. 2009;127:749-56.
17. Burnstein Y, Ellish NJ, Magbalon M, et al. Comparison of frequency doubling perimetry with humphrey visual field analysis in a glaucoma practice. Am J Ophthalmol. 2000;129:328-33.
18. Anderson AJ, Johnson CA. Frequency-doubling technology perimetry. Ophthalmol Clin North Am. 2003;16:213-25.
19. Turpin A, McKendrick AM, Jhonson CA, Vingrys AJ. Development of efficient threshold technology perimetry using computer simulation. Invest Ophthalmol Vis Sci. 2002;43:322-31.
20. Turpin A, McKendrick AM, Johnson CA, Vingrys AJ. Properties of perimetric threshold estimates from full threshold, ZEST, and SITA-like strategies, as determined by computer simulation. Invest Ophthalmol Vis Sci. 2003;44(11):4787-95.
21. Cello KE, Nelson-Quigg JM, Johnson CA. Frequency doubling technology perimetry for detection of glaucomatous visual field loss. Am J Ophthalmol. 2000;129(3):314-22.
22. Johnson CA, Cioffi GA, Van Buskirk EM. Frequency doubling perimetry using a 24-2 stimulus presentation pattern. OptomVis Sci. 1999;76:571-81.
23. Spry PGD, Hussin HM, Sparrow JM. Clinical evaluation of frequency doubling technology perimetry using the Humphrey matrix 24-2 threshold strategy. Br J Ophthalmol. 2005;89:1031-5.
24. Artes PH, Hutchison DM, Nicolela MT, LeBlanc RP, Chauhan BC. Threshold and variability properties of Matrix

frequency-doubling technology and standard automated perimetry in glaucoma. Invest Ophthalmol Vis Sci. 2005;46:2451-7.
25. Blumenthal EZ, Haddad A, Horani A, Anteby I. The reliability of frequency-doubling perimetry in young children. Ophthalmology. 2004;111(3):435-9.
26. Allen CS, Sponsel WE, Trigo Y, Dirks MS, Flynn WJ. Comparison of the frequency doubling technology screening algorithm and the Humphrey 24-2 SITA-FAST in a large eye screening. Clin Experiment Ophthalmol. 2002;30(1):8-14.
27. Wall M, Neahering RK, Woodward KR. Sensitivity and specificity of frequency doubling perimetry in neuro-ophthalmic disorders: a comparison with conventional automated perimetry. Invest Ophthalmol Vis Sci. 2002;43(4):1277-83.
28. Boden C, Pascual J, Medeiros FA, Aihara M, Weinreb RN, Sample PA. Relationship of SITA and full-threshold standard perimetry to frequency-doubling technology perimetry in glaucoma. Invest Ophthalmol Vis Sci. 2005;46(7):2433-9.
29. Medeiros FA, Sample PA, Weinreb RN. Frequency doubling technology perimetry abnormalities as predictors of glaucomatous visual field loss. Am J Ophthalmol. 2004;137(5):863-71.
30. Landers JA, Goldberg I, Graham SL. Detection of early visual field loss in glaucoma using frequency-doubling perimetry and short-wavelength automated perimetry. Arch Ophthalmol. 2003;121(12):1705-10.
31. Kogure S, Toda Y, Crabb D, Kashiwagi K, Fitzke FW, Tsukahara S. Agreement between frequency doubling perimetry and static perimetry in eyes with high tension glaucoma and normal tension glaucoma. Br J Ophthalmol. 2003;87(5):604-8.
32. Lamparter J, Aliyeva S, Schulze A, Berres M, Pfeiffer N, Hoffmann EM. Standard automated perimetry versus matrix frequency doubling technology perimetry in subjects with ocular hypertension and healthy control subjects. PLoS One. 2013;8(2):e57663.
33. Kim SA, Park CK, Park HL. Comparison between frequency-doubling technology perimetry and standard automated perimetry in early glaucoma. Sci Rep. 2022;12(1):10173.
34. Bradvica M, Biuk D, Štenc Bradvica I, Vinković M, Cerovski B, Barać I. The role of frequency doubling technology perimetry in early detection of diabetic retinopathy. Acta Clin Croat. 2020;59(1):10-18.
35. Richardson QR, Kumar RS, Ramgopal B, Rackenchath MV, A V SD, Mannil SS, et al. Diagnostic Accuracy of Frequency-Doubling Technology and the Moorfields Motion Displacement Test for Glaucoma. Ophthalmol Glaucoma. 2023;6(3):239-46.

CHAPTER 13

Short-wavelength Automated Perimetry

Rengaraj Venkatesh, Palaniswamy Krishnamurthy

■ INTRODUCTION

When compared to traditional white-on-white (W-W) perimetry (standard automated perimetry, or SAP), short-wavelength automated perimetry (SWAP) has been proposed as a potential investigative modality for detecting the presence of visual field defects as well as for detecting progressive field defects before W-W perimetry.

According to histologic studies, ganglion cell loss may be significant, up to 50% before visual abnormalities appear on SAP. Due to significant neural pathway redundancy and the nonselective character of traditional perimetry,[1,2] visual abnormalities could not accurately reflect the underlying neuronal injury. There is evidence that large diameter ganglion cells are lost first in early glaucoma.[2,3] An alternate theory involving redundancy in the visual pathways proposes that the sensitivity to identify early functional loss may be enhanced by selectively targeting a certain group of sparsely distributed ganglion cells.[4-6] These theories have led to the development of newer technologies such as SWAP and frequency doubling technology (FDT) perimetry.

There are various types of retinal ganglion cells such as parvocellular, magnocellular, and koniocellular.[7-9] The parvocellular cells, which make up the majority (80%), transmit mostly information regarding form and color. The koniocellular pathway (5%) is engaged in the transmission of short or blue wavelengths, whereas the magnocellular pathway (15%) is in charge of transmitting information about flicker or motion. The tiny bistratified ganglion cells that terminate in the interlaminar zones of the parvocellular region of the lateral geniculate nucleus (LGN) are thought to be the mediating cells for the processing of the blue stimulus in SWAP.[10] The koniocellular pathways are hypothesized to act as a conduit for the transfer of blue stimuli.

■ TWO-COLOR INCREMENT THRESHOLD

Short-wavelength automated perimetry is the clinical application of the technique developed by Stiles (Stiles WS 1959) to assess the blue-yellow [short-wavelength sensitive (SWS)] chromatic channel.

- *Principle:* On a yellow background with high brightness, a blue stimulus is provided whose peak wavelength is similar to the peak response of blue cones (also known as S-cones). The green, or medium-wavelength sensitive (MWS) cones, and the red, or long-wavelength sensitive (LWS) cones, are saturated (i.e., have a reduced response), and rod activity is simultaneously suppressed while the S-cones are largely unaffected by the high luminance yellow background. As a result, a certain amount of "pure" SWS pathway response can be isolated that is not mediated by either the MWS or the LWS pathways. The koniocellular pathways are hypothesized to act as a conduit for the transmission of this short wavelength.
- *Stimulus and stimulus size:* SWAP utilizes a Goldmann size V (1.8° visual angle) blue stimulus with a narrow band short wavelength interference filter (440-nm peak transmission, with a 15-nm bandwidth), 27-nm half-peak width (HPW) for the Humphrey field analyzer (HFA) and 15-nm HPW for the Octopus.
- *Stimulus duration:* 200 ms
- *Background color:* Yellow background (OG530 Schott filter—a 530-nm short wavelength cut off filter), 100 cd/m^2
- *Stimulus luminance:* HFA—65 apostilbs; Octopus—16 apostilbs
- *Shape of the normal hill of vision:* Slope of the normal hill of vision with age is steeper for SWAP than that of W-W perimetry probably due to reductions in foveal cone pigment, photoreceptor density and ganglion cell density, and morphology. The inferior field of SWAP exhibits higher sensitivity compared to superior field.

- *Gray scale*: Lower sensitivity of the superior field coupled with a greater age-related decline in sensitivity for SWAP leads to a darker appearance of superior field gray scale in SWAP which can mimic an arcuate defect.

Presently amongst the commercially available perimeters, SWAP is available on HFA 850, 860, and Octopus 900 perimeters.

Short-wavelength automated perimetry is essentially a static threshold perimetry in which Goldmann stimuli are delivered in the usual way to calculate threshold values using the full threshold algorithm. The only differences are a different color stimulus and the yellow background. STATPAC is used to analyze the data, and the single-field analysis layout is used to print the findings of the analysis. The glaucoma hemifield test and pattern threshold deviation plot, which are more sensitive indicators of localized glaucomatous damage and unaffected by generalized reduction, have been recommended as key indicators when interpreting the results.

Advantages

- Short-wavelength automated perimetry can detect glaucomatous visual field deficits earlier than standard (W-W) automated perimetry.
- Short-wavelength automated perimetry defects is frequently larger and usually progresses faster.
- Short-wavelength automated perimetry can predict the location of future glaucomatous visual field defects.

Disadvantages

- Higher test–retest variability than SAP.
- More affected by media opacities, making the test less suitable in patients with coexisting cataract or lenticular changes.[11]
- Compared to full threshold of SAP, SWAP requires 2–3 minutes more, which can be associated with patient fatigue and reduced efficiency in clinic patient flow.

Tips for getting better Short-wavelength automated perimetry results are given in **Box 1**.

BOX 1: Tips to increase reliability of short-wavelength automated perimetry test.

- Instructions similar to that of routine perimetry are given to the patient
- Patient given adequate time (few minutes) to adjust to the intense yellow background prior to starting the test
- Patient instructed to press the response button when they see a blue light anywhere in the bowl
- Inform patient that the stimulus may appear slightly different from blue color and could be bluish purplish
- Short trial before the actual test
- Constant monitoring by the technician

Short-wavelength automated perimetry has been found to be useful in the visual field evaluation of patients with diabetic retinopathy and other retinal diseases[12-21] optic neuropathies, prechiasmal, chiasmal, and post chiasmal deficits[22-24] and migraine.[25,26]

The advantages of SWAP testing are enhanced by Swedish interactive threshold algorithm (SITA) SWAP, which incorporates the effective testing methodology of SITA, resulting in considerable reduction of test time (3– 6 minutes per eye).[27,28] It is available only on the 24-2 program. SITA SWAP has its own normative data, and in a small number of eyes tested, it revealed less intersubject variability and increased dynamic range of the procedure. However, these results have not yet been validated in a larger sample.

ROLE OF SWAP IN GLAUCOMA

Compared to traditional (W-W) automated perimetry, SWAP can detect glaucomatous visual field abnormalities earlier,[5,9,29-42] detecting deficiencies in roughly 20–25% of patients at risk of glaucoma who have consistently had normal visual fields outcomes for routine automated perimetry. The pattern of visual field loss corresponds to those that would be expected to occur as a consequence of retinal nerve fiber bundle deficits in glaucoma.[43,44] Furthermore, the extent of SWAP defects is frequently larger than that seen with SAP,[4,45-47] and the progression of SWAP deficits is typically faster than SAP. The ability of SWAP to predict the onset and location of future glaucomatous visual field defects by 3–5 and probably by 10 years is perhaps its biggest advantage.[29-42]

When differentiating glaucomatous optic neuropathy from nonglaucomatous eyes, SWAP demonstrated a very high specificity compared to most of the SDOCT parameters. This would imply that as compared to SDOCT, the SWAP would identify more true normals as nonglaucomatous.[48]

The visual system assessed by SWAP has limited resolution and responds slowly, which may be why many patients still find the test challenging. Even with the best refractive correction, the stimulus frequently appears hazy and does not appear to turn on and off clearly. It is not surprising that there is frequently a learning effect when patients are introduced to SWAP testing, even among people who have extensive experience with SAP testing, because patients are not used to seeing under these circumstances. In addition, compared to evaluating the white cone system, testing the blue cone system results in increased intra- and intertest variability.[49,50]

ROLE OF SWAP IN DIABETIC RETINOPATHY

Short-wavelength automated perimetry is considered an earlier indicator of function loss in ischemic change in DR than SAP. SWAP has been shown to yield more extensive visual field loss than SAP in diabetic changes. This may be based on finding of wild[41] that the blue cone is more susceptible to damage in diabetes. SWAP is a functional test to detect visual field abnormality in patients at high risk of developing Diabetic Retinopathy (DR) where W-W (SAP) still within normal range.[33]

In diabetic patients without retinopathy, SWAP is more sensitive than SAP in detecting more abnormalities. The only variable that influences the mean deviation (MD) of SWAP in diabetic patients is diabetic control, which is reflected by level of glycated hemoglobin (HbA1c).[51] Hence, when overt clinical symptoms of DR are still lacking, SWAP is a better approach compared to SAP.

SWAP—OTHER CLINICAL APPLICATIONS

Neuro-ophthalmology

Compared to SAP, SWAP has manifested more extensive defects in eyes with optic neuritis, multiple sclerosis, and pseudotumor cerebri.[24] In autosomal dominant optic atrophy (ADOA), the blue-target deficits are typically peripheral, which is the difference between SAP and SWAP perimetry and could be a robust indicator of ADOA in both early and late stages of this disease.[22]

Age-related Macular Degeneration

Age-related macular degeneration (AMD) patients with soft drusen had significantly lower sensitivity than those without. Sensitivity was also reduced in those eyes with fellow eyes having a sight threatening complication of AMD. SWAP sensitivity loss is associated with common risk factors for progression to AMD.[19]

Central Serous Chorioretinopathy

In central serous chorioretinopathy (CSC) eyes, difference between retinal sensitivities outside and inside of the serous retinal detachment region was greater in SWAP than W-W perimetry, suggesting that SWAP is more sensitive in detecting structural changes in retina in CSC eyes.[52]

Tamoxifen Toxicity

Years before to the conclusion of the typical 5-year usage regimen, SWAP may exhibit tamoxifen field effects.[53]

REFERENCES

1. Kerrigan-Baumrind LA, Quigley HA, Pease ME, Kerrigan DF, Mitchell RS. Number of ganglion cells in glaucomatous eyes compared with threshold visual field tests in the same persons. Invest Ophthalmol Vis Sci. 2000;41:741-8.
2. Quigley HA, Dunkelberger GR, Green WR. Chronic human glaucoma causing selectively greater loss of large optic nerve fibers. Ophthalmology. 1988;95:357-63.
3. Glovinsky Y, Quigley HA, Dunkelberger GR. Retinal ganglion cell loss is size dependent in experimental glaucoma. Invest Ophthalmol Vis Sci. 1991;32:484-91.
4. Johnson CA, Adams AJ, Casson EJ, Brandt JD. Progression of early glaucomatous visual field loss for blue-on-yellow and standard white-on white automated perimetry. Arch Ophthalmol. 1993;111:651-6.
5. Johnson CA, Adams AJ, Casson EJ, Brandt JD. Blue-on-yellow perimetry can predict the development of glaucomatous visual field loss. Arch Ophthalmol. 1993;111:645-50.
6. Johnson CA, Samuels SJ. Screening for glaucomatous visual field loss with frequency-doubling perimetry. Invest Ophthalmol Vis Sci. 1997;38:413-25.
7. Kaplan E, Benardete E. The dynamics of primate retinal ganglion cells. Prog Brain Res. 2001;134:17-34.
8. Curcio CA, Allen KA. Topography of ganglion cells in human retina. J Comp Neurol. 1990;300:5-25.
9. Johnson CA. Selective versus nonselective losses in glaucoma. J Glaucoma. 1994;3:532-44.
10. Martin PR, White AJ, Goodchild AK, Wilder HD, Sefton AE. Evidence that blue-on cells are part of the third geniculocortical pathway in primates. Eur J Neurosci. 1997;9(7):1536-41.
11. Horn FK, Brenning A, Jünemann AG, Lausen B. Glaucoma detection with frequency doubling perimetry and short-wavelength perimetry. J Glaucoma. 2007;16:363-71.
12. Gilmore ED, Hudson C, Nrusimhadevara RK, Harvey PT. Frequency of seeing characteristics of the short wavelength sensitive visual pathway in clinically normal subjects and diabetic patients with focal sensitivity loss. Br J Ophthalmol. 2005;89:1462-7.
13. Razeghinejad MR, Torkaman F, Amini H. Blue-yellow perimetry can be an early detector of hydroxychloroquine and chloroquine retinopathy. Med Hypotheses. 2005;65:629-30.
14. Jacobson SG, Marmor MF, Kemp CM, Knighton RW. SWS (blue) cone hypersensitivity in a newly identified retinal degeneration. Invest Ophthalmol Vis Sci. 1990;31:827-38.
15. Sakai T, Iida K, Tanaka Y, Kohzaki K, Kitahara K. Evaluation of S-cone sensitivity in reattached macula following macula-off retinal detachment surgery. Jpn J Ophthalmol. 2005;49:301-5.
16. Han Y, Adams AJ, Bearse MA, Schneck ME. Multifocal electro-retinogram and short-wavelength automated perimetry measures in diabetic eyes with little or no retinopathy. Arch Ophthalmol. 2004;122:1809-15.
17. Afrashi F, Erakgun T, Kose S, Ardic K, Mentes J. Blue-on-yellow perimetry versus achromatic perimetry in type I diabetes patients without retinopathy. Diabetes Res Clin Pract. 2003;61:7-11.
18. Remky A, Weber A, Hendricks S, Lichtenberg K, Arend O. Shot-wavelength automated perimetry in patients with diabetes mellitus without macular edema. Graefes Arch Clin Exp Ophthalmol. 2003;241:468-71.
19. Remky A, Lichtenberg K, Elsner AE, Arend O. Short-wavelength automated perimetry in age-related maculopathy. Br J Ophthalmol. 2001;85:1432-6.
20. Remky A, Arend O, Hendricks S. Short-wavelength automated perimetry and capillary density in early diabetic maculopathy. Invest Ophthalmol Vis Sci. 2000;41:274-81.
21. Hudson C, Flanagan JG, Turner GS, Chen HC, Young LB, McLeod D. Short-wavelength sensitive visual field loss in patients with clinically significant diabetic macular oedema. Diabetologia. 1998;41:918-28.
22. Walters JW, Gaume A, Pate L. Short wavelength automated perimetry compared with standard achromatic perimetry in

autosomal dominant optic atrophy. Br J Ophthalmol. 2006; 90:1267-70.
23. Corallo G, Cicinelli S, Papadia, M, Bandini F, Uccelli A, Calabria G. Conventional perimetry, short-wavelength automated perimetry, frequency doubling technology and visual evoked potentials in the assessment of patients with multiple sclerosis. Eur J Ophthalmol. 200515:730-8.
24. Keltner JL, Johnson CA, Short Wavelength Automated Perimetry (SWAP) in neuro-ophthalmologic disorders. Arch Ophthalmol. 1995;113:475-81.
25. Yenice O, Temel A, Incili B, Tuncer N. Short wavelength automated perimetry in patients with migraine. Grafes Arch Clin Exp Ophthalmol. 2006;244:589-95.
26. McKendrick AM, Cioffi GA, Johnson CA, Short-wavelength sensitivity deficits in patients with migraine. Arch Ophthalmol. 2002;120:154-61.
27. Bengtsson B. A new rapid algorithm for short-wavelength automated perimetry. Invest Ophthalmol Vis Sci. 2003;44:1388-94.
28. Bengtsson B, Heijl A. Normal intersubject threshold variability and normal limits of the SITA SWAP and full threshold SWAP perimetric programs. Invest Ophthalmol Vis Sci. 2003;44:5029-34.
29. Sit AJ, Medieros FA. Weibren RN. Short-wavelength automated perimetry can predict glaucomatous standard visual field loss by ten years. Semin Ophthalmol. 2004;19:122-4.
30. Mansberger SL, Sample PA, Zangwill LM, Weinreb RN. Achromatic and short-wavelength automated perimetry in patients with glaucomatous large cups. Arch Ophthalmol. 1999;117:1473-7.
31. Johnson CA. The diagnostic value of short wavelength automated perimetry (SWAP). Curr Opin Ophthalmol. 1996;7:54-8.
32. Demirel S, Johnson CA. Short wavelength automated perimetry (SWAP) in ophthalmic practice. J Am Optom Assoc. 1996;67:451-6.
33. Demirel S, Johnson CA. Incidence and prevalence of short wavelength automated perimetry deficits in ocular hypertensive patients. Am J Ophthalmol. 2001;131:709-15.
34. Johnson CA, Brandt JD, Khong AM, Adams AJ. Short wavelength automated perimetry (SWAP) in low, medium and high risk ocular hypertensives: Initial baseline findings. Arch Ophthalmol. 1995;113:70-6.
35. Casson EJ, Johnson CA, Shapiro LR. A longitudinal comparison of temporal modulation perimetry to white-on-white and blue-on-yellow perimetry in ocular hypertension and early glaucoma. J Opt Soc Am A Opt Image Sci Vis. 1993;10:1792-806.
36. Sample PA, Weinreb RN. Color perimetry for assessment of primary open angle glaucoma. Invest Ophthalmol Vis Sci. 1990;31:1869-75.
37. Landers J, Goldberg I, Graham S. A comparison of short wavelength automated perimetry with frequency doubling perimetry for the early detection of visual field loss in ocular hypertension. Clin Experiment Ophthalmol. 2000;28:248-52.
38. Johnson CA. Recent developments in automated perimetry in glaucoma diagnosis and management. Curr Opin Ophthalmol. 2002;13(2):77-84.
39. Sample PA, Medieros FA, Racette L, Pascual J, Boden C, Zangwill LM, et al. Identifying glaucomatous vision loss with visual function specific perimetry in the diagnostic innovations in glaucoma study. Invest Ophthalmol Vis Sci. 2006;47:3381-89.
40. Lewis RA, Johnson CA, Adams AJ. Automated static visual field testing and perimetry of short-wavelength-sensitive (SWS) mechanisms in patients with asymmetric intraocular pressures. Graefe's Arch Clin Exp Ophthalmol. 1993;231:274-8.
41. Wild JM. Short wavelength automated perimetry. Acta Ophthalmol Scand. 2001;79:546-59.
42. Racette L, Sample PA. Short wavelength automated perimetry. Ophthalmol Clin North Am. 2003;16:227-36.
43. Adams AJ, Johnson CA, Lewis RA. S cone pathway sensitivity loss in ocular hypertension and early glaucoma has nerve fiber bundle pattern. In: Drum, Moreland, Serra, (Eds). Proceedings of the 10th Symposium of the International Research Group on Colour Vision Deficiencies. The Netherlands: Kluwer Academic Publishers; 1991. pp. 535-42.
44. Landers J, Sharma A, Goldberg I, Graham S. Topography of the frequency doubling perimetry visual field compared with that of short wavelength and achromatic automated perimetry visual fields. Br J Ophthalmol. 2006;90:70-4.
45. Landers JA, Goldberg I, Graham SL. Detection of early visual field loss in glaucoma using frequency-doubling perimetry and short-wavelength automated perimetry. Arch Ophthalmol. 2003;121:1705-10.
46. Bayer AU, Erb C. Short wavelength automated perimetry, frequency doubling technology perimetry, and pattern electroretinography for prediction of progressive glaucomatous standard visual field defects. Ophthalmology. 2002; 109(5):1009-17.
47. Soliman MA, de Jong LAMS, Ismaeil AAA, van den Berg TJT, de Smet MC. Standard achromatic perimetry, short wavelength automated perimetry, and frequency doubling technology for detection of glaucoma damage. Ophthalmology. 2002;109(3): 444-54.
48. Kalyani VK, Bharucha KM, Goyal N, Deshpande MM. Comparison of diagnostic ability of standard automated perimetry, short wavelength automated perimetry, retinal nerve fiber layer thickness analysis and ganglion cell layer thickness analysis in early detection of glaucoma. Indian J Ophthalmol. 2021;69(5):1108-12.
49. Blumenthal EZ, Sample PA, Zangwill L, Lee AC, Kono Y, Weinreb RN. Comparison of long-term variability for standard and short-wavelength automated perimetry in stable glaucoma patients. Am J Ophthalmol. 2000;129(3):309-13.
50. Kwon YH, Park HJ, Jap A, Ugurlu S, Caprioli J. Test-retest variability of blue-on-yellow perimetry in normal subjects. Am J Ophthalmol. 1998;126(1):29-36.
51. Zico OA, El-Shazly AA, Abdel-Hamid Ahmed EE. Short wavelength automated perimetry can detect visual field changes in diabetic patients without retinopathy. Indian J Ophthalmol. 2014;62:383-7.
52. Zhou HP, Asaoka R, Inoue T, Asano S, Murata H, Hara T, et al. Short wavelength automated perimetry and standard automated perimetry in central serous chorioretinopathy. Sci Rep. 2020;10:16451.
53. Eisner A, Austin DF, Samples JR. Short wavelength automated perimetry and tamoxifen use. Br J Ophthalmol. 2004;88(1):125-30.

CHAPTER 14

Integrating Technologies: Current Status

Shibal Bhartiya, Parul Ichhpujani, Oscar Albis-Donado, Faisal TT

INTRODUCTION

The word *"integration"* comes from the Latin word integer, which means "to complete" and "integrated" implies "reunited parts of a whole". Integrating or bringing together of elements or separate components, which include processes and technologies that simplify and improve healthcare delivery, is a step toward revolutionizing existing health systems, and patient-care outcomes.

INTEGRATION OF TECHNOLOGY IN PATIENT CARE

Health systems and healthcare institutions are complex entities; therefore, integration involves a coherent set of methods for not only funding, administration and organizational service delivery but also at clinical levels. Integration of all these processes endeavors to create connectivity, alignment, and collaboration within and between the cure and care sectors that, together with feedback loops, is the need of the hour.

Although it has been stressed by many authors and consensus that any functional change in glaucoma needs to be correlated by a structural change, it has not been a universal practice, especially because the correlation is not always easy to perform. Anatomical variation in the shape and size of the optic nerve tends to introduce a lot of noise and variation when an integrated interpretation is attempted, both clinically and with imaging. An additional correlation with changes in the ganglion cell layer or complex can be sought, but this area will only reflect changes in the central 20° of the visual field.[1-6]

A standardized manual system or method for performing a structural-functional correlation has not been available, although several have been attempted with Heidelberg Retinal Tomography (HRT) with variable degrees of success.

An experienced practitioner may be able to achieve this integration with a reasonable degree of success for most of his/her patients, but always keeping in mind the degree of test-retest variability for both types of studies.

The goal of integrating technologies is to enhance quality of care, consumer satisfaction, and system efficiency for both patients and physicians.

A technology that can improve functional-structural correlation should also be able to integrate to the existing health record system, and should be able to improve the diagnostic and prognostic efficiency of the practice.[1-13]

Logic

Better Efficiency

An automated glaucoma practice system not only improves an office's day-to-day efficiency, but also elevates the quality-of-care clinicians deliver to their patients. It also optimizes utilization of resources—both technological and manpower, thereby proving to be cost-effective in the long term.

Checks and Balances

Maintaining patient data on paper charts is cumbersome, time consuming, and often inefficient. Other tedious tasks involved in recordkeeping include recording routine examinations, generating prescriptions for medications as well as glasses, sending referral letters to primary care physicians and other specialists, as well as responding to patient emergency queries on phone. It is worse for multilocation practices as they spend a lot of resources, in addition to time, to send paper records from one location to another.

Electronic health records (EHR) are efficient solutions for this, they decrease the data capture time from diagnostic devices, and provide accurate, quick, and paperless documentation. They also ensure superior ICD coding levels, clinical decision support systems, and alerts. In addition to this, EHRs also generate accurate, legible medication prescriptions, follow-up schedules, as well as insurance-related data, making the patient journey seamless and easy.[5,6]

Compliance and Adherence

An integrated system can help to identify which glaucoma patients are not regular with follow-up appointments and send them reminders from within the system. In countries, where electronic prescribing to pharmacies is the trend, it has not only helped in making the practice paperless, they also increase both efficiency and convenience for clinic staff, and patients alike. They also help monitor compliance and adherence—the clinician can track if the patient has filled a prescription on schedule or not.

Follow-up Reminders

Glaucoma is a chronic, slowly progressing disease, and typically in the elderly, with issues of compliance and adherence plaguing almost every practice across the globe, electronic reminders and monitoring can have a positive impact on patient outcomes.

Keeping track of scheduled appointments and reminders has been a successful strategy in improving patient compliance and also in improving doctor/patient rapport, since the patient feels a sense of commitment by the doctor and/or by the practice.

Electronic Medical Records/Electronic Health Records

Electronic medical records (EMRs) or EHRs are web-based or intranet-based computer platforms or software packages designed to partially or completely eliminate paper records. Glaucomatologists need intensive image management with visual fields, Optical Coherence Tomography (OCT), Heidelberg retinal tomography (HRT), optic nerve pictures, etc. The EMR, therefore, can enable integrated image acquisition, helping the various devices to "talk" to each other, whereby the data from each of these sources can be interpreted synchronously. These therefore essentially must provide both equipment interfaces and image viewing and integration systems.

These systems run directly within an internet browser with extremely low bandwidth requirements, with data on a series of servers in a remote location. Large "server farms," or clouds, are instrumental is providing an increased efficiency, data safety, and reliability. These systems may be used with any computing devices including computers, tablets, and any operating system including Windows, Mac OS, or Android.

Cost Benefit[6]

- *Patient perspective:* Glaucoma is a chronic asymptomatic disease that slowly progresses; and the progression is difficult to demonstrate to a patient as there are no symptoms. If the physician is able to show a patient concrete evidence in the form of say, serial visual field changes or disc photos, the patient can understand the progression better. The serial follow-up pictures can help the patient to understand the changes in the optic nerve head (structural) or visual fields (functional). Patient comprehension additionally may help to encourage patient adherence with medication use.
- *Clinicians' perspective:* Since glaucoma is a disease characterized by asymptomatic progression of structural and functional damage, the serial follow-ups on visual display can help the doctor in formulating clinical decisions. The overview of intraocular pressure (IOP) overtime, peak, target, and fluctuation of IOP and can be represented graphically over the glaucoma progression timeline. It streamlines practice compared to thumbing through paper files to compare numbers, saving time, and increasing efficiency.

Intranet and Medical Records

Efficient user interface designs in the EMR/EHR eliminate visual "noise" because too much information on the screen leads to waste of time when one is searching for that a particular piece of information that is really needed at that moment. Certain systems have a built-in IOP adjustment for pachymetry, displaying both recorded IOPs, and those with corneal correction; since all IOP readings also record the time at which it was recorded, diurnal phasing or variation of IOP can also be ascertained.

The screen depicts the dates and results of previous glaucoma investigations and a summary of all the results. The system may also plot the graphs for IOP, with or without a synchronous plot of medications, and treatments (laser or surgical).

■ GLAUCOMA MANAGEMENT PARADIGM

Most diagnostic devices were not capable of integration with EMR systems. The cumbersome process of print outs which are to be uploaded to the patient's file after scanning, can now be substituted by a single integrated system. With progression analyses being built into most glaucoma investigations including visual fields and retinal nerve fiber layer (RNFL) OCT, documenting and monitoring progression have become simpler, easier, and more objective.

Use of Macros

A macro is a small computer program, made a part of any software. It can be used to trigger a response when some events take place, or some conditions are met. Recently, macros are being used in the system to highlight patient defaults, to prepopulate laser settings for procedures such as trabeculoplasty, and standardize postoperative medication charts. Say, a middle age, one eyed, primary open angle glaucoma patient, has increasingly high IOP on three medications, the system will potentially flag him for possible selective laser trabeculoplasty (SLT), if IOP is climbing on current treatment.

■ VISUAL FIELD PROGRESSION

- *Glaucoma progression analysis (GPA) and EyeSuite:* Computer-assisted analysis programs have been developed with the intent of improving progression assessment. It is believed that these programs correct the "noise" and the distraction of variability in visual field data. This in turn can reveal changes within the data that indicate true progression, which would otherwise be difficult for a skilled human analyzer to detect.
- *Glaucoma progression analysis:* The GPA software enables the serial evaluation of visual fields by identifying areas of progression.

Unlike the older HFA algorithm, the GPA uses pattern deviation plot values and not the total deviation. The delta in the latter is often influenced by factors other than glaucoma (including cataract progression and reduced size of the pupils). The GPA , therefore, specifically delineates the localized change associated with glaucoma, not representing any diffuse glaucomatous change.

Any new localized glaucomatous defects or the expansion and deepening of existing defects are best delineated using the GPA.

An open triangle marks the location of change in a follow-up visual field. The GPA software is capable of assessing the next visual fields for the repeatability of the change, automatically. If the change is found to be present and consistent on two consecutive tests, it is represented by a half-filled triangle. In case the change is repeatable even on three consecutive tests, it is represented by a closed triangle.

The repeatability of three or more points is then tested and the GPA Alert report of *"possible progression"* is given if two consecutive fields show the same three or more points changed from baseline. In case, three consecutive fields show change at the same three or more points the machine flags it as *"likely progression"*.

Advantages

- **Quick Summary:** The Visual Field Index™ (VFI), summarizes the visual field status expressed as a percentage of the presumed normal age-adjusted visual field.[3] So as to correlate with ganglion cell density and visual function, it is weighted more at the center, and therefore, is not affected by cataract and other media changes as much. The VFI is represents the rate of progression, and is plotted relative to patient age, so that the rate of functional loss may be calculated. The VFI Plot, therefore, enables linear regression analysis of the VFI overtime. This analysis, however, requires at least five tests over 3 years. The VFI bar also projects the rate of progression up to a maximum of 5 years, depending on the available GPA data.
  - *EyeSuite:* With EyeSuite Perimetry, trend analysis can be obtained with specific and comprehensive graphs. Other advantages of using EyeSuite include global and cluster progression rates, with a quick overview which displays a series for both eyes. The printout is more intuitive with a color code for significant change making for easier and faster understanding of the change. It also provides a structure and function correlation and cluster analysis, as well as a trend analysis for specific areas of the visual field/display of both eyes. The EyeSuite can import and convert Humphrey visual field data both for progression analysis versus Octopus data, and for structure-function (S-F) correlation.
  - *Serial disc photography:* Stereoscopic analysis of disc photographs will soon be standard of care. Software that permits analysis by flicking between old and new stereo photographs has become available and has demonstrated to be a valuable tool for improving detection of change by observers.
- *Visual field and OCT (S-F) correlation:*
  - *Forum glaucoma workplace:* Carl Zeiss Meditec has introduced a new image management system software product, FORUM Viewer. This PC program holds and displays many types of printouts and images from a variety of imaging devices **(Fig. 1)**. It centralizes images from OCT, fundus and anterior segment cameras, perimeters, and other devices **(Figs. 2 to 4)**. The FORUM Glaucoma Workplace application automatically combines structure and function numerical data from the HFA perimeter and Cirrus OCT; it streamlines assessment by improving clinical case visualization. The GPA summary automatically allows analysis of progression.

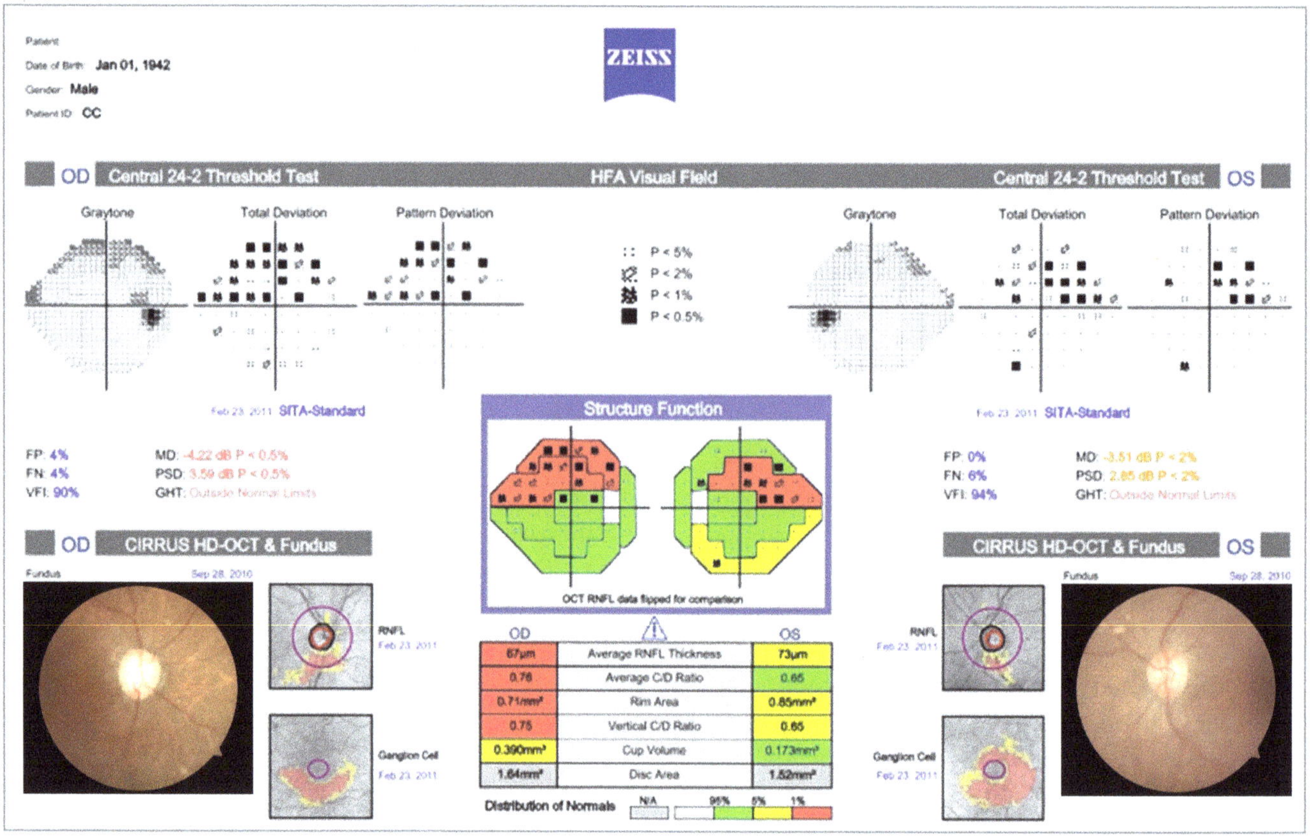

Fig. 1: Structure-function correlation.

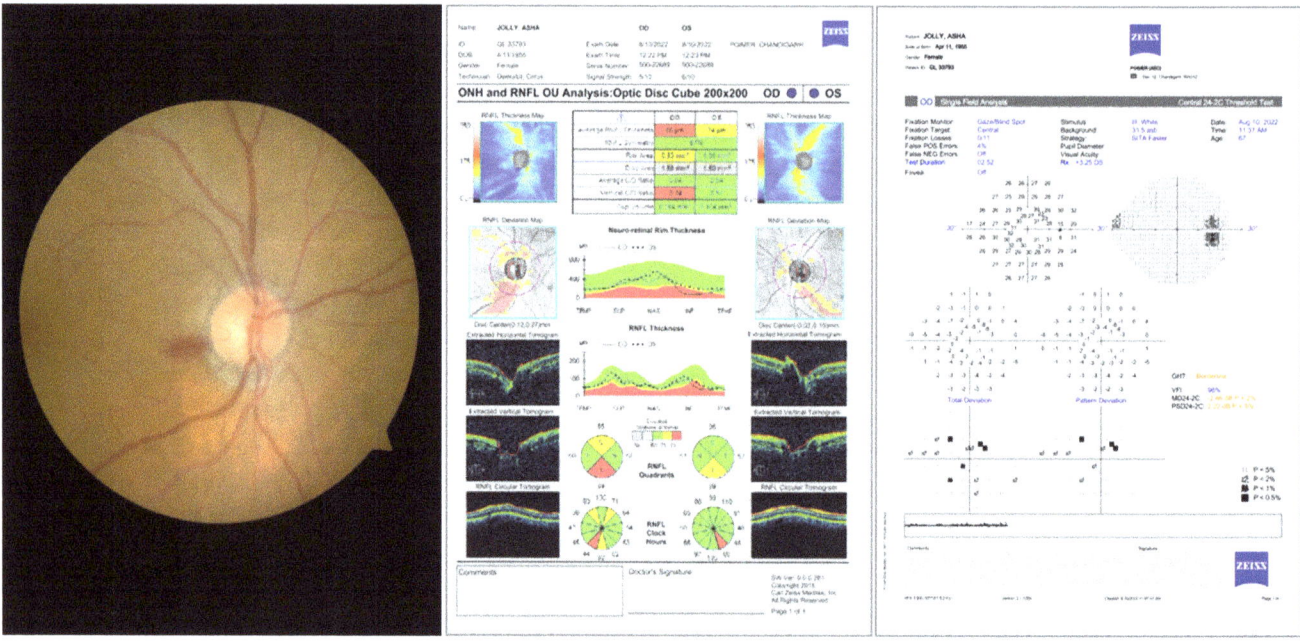

Fig. 2: Showing optic disc photo, OCT and Humphry automated visual field of the same eye in a single window of FORUM workplace.

Baseline examinations can be chosen manually and any outliers removed from the analysis. Moreover, the serial overview of visual field examinations also helps in clinical decision making.

Retinal nerve fiber layer segmental deviation maps are combined with pattern deviation results from HFA visual fields using a methodology published by Garway-Heath et al.[7]

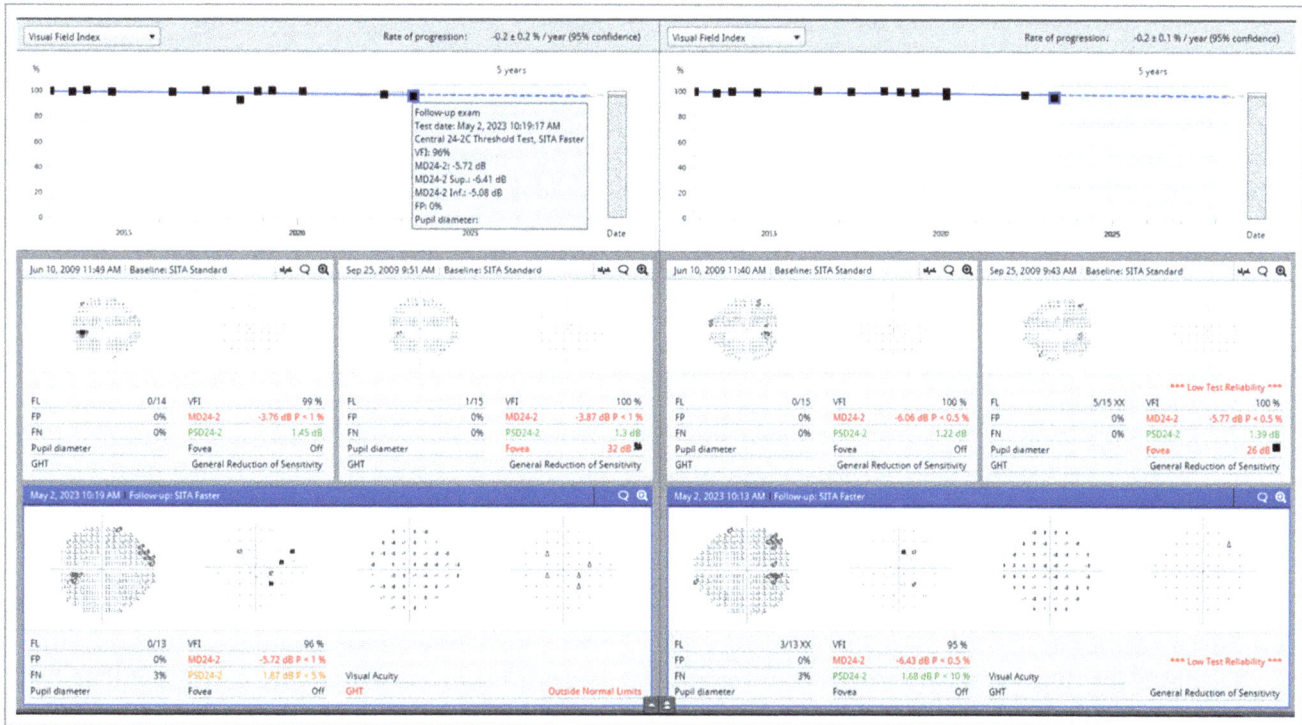

Fig. 3: Drop box contains various test details on keeping cursor at a particular test visit. Top row shows VFI data, middle row shows global indices with SITA Standard strategy while bottom row shows data with switch to a newer strategy, SITA Faster. (SITA: Swedish interactive threshold algorithm; VFI: visual field index)

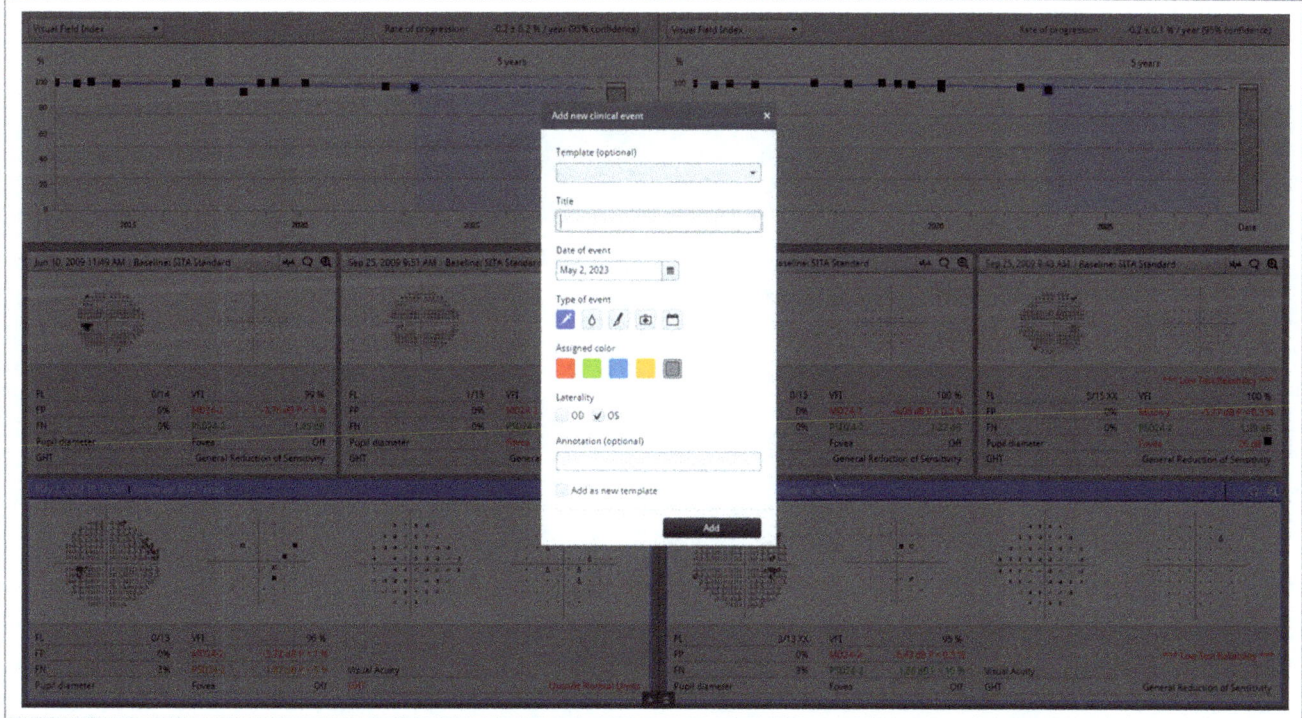

Fig. 4: Showing comment box for adding various clinical events at a particular visit.

A recent study has shown that the applicability of a S-F analysis combining Spectral-Domain (SD)-OCT and standard automated perimetry (SAP) has improved diagnostic values of glaucoma screening.

- *SPECTRALIS platform:* SPECTRALIS has enhanced the role of SD-OCT by integrating it with confocal scanning laser ophthalmoscopy (CSLO). The combination of these two technologies has enabled new imaging capabilities providing clinicians with unique views of the structure and function of the eye along with noise reduction, and an upgradable hardware platform.

HEYEX 2 is the image management software module of Heidelberg Eye Explorer that connects and operates all Heidelberg Engineering products, SPECTRALIS, ANTERION, and HRT.[9] Every workstation provides access to the clinical tools available at the acquisition station, and instant access to images and patient data.

- *Topcon platform:* Topcon Harmony connects all diagnostic instruments, regardless of manufacturer, in one secure, web-based platform. It supports both artificial intelligence integrations and analytics along with telehealth **(Fig. 5)**.[10]

Each platform has special features and strengths that enable the importing of images from other sites. While the Carl Zeiss's Forum provides superior field analytics, the Topcon Harmony offers better cloud features enabling superior shared care.

- *Human error:* Automated data entry directly from the diagnostic devices, along with clinical decision support systems and alerts for critical medication decrease human error. When comparing two different time points of OCT data printouts at times, it is difficult to read on smaller screens. The larger screens allow for better resolution, legibility, and understanding.
- *Paperless workplace:* Since the integrating platforms capture images digitally, and store them on servers (often cloud based), they can be accessed anywhere using the internet. This enables secure data sharing and storage across facilities and geographies.
- *Single worksheet* which enables the clinician to have all the record on file in an easy to interpret, and easy to demonstrate, and accessible format.
- *Cross referrals:* Most EMR systems also generate letters and prescriptions for primary care and referring physicians, as well as pharmacies, opticians, and other care providers. These letters can be transmitted via Health Insurance Portability and Accountability Act (HIPAA) compliant emails in real time, or as letters sent after printing.

CHALLENGES AND THE FUTURE

Over the next few years, the integrating platforms will have an improved Digital Imaging and Communications in Medicine (DICOM) compliance. DICOM is a standard for handling, storing, printing, and transmitting information in medical

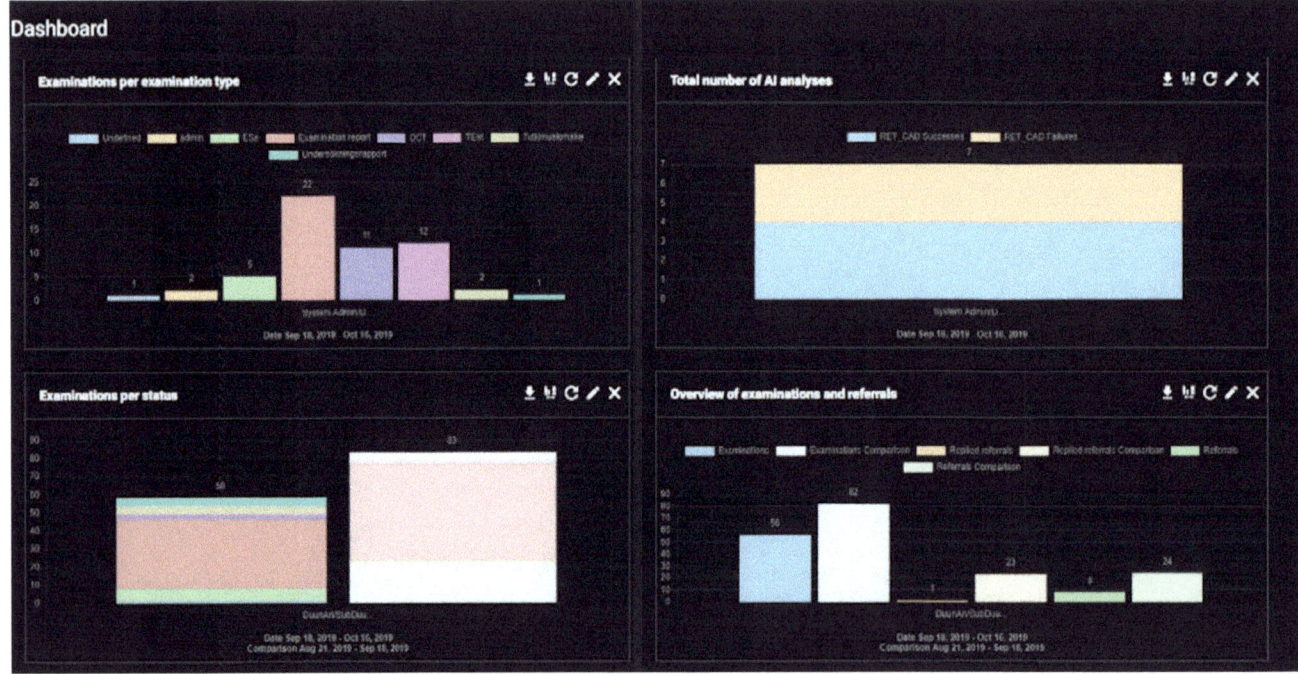

Fig. 5: Topcon Harmony Health analytics.
Source: https://topconhealthcare.in

imaging. Critical to DICOM are the file format definition and network communications protocols. The latter is an application protocol that uses TCP/IP to communicate between various devices that are otherwise incompatible. DICOM files can be exchanged between any two devices that have the technology to receive patient data, including images, in DICOM format. Most diagnostic equipment in ophthalmology have been ratified for DICOM standards and several manufacturers are attempting to incorporate the same. This includes enabling connectivity into the hardware and DICOM-compliant output into the software. For now, their use in current glaucoma practice is only limited by their costs: as the devices become cheaper, integrated technologies are fast becoming the standard of care.[11-13]

CONCLUSION

Artificial intelligence has captured the imagination of clinicians and patients alike, with the simultaneous maturation of digital and telecommunications technologies. The integration of various diagnostic device outputs, therefore, is critical for the automated processing of large data sets, including the classification, segmentation, and enhancement of ocular images, and synchronous processing of other clinical parameters. This along with autonomous deep learning algorithms, has the potential to revolutionize detection and monitoring of disease patterns, as well as prognosticate glaucoma progression.[12,13]

REFERENCES

1. Myung JS, Gelman R, Aaker GD, Radcliffe NM, Chan RV, Chiang MF. Evaluation of vascular disease progression in retinopathy of prematurity using static and dynamic retinal images. Am J Ophthalmol. 2012;153(3):544-51.e2.
2. Liu J, Zhang Z, Wong DW, Xu Y, Yin F, Cheng J, et al. Automatic glaucoma diagnosis through medical imaging informatics. J Am Med Inform Assoc. 2013;20(6):1021-7.
3. Bengtsson B, Heijl A. A visual field index for calculation of glaucoma rate of progression. Am J Ophthalmol. 2008;145(2):343-53.
4. Leung CK, Cheung CY, Weinreb RN, Qiu K, Liu S, Li H, et al. Evaluation of retinal nerve fiber layer progression in glaucoma: a study on optical coherence tomography guided progression analysis. Invest Ophthalmol Vis Sci. 2010;51(1):217-22.
5. Silverstone DE, Paek HM, Kogan Y, Essaihi A, Shiffman RN. Incorporation of clinical practice guidelines for glaucoma into an ophthalmology electronic medical record. AMIA Annu Symp Proc. 2005;2005:1115.
6. Barlow S, Johnson J, Steck J. The economic effect of implementing an EMR in an outpatient clinical setting. J Healthc Inf Manag. 2004;18(1):46-51.
7. Garway-Heath DF, Poinoosawmy D, Fitzke FW, Hitchings RA. Mapping the visual field to the optic disk in normal tension glaucoma eyes. Ophthalmology. 2000;107(10):1809-15.
8. Karvonen E, Stoor K, Luodonpää M, Hägg P, Leiviskä I, Liinamaa J, et al. Combined structure–function analysis in glaucoma screening. Br J Ophthalmol. 2022;106:1689-95.
9. Heidelberg Engineering. (2023). HEYEX 2. [online] Available from: https://business-lounge.heidelbergengineering.com/us/en/products/heidelberg-eye-explorer/heyex-2/ [Last accessed July, 2023]
10. Topcon Healthcare Solutions. (2022). Discover Harmony. [online] Available from: https://topconhealthcare.jp/wp-content/uploads/2022/12/M000031E-5AP_Topcon-Harmony-12-page-brochure-ENG-for-web.pdf (Last accessed July, 2023].
11. Haider D. (2020). Transferring imaging from primary to secondary care (part 2). [online] Available from: https://www.eyenews.uk.com/reviews/tech-reviews/post/transferring-imaging-from-primary-to-secondary-care-part-2 [Last accessed July, 2023]
12. Mursch-Edlmayr AS, Ng WS, Diniz-Filho A, Sousa DC, Arnold L, Schlenker MB, et al. Artificial Intelligence Algorithms to Diagnose Glaucoma and Detect Glaucoma Progression: Translation to Clinical Practice. Transl Vis Sci Technol. 2020;9(2):55.
13. Bhartiya S. Glaucoma Screening: Is AI the Answer? J Curr Glaucoma Pract. 2022;16(2):71-3.

CHAPTER 15A

Recent Advances in Perimetry

Parul Ichhpujani, Hennaav Dhillon

■ INTRODUCTION

Testing of the visual fields (VF) is the only method to quantify the extent of functional loss in glaucoma patients. Standard automated perimetry (SAP) using the Humphrey field analyzer (HFA) Swedish interactive threshold algorithm (SITA) Standard and SITA Fast program are widely accepted as gold standard. However, due to inherent disadvantages such as bulky nature and limited portability in addition to being costly and requiring trained personnel to run it, portable virtual reality (VR) headset perimetry and tablet perimetry tests are gaining popularity as an alternate form of VF testing.

■ VIRTUAL REALITY PERIMETRY

In 1962, Morton Heilig created the first true VR system, the multimodal theater system, "*Sensorama*".[1] In the era of multidimensional viewing and VR, several technology enthusiasts and innovators have joined hands with ophthalmologists to develop various devices.

Virtual reality is an upcoming field in ophthalmology and is gaining significant importance in the aspects of ophthalmic surgical training especially microsurgical procedures (Eyesi Surgical Trainer, VRmagic, Mannheim, Germany[2] and MicroVisTouch, ImmersiveTouch, Chicago, Illinois),[3] as a teaching tool such as VR ophthalmoscopy (Eyesi Direct and Indirect Ophthalmoscope),[4,5] amblyopia and strabismus diagnosis and management (Oculus Rift VR headset, FOVE VR Headset),[6,7] perimetry (head mounted perimeters,[8,9] and low visual aids (Microsoft HoloVision).[10]

■ PROCEDURE FOR VIRTUAL REALITY PERIMETRY

The patient is made to wear the VR headset while being comfortably seated or lying down and holds a wireless clicker to respond to visual stimuli. The operator activates the head set from their controls on a tablet. This displays a visual acuity, and the VFs are started. The patient keeps both eyes open and looks at the fixation point while the stimuli are displayed in the periphery. The patient is supposed to press the clicker button when the patient sees the stimuli with the live result being display on the tablet continuously. Once, the test for both the eyes is completed, the final report is displayed and can be exported/printed as a PDF file. The test can be paused by removing the headset at any time.

The overview of the VR perimetry devices is given in **Table 1**.

■ COMPARISON OF VR PERIMETRY WITH SAP (HUMPHREY VISUAL FIELD)

Matsumoto C et al., used the head mounted VR perimeter "imo" and found that the mean sensitivity obtained by the Humphrey visual field (HVF) analyzer highly correlated with the mean sensitivity by the "imo" monocular test device (R:r = 0.96, L:r = 0.94, $p < 0.001$). The mean sensitivity value by the monocular and binocular random single eye tests also highly correlated (R:r = 0.96, L:r = 0.95, $p < 0.001$).[14] They concluded that "imo" had highly comparable results with HVF in patients with established glaucoma.

In another study, on C3FA, Mees et al. observed that the number of stimuli missed on the C3FA correlated with the HVF mean deviation (r = 0.62, $p < 0.001$) and with pattern standard deviation (r = 0.36, $p < 0.001$). They concluded that the C3FA did not reliably identify deficits that matched the HVF, but was moderately effective at identifying glaucoma subjects.[8]

Tablet Perimetry

With the advent of improved technology in the newer tablets, viz., high spatial resolution, large dynamic luminance range, and 8-bit luminance control, the tablets can now be used for perimetry test.

TABLE 1: Overview of the VR perimetry devices.			
S. No.	Device name	Manufacturer	Features
1.	Periscreener[11]	Aravind Eye Hospital and Vellore Institute of Technology	• Low-cost Google cardboard headset, two Android smartphones, bluetooth wireless clicker • Only suprathreshold testing • Prototype device
2.	Virtual Eye[12]		• Eye tracking perimeter—VisualGrasp • Equivalent to 24-2 threshold field
3.	VIP Visual Fields[13]	Arieh Solomon, Tel Aviv, Israel	• Only suprathreshold testing • Prototype device
4.	Vivid Vision Perimetry[14]	Matsumoto et al. Vivid Vision Inc, imo.	• Oculokinetic perimetry • VVP Swift test can generate reproducible results as Humphrey visual field 24-2 • Platform independent • https://www.perimetry.seevividly.com/
5.	VF2000 NEO	Micro Medical Devices Inc.	• Full and fast thresholds VF testing plus neuro and ptosis • FDT testing • Stereopsis testing • Contrast sensitivity testing • https://micromedinc.com/vf2000-visual-field-analyzer/
6.	Virtual Field[12]	Virtual Field Inc.	• https://www.virtualfield.io/
7.	Advanced Vision Analyser[12]	AVA; Elisar Vision Technology	• Optical system is dichoptic • Monocular field of view for each eye is 60° • Uses Elisar standard algorithm • https://www.elisar.com/
8.	Visual Field Visualizer[15]	Nyugen et al.[15]	• Only Suprathreshold testing • home.virtualfield.io
9.	Telemedicine visual field test	Tsapakis et al.[16]	• Low cost, fast threshold 3 dB step staircase algorithm for central 24° field (52 points) • Uses web camera as a "virtual photometer" and requires an Android phone with 6-inch screen • Based on Microsoft's. NET technology as well as on Google's Android platform • Free software: info@visual-field.com
10.	Mobile Virtual Perimetry (MVP)	Karma Alawa et al.[9]	• Frequency doubling technology with the C-20 testing pattern • Comparable to Humphrey Matrix
11.	C3FA-C3 Field Analyzer[17]	Alfaleus Technology Pvt. Ltd, India with Remidio	• Threshold field testing • Rechargeable battery pack with no external power supply and internet need
12.	Pupil Perimetry[8]		• Measures amplitude or latency of pupillary responses using infrared pupillometry • Use VEPs that give an objective patient response
13.	nGoggle[18]	Ngoggle, Inc, San Diego, California, USA	Uses a brain–computer interface (BCI) using electroencephalogram (EEG) multifocal steady state VEP to detect patient response to eliminate errors like false positives and negatives to improve test reliability

Visual Fields Easy

Visual Fields Easy (VFE) application is the first free, iPad (Apple, Cupertino, CA) suprathreshold perimetric screening application. The VFE program tests 96 VF locations within the central 30°, using a background luminance of 31.5 apostilbs (10 cd/m^2), a size V target (when placed at 33 cm test distance) and a 16 dB suprathreshold static perimetry target (**Figs. 1A and B**). A red fixation point is presented to one corner of the display and one VF quadrant is assessed, followed by movement of the fixation point to the other corners of the display to test the other three quadrants. Participants respond to detection of a stimulus by touching the display screen. Testing with the VFE app can be

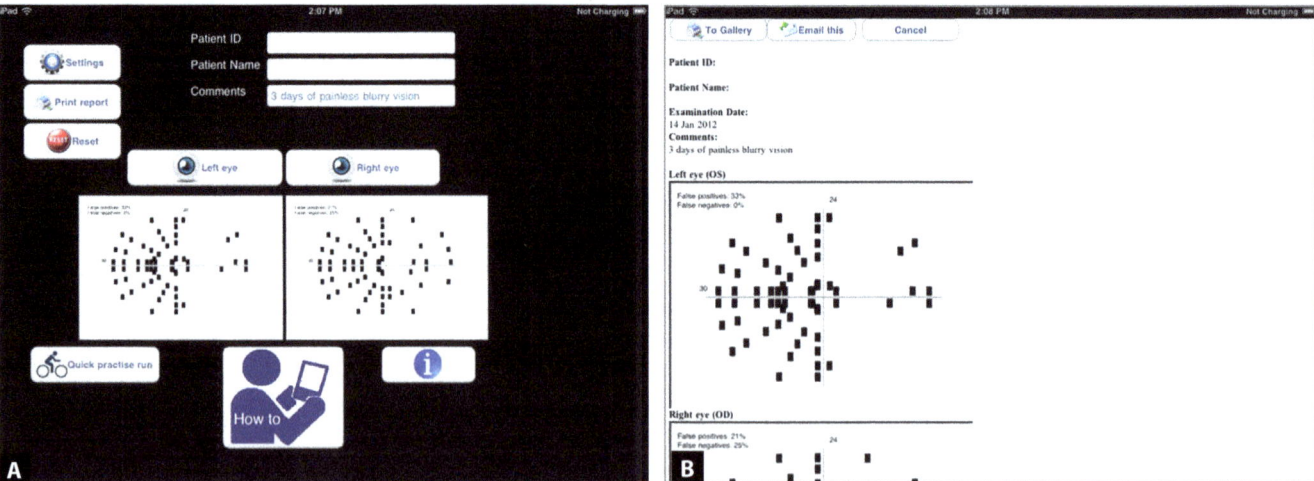

Figs. 1A and B: Visual Fields Easy application screening test.

completed in <3.5 minutes per eye, and preliminary results indicate good screening performance for moderate and advanced glaucoma.[19]

Melbourne Rapid Fields

The Melbourne Rapid Fields (MRF) application allows assessment in two modes—(1) a full threshold test of 4-5 minutes duration per eye and (2) a screening test of approximately 90 seconds duration. The MRF perimeter software uses a modified 24-2 grid, or a full test centered at fixation, which tests 30° × 20° of the VF, equivalent to the HFA 24-2 program. MRF uses blind spot monitoring by presenting stimuli to the blind spot to estimate fixation accuracy during central fixation testing. The software controls the difference in number and location as per the selected test.[20]

As the screen size of an iPad is small (around 15 × 12°), the patient must fixate in the four corners of the screen at different times to gain eccentricities to 30°. The spot size is increased with eccentricity to account for the tangent effect of the flat screen and to produce a fixed threshold across the central field. Targets are presented for 300 ms. It also provides audio commands to remind the participants to maintain fixation.

Fixation monitoring is done using a blind spot monitor with a large stimulus, 19 dB stimulus (nearly 40% larger in area than the Goldmann size II spot). Testing is performed by charting the blind spot at the beginning of each test, and a stimulus is presented in that location throughout the test using central fixation. False positive checks are conducted by interspacing periods (1,000–1,400 ms) throughout the test. **Figure 2** shows output obtained by MRF.

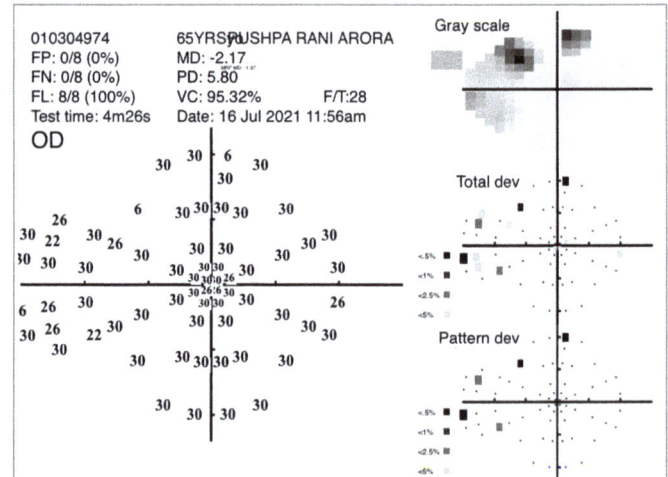

Fig. 2: Outcome of perimetry obtained with MRF glaucoma.

Kumar et al. have shown that the test time of the MRF is approximately 30 s/eye shorter than the HFA 24-2 SITA-Standard (conducted on 9.7-inch iPad).[21]

Peristat Online Perimetry

Peristat online perimetry (POP) was first developed in 2002 by two resident doctors of Doheny Eye Institute (University of Southern California), Dr Ianchulev and Dr Peter Pham.

Peristat online perimetry is delivered via the KYS telemedicine platform (https://kysvision.com/peristat-test/).

Peristat online perimetry allows perimetry testing of up to 24° of VF from fixation horizontally and 20° vertically using four levels of standardized threshold stimuli. POP testing is performed with dimmed ambient light and no direct light sources over the screen. The red, green, and blue range for the target is between 64 and 225 with a differential light intensity between 30 and 300 lux. Target is presented for 0.2 seconds, and an additional grace period of 1.8 seconds is given to the patient to respond. The appropriate working distance is determined by adjusting positioning until the flashing light temporal to the fixation point disappears in the blind spot. Gaze fixation assurance and false-positives/false-negative registration is also present. Patient responses can then be composed into a grayscale VF image. Earlier, POP was available for use by any patient across the globe, but now it is available only for registered practices in the united States.[22]

Eyecatcher

Eyecatcher is an inexpensive, near infrared, and remote eye tracker which allows a precision of >0.6°. The stimuli are displayed on a tablet computer and the eye movements are recorded using a Tobii EyeX eye-tracker (Tobii Technology, Stockholm, Sweden).

Jones et al. compared the results of Eyecatcher with SAP using HFA in glaucoma patients and healthy controls. They found that the application was able to distinguish between the glaucomatous and normal eyes and between eyes with mild and advanced glaucomatous impairment.

Jones et al. conducted another study to assess the accuracy and adherence of VF home monitoring in 20 glaucoma patients using this application over 6 months. They found a good concordance between VFs measured at home and in the clinic (r = 0.94, $p < 0.001$).[23]

Advantages for VR and Tablet Perimetry

- As a portable and cost-effective screening tool in camps.
- For perimetry in intensive care unit (ICU), bed ridden and postoperative patients with limited mobility.
- Home-based perimetry for telemedicine and follow-ups.

Disadvantages of VR Perimetry and Tablet Perimetry

- Sensitivity is not as good as SAP, so early stages of glaucoma may be missed.
- Normative databases are still new and need to be updated.
- Gaze tracking is not available in most cases hence reliability is questionable.
- It is not possible to know if the screen is at the right distance from the patient's eyes for the stimuli to appear in the patient's VF at the location that we plan to test.
- Ambient lighting conditions during the test cannot be controlled.

- The screen resolution, or the background luminance cannot be ascertained during the test. Additionally, these can be significantly different from device to device.

To conclude, these new VF-testing modalities are still evolving but in near future will definitely have a useful complementary role to SAP.

CONCLUSION

Tablet based perimetry and VR perimetry has opened up new possibilities and are therefore a promising new step into a future which can complement the current "gold standard" SAP.

REFERENCES

1. Iskander M, Ogunsola T, Ramachandran R, McGowan R, Al-Aswad L. Virtual reality and augmented reality in ophthalmology: A contemporary prospective. Asia Pac J Ophthalmol. 2021;10(3):244-52.
2. Thomsen ASS, Subhi Y, Kiilgaard JF, la Cour M, Konge L. Update on simulation-based surgical training and assessment in ophthalmology: A systematic review. Ophthalmology. 2015;122:1111-30.
3. Lee R, Raison N, Lau WY, Aydin A, Dasgupta P, Ahmed K, et al. A systematic review of simulation-based training tools for technical and non-technical skills in ophthalmology. Eye. 2020;34:1737-59.
4. Wilson AS, O'Connor J, Taylor L, Carruthers D. A 3D virtual reality ophthalmoscopy trainer. Clin Teacher. 2017;14:427-31.
5. Rai AS, Rai AS, Mavrikakis E, Lam WC. Teaching binocular indirect ophthalmoscopy to novice residents using an augmented reality simulator. Canad J Ophthalmol. 2017; 52:430-4.
6. Miao Y, Jeon JY, Park G, Park SW, Heo H. Virtual reality-based measurement of ocular deviation in strabismus. Comput Methods Progr Biomed. 2020;185:105132.
7. Panachakel JT, Ramakrishnan AG, Manjunath KP. VR glasses-based measurement of responses to dichoptic stimuli: a potential tool for quantifying amblyopia? Annu Int Conf IEEE Eng Med Biol Soc. 2020;2020:5106-10.
8. Mees L, Upadhyaya S, Kumar P, Kotawala S, Haran S, Rajasekar S, et al. Validation of a head-mounted virtual reality visual field screening device. J Glaucoma. 2020;29:86-91.
9. Alawa KA, Nolan RP, Han E, Arboleda A, Durkee H, Sayed MS, et al. Low-cost, smartphone-based frequency doubling technology visual field testing using a head-mounted display. Br J Ophthalmol. 2021;105:440-4.
10. Deemer AD, Swenor BK, Fujiwara K, Deremeik JT, Ross NC, Natale DM, et al. Preliminary evaluation of two digital image processing strategies for head-mounted magnification for low vision patients. Transl Vision Sci Technol. 2019;8:23-123.
11. Aravind Eye Hospital Pondicherry—AUROTUBE. (2020). Peri-Screener. [online] Available from https://www.youtube.com/watch?v=Vink4PCBfLI [Last accessed July, 2023].
12. Akkara JD, Kuriakose A. Review of recent innovations in ophthalmology. Kerala J Ophthalmol. 2018;30(1):54.

13. Solomon A. (1999). Method and apparatus for evaluating and mapping visual field. [online] Available from https://patents.google.com/patent/US5880812A/en [Last accessed July, 2023].
14. Matsumoto C, Yamao S, Nomoto H, Takada S, Okuyama S, Kimura S, et al. Visual Field Testing with Head-Mounted Perimeter 'imo.' PLoS one. 2016;11(8):e0161974.
15. Nyugen NT, Nanayakkara S, Lee H. Visual Field Visualizer: Easier & Scalable Way to Be Aware of the Visual Field. Proceedings of the 9th Augmented Human International Conference. AH '18. 2018;31:1-31.
16. Tsapakis S, Papaconstantinou D, Diagourtas A, Kandarakis S, Droutsas K, Andreanos K, et al. Home-based visual field test for glaucoma screening comparison with Humphrey perimeter. Clin Ophthalmol. 2018;12:2597-606.
17. Nakanishi M, Wang YT, Jung TP, Zao JK, Chien YY, Diniz-Filho A, et al. Detecting glaucoma with a portable brain-computer interface for objective assessment of visual function loss. JAMA Ophthalmol. 2017;135(6):550-7.
18. Nakanishi M, Wang YT, Daga FB, Jung TP, Zao J, Ogata NG, et al. Detecting Preperimetric Glaucoma with the nGoggle, a Portable Brain-Computer Interface for Assessing Neural Damage. Invest Ophthalmol Vis Sci. 2017;58.
19. Ichhpujani P, Thakur S, Sahi RK, Kumar S. Validating tablet perimetry against standard Humphrey Visual Field Analyzer for glaucoma screening in Indian population. Indian J Ophthalmol. 2021;69(1):87-91.
20. Harris PA, Johnson CA, Chen Y, Fann H, Gafford G, Kim YJ, Mezgebu ED. Evaluation of the Melbourne Rapid Fields Test Procedure. Optom Vis Sci. 2022;99(4):372-82.
21. Kumar H, Thulasidas M. Comparison of Perimetric Outcomes from Melbourne Rapid Fields Tablet Perimeter Software and Humphrey Field Analyzer in Glaucoma Patients. J Ophthalmol. 2020;2020:8384509.
22. Ichhpujani P, Dhillon H. Spotlight on iPad Visual Field Tests Efficacy. Clin Ophthalmol. 2022;16:2179-85.
23. Jones PR, Lindfield D, Crabb DP. Using an open-source tablet perimeter (Eyecatcher) as a rapid triage measure for glaucoma clinic waiting areas. Br J Ophthalmol. 2021;105(5):681-6.

CHAPTER 15B

Brief Overview of Various Types of Head-mounted Virtual Reality Perimeters

Prasanna Venkatesh Ramesh, Shruthy Vaishali Ramesh, Vivek Velumani, Aji Kunnath Devadas

INTRODUCTION—THE INCEPTION OF HEAD-MOUNTED PERIMETER

Standard automated perimetry (SAP) is the gold standard and an internationally accepted device for evaluating the presence of visual field defects (VFDs) in glaucoma patients. Nevertheless, it needs some unavoidable conditions, such as prolonged attention, stable fixation, and space restriction. Moreover, it was nearly impossible to assess glaucoma patients during the coronavirus disease 2019 (COVID-19) pandemic with the option of using SAP due to bowl contamination and mask-induced artifacts. Therefore, a novel approach of virtual visual field testing has gained popularity as a complementary technique to SAP in glaucoma settings to treat the patient effectively. In addition, it has shown much promise in this scenario in terms of freedom of head movement, comfort, and portability. In this chapter, a brief overview of various head-mounted virtual reality perimeters is highlighted with novel practical experiences for the assessment of functional glaucomatous loss and progressive damage.

Visual fields play a significant role in diagnosing, monitoring, and predicting the course of glaucoma.[1] The first record of visual field testing was documented in the Hippocratic Corpus in the 5th century BC.[2-4] The circular form of the visual field was first noted by Ptolemy in 150 BC. Since then, quantum leaps have been made in the field of ophthalmology to quantify and qualify the visual field. SAP remains the gold standard for visual field analysis. However, most of these conventional SAPs need to be used in a dim testing room, requiring a fixed testing position for long periods during the examination. Additional issues such as portability, space restrictions, inaccessibility to wheelchair patients, hyperkinetic patients with neurological or psychiatric disorders, or patients with sarcopenia can lead to increased difficulty or discomfort. Therefore, a patient-oriented perimeter with better flexibility in performing the test is a pressing need, and a head-mounted perimeter acknowledges all these setbacks. The inception of the head-mounted virtual reality perimeter was done in 1999 by Chan et al.[5]

PROS OF HEAD-MOUNTED DEVICES

- *Comfort:* With improved ergonomics, the patient does not need to sit in a stationary machine for an extended period.
- *Portability:* It can be used in a variety of settings, including clinics, hospitals, and even in a patient's home. It has the advantage of evaluating a bedridden patient.
- *Compact:* It does not require a separate dark room or a large area for testing or storage, like the bowl perimetry.
- *Cost-efficient:* Head-mounted visual field analyzers are typically less expensive than traditional visual field analyzers, which make them a more cost-effective option for smaller clinics or practices.
- *Teleophthalmology and screening:* Due to its compact and portable nature, it can function as an effective tool for teleglaucoma services.

CONS OF HEAD-MOUNTED DEVICES

- Less sensitivity than SAP
- It may be difficult for claustrophobic patients
- Need for an updated normative database
- Gaze tracking is not available on all devices

TYPES OF HEAD-MOUNTED VIRTUAL REALITY PERIMETERS

Currently, there are a few head-mounted perimeters readily available for use in the market **(Table 1)**. They are described here.

TABLE 1: Comparison of perimeters available in the market.

Model	Company	Stimulus duration	Gaze tracking	Stimulus color	Stimulus size	Screening test strategies	Central pattern	Temporal range
C3 Field Analyzer (0.6 kg)	Remidio	200 ms	Heijl–Krakau	WoW	Goldmann III	CFA suprathreshold	10-2 and 24-2	27°
Vivid Vision	Vivid Vision	300 ms	Heijl–Krakau	BoW	Goldmann III	Full threshold	24-2	43°
Olleyes VisuALL (0.3 kg)	Macro Advancing Eyecare	200 ms	Heijl–Krakau	WoW	Goldmann III	Full Threshold, Fast Threshold Proprietary	10-2 and 24-2	24°
AVA (0.5 kg)	Elisar Vision Technology	200 ms	Heijl–Krakau	WoW	Goldmann III	Suprathreshold, Full Threshold, Elisar Standard, Elisar Fast	10-2, 24-2, and 30-2	30°
Imo (0.85 kg)	CREWT Medical Systems	200 ms	Heijl–Krakau	WoW	Goldmann I, II, III, IV, and V	Full Threshold, AIZE, AIZE-Rapid, AIZE-EX, AIZE-Rapid EX	10-2, 24-2, and 30-2 24plus (1-2), 24plus (1)	30°
HERU re:Vive	Heru	200 ms	Heru Active Eye Track	WoB	Goldmann III	re:Imagine (re:I) Threshold	24-2	N/A
Virtual Field (0.49 kg)	Virtual Field	N/A	N/A	N/A	Goldmann I, II, III, and IV	Esterman, Full Field 120	10-2, 24-2, and 30-2	N/A
Virtual Eye	Virtual Vision	N/A	N/A	N/A	Goldmann III and V (I–VI)	Full Threshold, Standard, Fast, Suprathreshold, Screening	30-2, 24-2, Superior 64 (ptosis), and Esterman	N/A

(AVA: advanced vision analyzer; BoW: black on white; CFA: C3 Field Analyzer; N/A: not available; WoB: white on black; WoW: white on white)

C3 Field Analyzer

C3 Field Analyzer (C3FA) was the world's first clinically validated portable visual field perimeter (0.6 kg). There is no need to occlude the patient's eye during testing with C3FA headset. A Bluetooth response clicker is used along with a tablet for test administration, and the reports are saved via cloud-based storage. White-on-white perimetry is used with a Goldmann III-sized stimulus. Fixation monitoring is done via the Heijl–Krakau method. The testing battery consists of 10-2 and 24-2 fast and suprathreshold strategies.[6,7] C3FA demonstrated 86.11% sensitivity and 80.26% specificity in the classification of early (mean deviation <6 dB) versus moderate (mean deviation between 6 and 12 dB) and advanced (mean deviation >12 dB) glaucoma, and 89.74% sensitivity and 88% specificity in the classification of early and moderate versus advanced glaucoma.

Advantages: Lightweight and no need for eye occlusion.

Vivid Vision Perimeter

Vivid vision perimeter (VVP) can be performed with commercially available virtual reality (VR) headsets. It does not need a dedicated computer and can be done on any device with an existing internet connection. The testing software incorporates a dynamic fixation marker that changes the location to which patients respond by moving their heads or a handheld pointer in the direction of the targets. It tests 69 spots per eye with a 1° target twice. Additionally, two other tests are included for vision screening and scotoma measurement. The VVP has been shown to provide reproducible visual field sensitivity measurements in both glaucoma suspects and patients. Its repeatability is consistent with SAP and can demonstrate the structure–function correlations demonstrated by SAP and optical coherence tomography.[4]

Advantages: Reliable visual fields and dynamic fixation marker is patient-friendly.

VisuALL Head-mounted Perimetry

The VisuALL perimetry is ergonomic and lightweight (0.3 kg). It does full-threshold perimetry in as fast as 4 minutes per eye and screening tests at a rate of 45 seconds per eye. It has two versions based on office and home use. Both versions consist of a head-mounted device, a tablet, a Bluetooth-enabled response button, and a cloud-based report storage. It has Heijl–Krakau gaze tracking technology. It consists of all the standard protocols (24-2 and 10-2); the 24-2 protocol implements a proprietary testing strategy called the Philadelphia Adaptive Threshold Algorithm. This device has shown high diagnostic performance and comparable performance with SAP. Additionally, a single technician can perform tests on multiple patients at the same time.[8]

Advantages: Ergonomic, lightweight, and reduced manpower requirement.

Advanced Vision Analyzer

The advanced vision analyzer (AVA) consists of a head-mounted device (0.5 kg), a patient response button, a test controller device, and a backend cloud server **(Fig. 1)**. It tests each eye separately and does not require an occluder. It tests up to 60° of field in each eye with white-on-white perimetry and a central fixation target. The battery of tests includes 30-2, 24-2, and 10-2 with the AVA-incorporated testing algorithms (Full Threshold, Elisar Standard, and Elisar Fast). It offers an operator eye tracking system; the image of the pupil is displayed on the screen, which allows for gaze tracking.[9] Studies have shown AVA to have functional equivalence to Humphrey field analyzer (HFA).

Advantages: Wider angle of imaging and consistent results at par with SAP.

Imo Perimeter

Imo perimeter comprises main perimeter unit, control tablet, and patient response button. A computer unit and a lithium-ion battery are built in the perimeter unit (0.85 kg). The control tablet and patient response button are connected by Bluetooth. The right and left optical systems in the perimeter unit are completely separated and stimulus presentation and pupil monitoring are independently performed for each eye. A telecentric optical system is introduced to equalize the central and peripheral light intensities.

Advantages: Conventional perimetry usually tests the right and left eyes separately. Imo not only can test the right and left eyes separately, but also presents the test target randomly to either eye under a nonocclusion condition without the examinee being aware of which eye is being tested.

Heru re: Vive Visual Field

The novel Heru re: Vive visual field technology strongly correlates with the Humphrey perimeter with a shorter testing time. In addition, the portable nature of the wearable device, along with features such as the patented Heru Active Track™, and no requirement of a dark room allow for more flexibility in visual field testing and may help expand the patient base and settings in which visual field testing can be performed.

Advantages: Lightweight and shorter testing time.

Virtual Eye

Virtual reality visual field (VRVF), a head-mounted eye-tracking perimeter, is a device designed by virtual vision. In addition to manual response of patients' click, it utilises a newer technique of visual grasp, where change in gaze is perceived as a stimulus. This mode utilizes the natural tendency to look at a new, moving, or transient visual stimulus. The hypothesis is that the M-cell system inputs to a reflex that, unsuppressed, drives an eye movement to acquire the novel target to the fovea. This mode does not require manual input from the patient and does not require the cortical processing and decision-making required for manual mode. There is a systematic bias of –4 –6 dB and an average standard deviation of 5 dB when compared to HFA. Fixation issues are noted with visual grasp mode.

Advantages: There is no need for manual input and cortical processing from the patient.

Virtual Field

Virtual Field (VVF, Virtual Field, Inc.) was launched in 2019. The system includes a VR headset, a trial lens adapter, and a clicker. The test parameters include the traditional 24-2, 10-2, 30-2, kinetic, and frequency doubling threshold tests. The stimuli are presented to each eye independently inside the headset. The results can be accessed from any laptop or mobile device via the company's Health Insurance

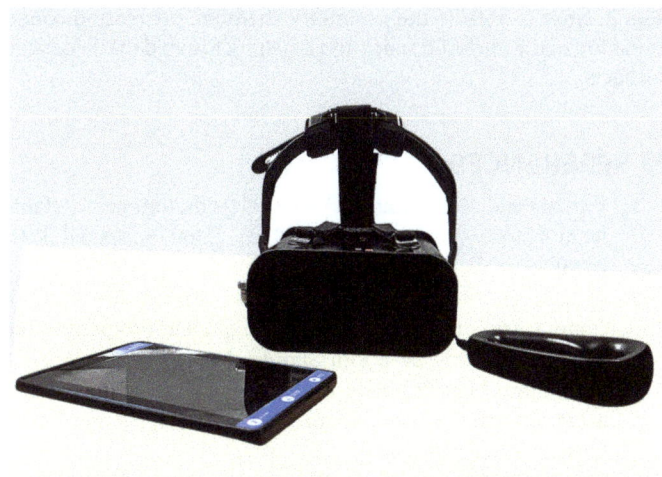

Fig. 1: Advanced vision analyzer (AVA, Elisar) with the tablet and the button for responding to the visual stimuli.

Portability and Accountability Act (HIPAA)-compliant website.[10,11] VVF yielded statistically fewer fixation losses as well as fewer false positives than the HFA. It has also shown an excellent correlation to HFA in terms of mean deviation, pattern deviation, and visual field index.

Advantages: Performance at par with SAP and reliable results.

Step-by-Step Functional Testing Procedure

The common procedure followed in virtual reality headsets is as follows:
1. The perimeter headset is mounted on the subject while they are seated comfortably. The subject can also even stand or lie down if it is more comfortable.
2. The subject is handed over the response button for responding to the visual stimuli.
3. The headset is activated by the user using the tablet's controls.
4. An appropriate visual field test is initiated.
5. The subject is asked to look straight at the fixation point, while the stimuli appear in the periphery keeping both eyes open.
6. When the subject sees the stimuli, he must press the response button.
7. The tablet or PC displays the real-time result of the test.
8. When the tests for both eyes are completed, the final report is displayed and can be exported as a PDF file.

■ UNDUE ADVANTAGE DURING COVID-19

During the global COVID-19 pandemic, the head-mounted visual field analyzer played an essential role in glaucoma diagnosis, progression assessment, and treatment, while limiting the risk of COVID-19 exposure. The testing can be done during the patient's waiting time at the waiting lounge, reducing the hours spent in the clinic **(Fig. 2)**. Another value added to this machine is that the test can be performed with or without a mask, as the nose will remain outside the machine **(Fig. 3)**, so it will avoid mask-induced artifacts and will not contaminate the machine, which was a major setback for bowl perimetry during the pandemic.[9,12-15]

■ CONCLUSION

Virtual reality perimetry is becoming an indispensable tool in the modern era of glaucoma diagnosis and management. These devices could be combined with home-based tonometry for patients with high intraocular pressure (IOP) fluctuation and questionable progression. The cloud-based storage of these devices, combined with their portability, makes VR head-mounted an important practical tool for the functional assessment of glaucomatous defects.

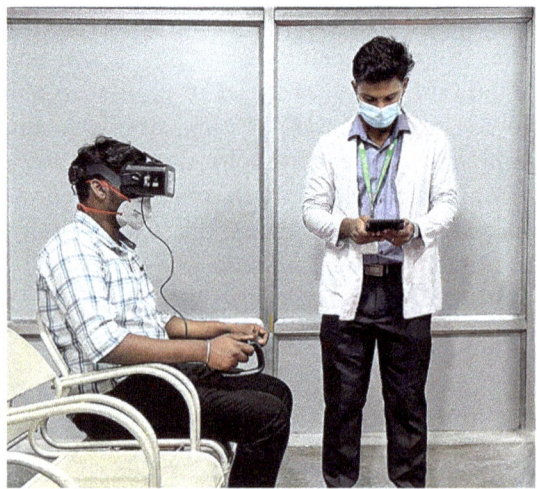

Fig. 2: Visual field test undergoing with the use of head-mounted visual field analyzer (Elisar) by following the protocols for coronavirus disease 2019 (COVID-19) in the outpatient department (OPD) waiting lounge.

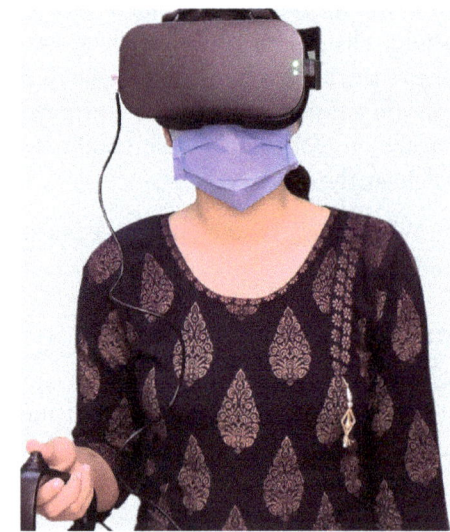

Fig. 3: Nose is outside the perimetry chamber, preventing contamination of the enclosed space and is helpful to avoid mask-induced artifacts.

■ REFERENCES

1. Virtual Field. Gold standard VR visual fields. [online] Available from https://home.virtualfield.io/ [Last accessed July, 2023].
2. Chiang H, Hoang A, Waldman C, Rubin JM. (2020). Comparison of a Virtual Reality Visual Field Program to the Zeiss Humphrey 24-2 Sita Standard in a Comprehensive Ophthalmology Practice. [online] Available from https://ascrs.confex.com/ascrs/20am/meetingapp.cgi/Paper/61842 [Last accessed July, 2023].
3. Deiner MS, Damato BE, Ou Y. Implementing and monitoring at-home virtual reality oculo-kinetic perimetry during COVID-19. Ophthalmology. 2020;127(9):1258.

4. Greenfield JA, Deiner M, Nguyen A, Wollstein G, Damato B, Backus BT, et al. Measurement reproducibility using Vivid Vision Perimetry: A virtual reality-based mobile platform. Invest Ophthalmol Vis Sci. 2020;61(7):4800.
5. Chan AD, Eizenman M, Flanagan JG, Trope GE. Head-mounted perimetry. In: Vision Science and its Applications. Optical Society of America. New Mexico: Optica Publishing Group; 1999. paper MB1.
6. Odayappan A, Sivakumar P, Kotawala S, Raman R, Nachiappan S, Pachiyappan A, et al. Comparison of a New Head Mount Virtual Reality Perimeter (C3 Field Analyzer) With Automated Field Analyzer in Neuro-Ophthalmic Disorders. J Neuro-ophthalmol. 2023;43(2):232-236.
7. Ophthalmology Management—Diagnosing glaucoma: COVID-19 and beyond. Ophthalmology Management. 2021 [cited 2023 Jul 31]. Available from: https://www.ophthalmologymanagement.com/issues/2021/march-2021/diagnosing-glaucoma-covid-19-and-beyond
8. Matsumoto C, Yamao S, Nomoto H, Takada S, Okuyama S, Kimura S, et al. Visual Field Testing with Head-Mounted Perimeter 'imo.' PLoS One. 2016;11(8):e0161974.
9. Ramesh P, Vaishali R, Ray P, Kunnath A, Ramesh M, Rajasekaran R. The curious cases of incorrect face mask positions in bowl-type perimetry versus enclosed chamber perimetry during the COVID-19 pandemic. Indian J Ophthalmol. 2021;69:2236-9.
10. Olleyes. Olleyes Virtual Visual Field Products. [online] Available from https://olleyes.com/ [Last accessed July, 2023].
11. Greenfield JA, Deiner M, Nguyen A, Wollstein G, Damato B, Backus B, et al. Relationship between ocular structure and visual sensitivity using virtual-reality perimetry. Invest Ophthalmol Vis Sci. 2020;61(7):PB0076.
12. Razeghinejad R, Shukla AG. In the field: How does a novel portable head-mounted perimeter compare with the gold standard in visual field testing? Ophthalmologist. 2020;47:34-7.
13. Razeghinejad R, Gonzalez-Garcia A, Myers JS, Katz LJ. Preliminary report on a novel virtual reality perimeter compared with standard automated perimetry. J Glaucoma. 2021;30(1):17-23.
14. Razeghinejad R, Gonzalez A, Myers JS, Katz LJ. Virtual reality perimetry with eye tracking compared with standard automated perimetry. J Glaucoma. 2018;29(2):2018.
15. Mees L, Upadhyaya S, Kumar P, Kotawala S, Haran S, Rajasekar S, et al. Validation of a head-mounted virtual reality visual field screening device. J Glaucoma. 2020;29(2):86-91.

16 Care and Maintenance of Perimeters

Shibal Bhartiya, Parul Ichhpujani

■ INTRODUCTION

Dynamic perimetry is a very valuable tool in the glaucoma surgeons' armamentarium, and has become the standard of care for monitoring and diagnosis of glaucoma. Proper care and maintenance of its equipment can ensure an error-free and hassle-free result each time.

In this chapter, emphasis is given to the care and maintenance of the Humphrey Field Analyzer and Octopus perimeter. These instruments were chosen because they are more widely used across the globe. Both the Humphreys and the Octopus perimeters are basically computers associated with a projection device, and an output device (printer). New machines continue to be made available with repeated improvements in both hardware and software but broad directives for care of the equipment remain the same, with minor variations in individual instruments.

■ GENERAL INSTRUCTIONS

- Switch off the device at night.
- Use the appropriate power supply and plugs.
- Keep the device in a dust-free, cool room.
- Cover the device when not in use.
- Make sure the device is gently wiped with a soft, lint-free cloth before use.
- Do not use strong oxidizing agents or solvents, as they could damage surface coatings.
- Make sure the printer is handled gently, and cartridges changed at appropriate intervals.
- Ensure periodic calibration of the device.
- Ensure that the disc is cleaned as specified, at appropriate intervals, depending on device usage.
- Contact the manufacturers for authorized and trained technicians for repairs and troubleshooting.
- Do not encourage the use of pendrives for accessing data to prevent virus in the machine.[1]

■ HUMPHREY'S VISUAL FIELD ANALYZER

Power Supply

- For a 120 V power supply/machine, a 4 Ampere plug should be used.[2]
- A 2 Ampere plug is recommended for a 220 V instrument and power supply.
- The power cord should not be plugged into the power supply at night while the machine is not in use.

Changing the Fuse

- In case a fuse change is needed, the instrument should first be switched off.
- After that, the power cord is removed, and the plastic slide moved to the left. This exposes the fuse release tab, pulling which releases the fuse.
- A new fuse may then be inserted, and the procedure reversed by sliding the plastic cover to the right.

Daily Maintenance

- The perimeter should be kept covered at night, and the outside of the machine dusted with a soft lint-free cloth.
- Static wipes may be used to clean the display terminal.
- The light pen tip may be cleaned with an alcohol swab, and the patient button with either the same, or soap and water.
- Care must be taken to prevent scratches on the machine, therefore, it is important to remove any jewelry or watches while cleaning the machine.

Calibration

- It is essential to examine the stimulus once a week for any blurred edges or inconsistencies.

- To calibrate the perimeter, the room light should be dimmed to what they are at the time of performing the test.

Disc Cleaning

The disc should be cleaned at least thrice a year, or more often in case the perimeter is used more extensively.

Printer Care

The power should be turned off before opening the printer for maintenance **(Fig. 1)**.

Printer Head Clogging

In case a document comes out of the printer with white lines running across the text or graphics that are missing ink, even though the cartridges are full, it implies that the printer heads are clogged and need to be cleaned. Printers will self-clean with just a few clicks but can also be cleaned manually with a soft lint-free cloth or using a small vacuum.

Paper Jam

In case of a paper jam gently use both hands to slowly pull the jammed paper out of the printer to avoid leaving ripped paper behind or damaging the internal parts of the printer.

Changing Cartridge

The printer requires a new cartridge once the print becomes light. To do so, with the machine switched off, the printer door should be opened. The top of the cartridge is pulled, and the right end lifted out, to remove the cartridge. To insert a new cartridge, the cartridge is inserted on the left slide first, and then the right end is lowered to snap in place. The door is then shut, and the printer is ready for use.

Changing the Bulbs

The machine gives error messages when the projection or background illumination bulbs need replacing.

- *Projection bulb:* The projection bulbs should be changed after switching off the power and opening the access panel of the machine and pulling the bulb out after the machine has cooled. New bulb should be put on with the protective envelope so that the fingerprints do not etch on the glass jacket.
- *Background bulb:* Background illumination bulbs are located near the front of the bowl **(Fig. 2)**. They are covered by a filter that can be rotated to expose the bulb. The bulb is slightly pushed in and then twisted for removal.

The background illumination assembly surface should also be kept dust free as shown in **Figure 3**.

Lens Holder

Lens holder should be folded completely when machine is turned off and covered. An incompletely folded lens holder can get misaligned **(Figs. 4A to C)**. Lens holder and surrounding area should be dust free and cleaned with a soft brush **(Fig. 5)**.

OCTOPUS PERIMETER

Cleaning Instructions

When the ocular lens and the headrest need cleaning, it is recommended to use a damp chamois leather wetted with alcohol, if necessary.[3]

Moving the Perimeter

- Remove all the cables from the plug panel.
- If the unit is transported in its original packaging, then adjust the height of the cross support to the lowest position.

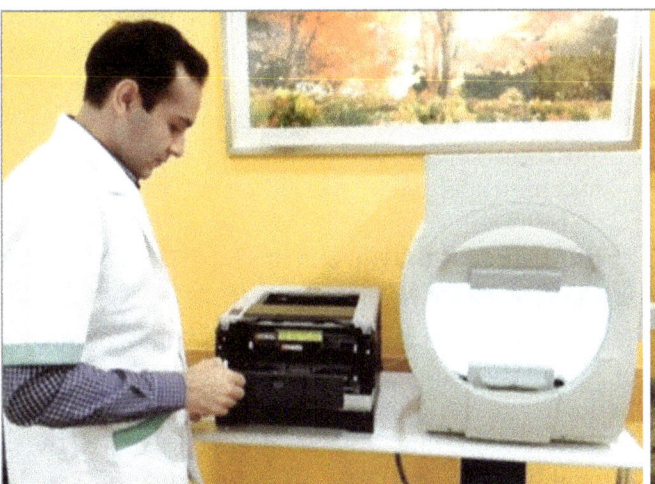 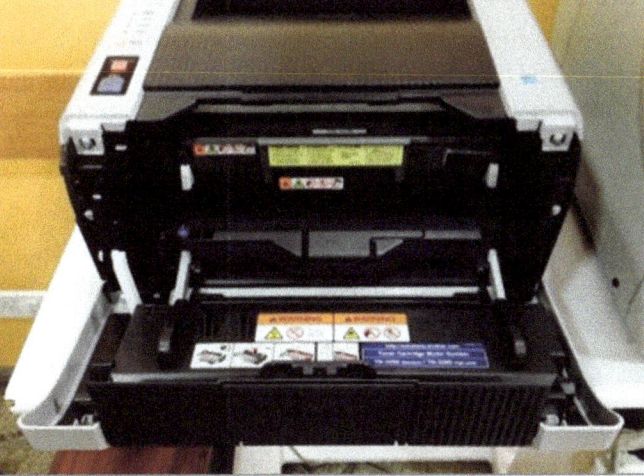

Fig. 1: Opening the printer.

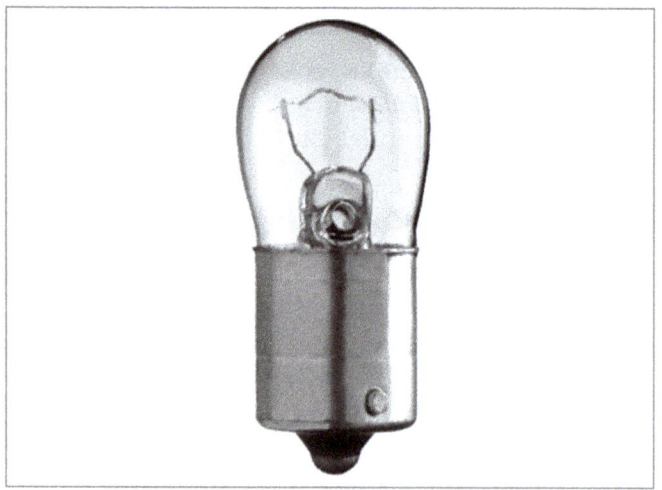

Fig. 2: Humphrey perimeter background bulb.

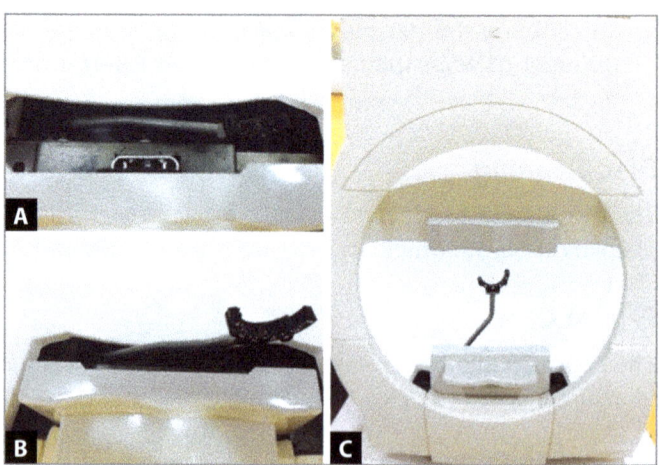

Figs. 4A to C: (A) Properly folded lens holder; (B) Partly folded lens holder; (C) Properly aligned and positioned holder (in use).

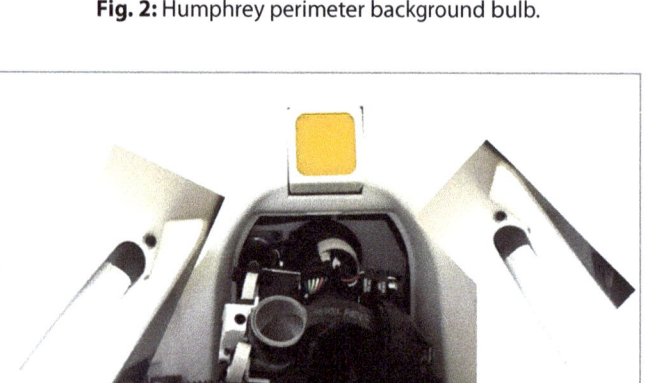

Fig. 3: View from inside the bowl of a Humphrey field analyzer showing the top lights illuminating the bowl and the central panel which is having a film of dust. It is imperative to keep this part dust free to provide adequate illumination of bowl.

- Always ensure that the cross support is firmly secured by fixing the two screws.

MEDMONT AUTOMATED PERIMETER

Medmont automated perimeters are used commonly in Australia. The fully electronic stimulator unit with no moving parts, together with standard computer hardware, results in minimal maintenance requirement.[4]

Cleaning Instructions

- These perimeters are equipped with a charge-coupled device (CCD) camera and require a soft optics brush with blower for cleaning.
- The vertical chinrest should be lubricated regularly to prevent dust entering the sliding mechanism and to prevent corrosion.
- Wind up the chinrest to the upper limit. Put a small amount of sewing machine oil onto a lint free cloth.

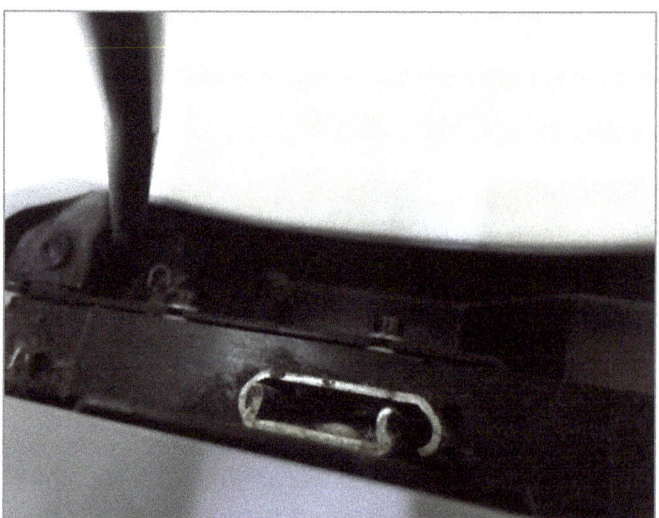

Fig. 5: Poorly cleaned lens holder.

Wipe the steel shaft on the rear side to remove any dust and contamination. A tiny drop of oil may also be applied to the rotating parts and joints of the lens holder mechanism. Wipe off excessive oil immediately.
- The frequency of the lubrication depends on the environment in which the device is kept but is recommended on a 3–6 monthly interval.

PERIMETER BOWL DISINFECTION DURING COVID-19 PANDEMIC

While there was a dramatic switch to alternate methods of perimetry, and several practitioners did not perform perimetry at all, international public health guidelines recommended that 70% isopropyl alcohol (IPA) or ultraviolet-C light (UV-C) at 254 nm may be used for disinfection of perimeter bowls. All patient and technician interface surfaces are to be wiped down with 70% IPA, after each patient. The bowl of the perimeter, however, needs to be sprayed with 70% IPA solution.[5-8]

It is suggested by the companies to use a fine spray onto the internal bowl surface whilst the perimeter lights are on and allow the spray to evaporate. The whole internal bowl surface must not be rubbed or wiped. One must not allow the disinfectant to drip, as this may damage the equipment.[8-12]

Despite >75,000 disinfection cycles for both, automatic verification tests have shown good tolerance with a reading error spread <1 dB for an attenuation range of 0–34 dB. Similarly, UV-C exposure bowl also caused a shift of <0.002 in chromaticity and 18 fL in luminance. Even though the plastic parts including chin rest, cover, and baffle were affected by UV-C, showing solarization, this did not impact the visual field stimulus, or test performance.[5]

■ CONCLUSION

Instructions for care and maintenance of individual perimeters, and particular models are available in the accompanying manual. When in doubt, it is best to ask for expert advice from authorized and trained technicians.

Always use the appropriate power supply and plugs, maintain all precautions as for electronic devices and computers.

Make sure the perimeter is installed in a dust free, cool room, and cleaned periodically. Ensure periodic calibration of the device to ensure optimal performance.

All patient and technician interface surfaces can be wiped down 70% IPA. Perimeter bowl disinfection with IPA spray or UV-C radiation does not affect test performance.

■ REFERENCES

1. Herrin MP. Instrumentation for eyecare paraprofessionals. United States: Slack Inc; 1999. pp. 59-61.
2. ZEISS Group. (2023). Humphrey's Field Analyser Manual. [online] Available from: www.zeiss.com [Last accessed July, 2023].
3. HAAG-STREIT USA. (2023). Octopus Manual. [online] Available from: www.haag-streit-usa.com [Last accessed July, 2023].
4. Medmont. (2023). User manual, automated perimeter. [online] Available from: www.medmont.com [Last accessed July, 2023].
5. Romero K, Bourque R, Callan T, Foote KG, Larson E, Sprowl R, et al. Perimeter bowl disinfection during the COVID-19 pandemic. Invest Ophthalmol Vis Sci. 2021;62(8):1747.
6. The Royal College of Ophthalmologists. (2020). Use of bowl perimeters for testing visual
7. field during COVID-19. [online] Available from: https://www.iapb.org/wp-content/uploads/2020/11/Use-of-perimeters-for-testing-visual-field-during-COVID19-300720-FINAL-FINAL-1.pdf [Last accessed July, 2023].
8. Carl Zeiss Meditec, Inc. (2020). Cleaning Guidance for the Humphrey Field Analyzer (HFA). [online] Available from: https://www.optometry.org.au/wp-content/uploads/Professional_support/COVID-19/HFA-COVID-Guidance_EN_31_025_0408I_HFA.12415_FINAL.pdf [Accessed July, 2023].
9. Parikh RS, George R, Parikh SR. Sanitization of glaucoma clinic instruments in COVID-19 era. Indian J Ophthalmol. 2020;68(6):1225.
10. Henson perimeters. [online] Available from: https://www.elektron-eye-technology.com/support/ [Last accessed July, 2023].
11. Octopus perimeters https://www.haag-streit.com/fileadmin/Haag-Streit_Diagnostics/_ALLGEMEINE_BILDER_UND_ICONS/Corona/PDFs/Cleaning_and_Disinfe ction_of_OCTOPUS_Perimeters_updated.pdf [Last accessed July, 2023].
12. Medmont perimeters. [online] Available from: https://www.medmont.com.au/media/52659/medmont-device-technical-bulletin_disinfecting-may-2020.pdf [Last accessed July, 2023].

CHAPTER 17

History of Perimetry

Harsha L Rao, Zia S Pradhan, Chris A Johnson

■ INTRODUCTION

Although there were attempts in history to evaluate the peripheral visual fields since the time of Hippocrates, the credit for introducing perimetry into clinical practice in the year 1856 goes to Albrecht von Graefe **(Fig. 1)**.[1,2] He plotted visual fields of patients using a blackboard as a tangent screen and white chalk as a test object. He also described various visual field defects such as ring scotoma, concentric constriction of the visual field, enlargement of the blind spot, and hemianopia.[1]

■ DEVELOPMENT OF PERIMETRY

Hermann Aubert and Richard Förster of Breslau, initially working with Von Graefe's tangent screen, recognized the importance of keeping the stimulus at a constant distance from the eye as it was positioned in different locations of the visual field. They went on to develop the first arc perimeter in 1869 **(Fig. 2)**.

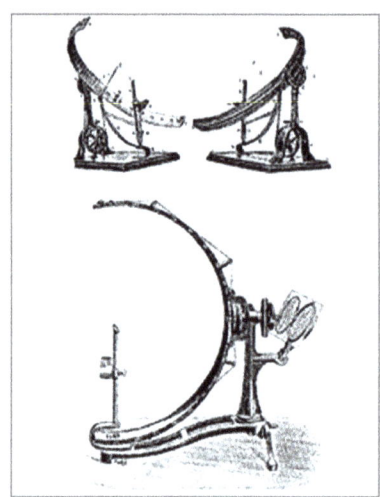

Fig. 2: Arc perimeter.

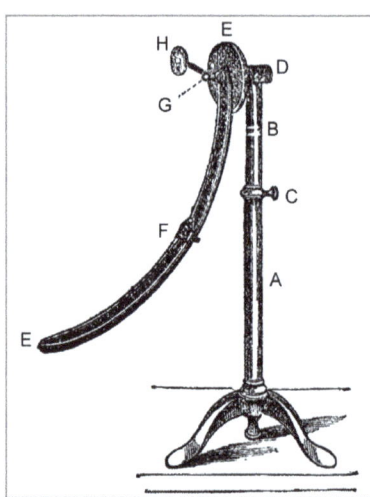

Fig. 3: Carter's arc perimeter. (A: hollow stem on tripod; B: height-adjustable second stem; C: screw; D: horizontal axis; E: quadrant/arc which moves in a complete circle; F: travelling slide to carry a spot of any color/size; G: fixation target; H: additional fixation target comprising of a disc with central perforation through which patient looks at distant object to obtain fixation without accommodation/fatigue.)

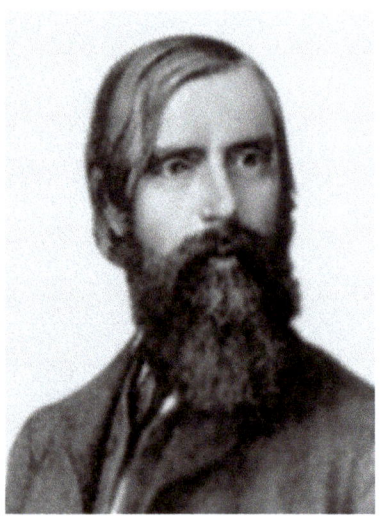

Fig. 1: Albrecht von Graefe.

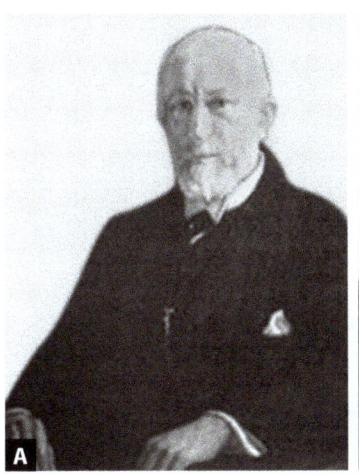 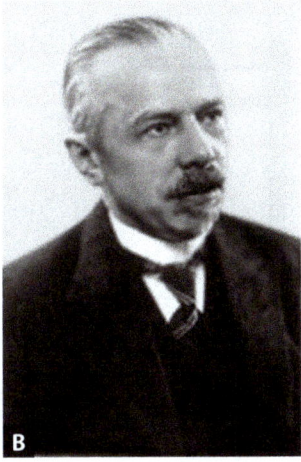 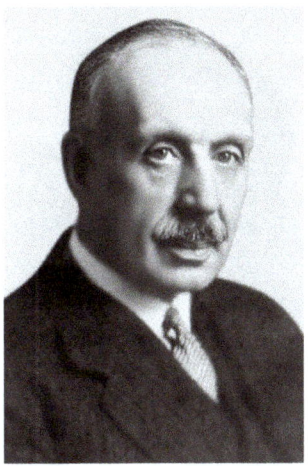

Figs. 4A and B: (A) Jannik Bjerrum; and (B) Henning Rønne.

Fig. 5: Harry Moss Traquair.

In 1873, Brudenell Carter simplified Förster's perimeter design to one with an arc occupying only one quadrant **(Fig. 3)**. This became popular and largely replaced Förster's perimeter in clinical practice. The predominant purpose of perimetry during this time was to identify the far periphery (the very outside limits) of the visual field with a single, relatively large stimulus. During this period, it was also generally accepted that the arc perimeter was satisfactory for mapping defects in the central visual field, leading to the misconception that there were no central field defects of clinical importance in glaucoma.

In spite of the popularity of arc perimeters, some practitioners continued to work with tangent screens. Julius Hirschberg was one of them, and he coined the term "campimetry" for the tangent screen technique in order to distinguish it from "perimetry." It was Jannik Peterson Bjerrum, Professor of Ophthalmology in Copenhagen, who reintroduced and popularized campimetry with his publications in 1889 **(Fig. 4A)**. Bjerrum felt that mapping the subtleties of the central 30° was far more useful than the routine evaluation of the far periphery of the visual field that was commonly being conducted in earlier studies. During the years 1909–1927, his assistant Henning Rønne emphasized the use of a graduated series of smaller test objects of more difficult visibility **(Fig. 4B)**. With these techniques, Bjerrum and Rønne were able to demonstrate the characteristics of early visual field loss in glaucoma, with which their names are still associated. Tangent screens returned and arc perimeters began to disappear from practice.

Another major contributor to the field of perimetry was Harry Moss Traquair of Edinburgh **(Fig. 5)**. Traquair worked with both arc perimeters and tangent screens and provided many astute insights into visual field interpretation. He provided the description of the visual field as "an island of vision in a sea of darkness."[3]

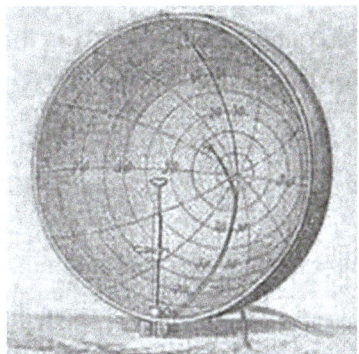 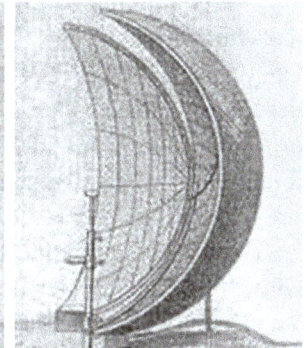

Fig. 6: Scherk's bowl perimeter.

One of the very first bowl perimeters was developed by Scherk in 1872 to eliminate the distracting background that was always present with an arc perimeter. It was, however, large, heavy, and expensive **(Fig. 6)**. Bowl perimeters became more popular in 1945, when Hans Goldmann of Bern devised a hemispheric bowl, with a self-illuminated projection perimeter, in which fixation, retinal adaptation, and stimulus size and intensity could be precisely controlled **(Figs. 7A and B)**. The visual field could be readily recorded by means of a pantograph.[1] This allowed elegant mapping of defect shape and depth and was easy for the perimetrist to use. The utility of the instrument further increased in 1971 when Mansour Armaly and Stephen Drance developed screening methods for glaucoma detection that included using suprathreshold static testing with Goldmann's perimeter. By concentrating test locations, where one expected field defects in glaucoma, the yield of finding visual field damage was substantially increased. This instrument, made by Haag-Streit of Bern, became the standard kinetic perimeter in clinical practice.

Although the advantages of static threshold perimetry were pointed out in 1933 by Louise L Sloan, the first perimeter designed to do static threshold perimetry was

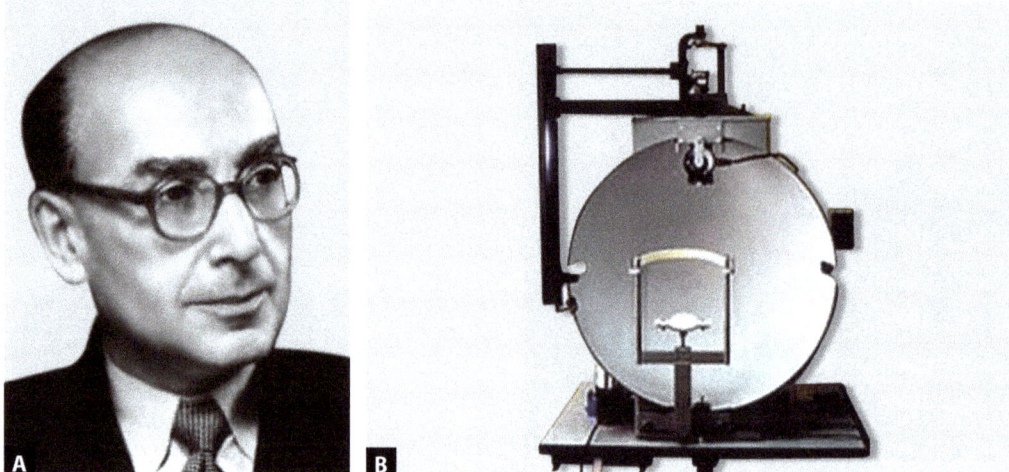

Figs. 7A and B: (A) Hans Goldmann; and (B) The Goldmann bowl.

developed by Elfriede Aulhorn and Heinrich Harms in the late 1950s. This was called the "Tübinger Perimeter" and was made by Oculus in 1959 **(Figs. 8A and B)**. Cross-sections or profiles of the "island of vision" could be determined by finding the threshold sensitivity at various locations along a single meridian.

The advent of automated perimetry began around 1970 with the perimeter developed by John Lynn and George Tate.[4] This got a significant boost with the development of the Octopus perimeter in the laboratory of Dr Fankhauser.[5] The others who have contributed significantly to the development and improvizations of automated perimetric techniques are Anders Heijl, Torsten Krakau, Stephen Drance, and Douglas Anderson. As with Goldmann perimetry, differential light sensitivity in static perimetry is tested over a 4 log unit (40 dB) range. Testing generally targets the central visual field using either a spaced Cartesian grid or a polar coordinate system weighted toward the central test locations. Automated perimetry has become the standard for visual field assessment in clinical practice today.

CONCLUSION

Various forms of visual field assessment have been conducted for the past 2000 years. However, in the last 200 years, almost all perimetric tests involved detection of a target on a uniform background allowing quantitative measurements of retinal sensitivities. The automation of this test led to the development of the standard automated perimeters which have been used in ophthalmic practice for the past 50 years. These same perimetric principles are currently being applied to different gadgets resulting in an era of tablet-based strategies and virtual-reality headsets for the use of visual field testing.[6] These devices hold the promise of allowing

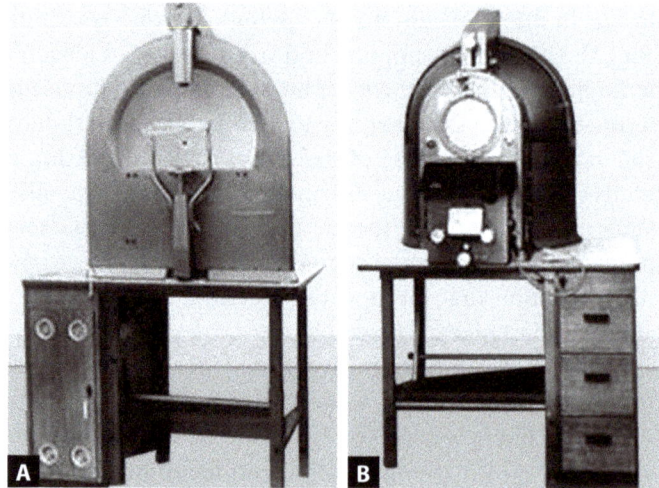

Figs. 8A and B: Tübinger perimeter.

perimetry to be conducted in remote area and potentially be used for home-testing along with telemedicine.

REFERENCES

1. Thompson HS, Wall M; Imaging and Perimetry Society (IPS). History of perimetry. [online] Available from: http://webeye.ophth.uiowa.edu/IPS/PerimetryHistory/index.htm [Last accessed July, 2023].
2. Johnson CA, Wall M, Thompson HS. A history of perimetry and visual field testing. Optom Vis Sci. 2011;88:E8-15.
3. Traquair HM (Ed). An Introduction to Clinical Perimetry. St Louis, MO: Mosby; 1927.
4. Tate GW, Lynn JR. Principles of Quantitative Perimetry: Testing and Interpreting the Visual Field. New York, NY: Grune and Stratton; 1977.
5. Bebie H, Fankhauser F, Spahr J. Static perimetry: Strategies. Acta Ophthalmol (Copenh). 1976;54:325-38.
6. Prager AJ, Kang JM, Tanna AP. Advances in perimetry for glaucoma. Curr Opin Ophthalmol. 2021;32(2):92-7.

Index

Note: Page numbers followed by '*b*' box; '*f*' figure; and '*t*' indicate table respectively.

A

Adjustment, method of 161
Age-related macular
      degeneration 96, 134, 171
Albrecht von Graefe 194, 194*f*
American Academy of Ophthalmology 134
Amsler grid 132
Anderson's criteria 96, 119
    diagnose glaucomatous visual field
      defect 96
Antiglaucoma medication
Antiretinal antibodies, circulating 134
Apostilb, equivalences of 36*t*
Apostilbs 92
Arc perimeter 194*f*
    popularity of 195
Arcuate field defect
    left eye of superior 164*f*
    superior 163*f*
Arcuate scotoma 10
Arcuate scotoma
    inferior 130*f*
    superior 31*f*, 96, 120*f*
Armamentarium, part of 3
Arterial occlusions typically 133
Autoimmune retinopathy 134
Automated eye tracking 16
Automated glaucoma practice system 173
Automated imaging devices 105
Automated macular perimeter, third-
      generation 132
Automated perimetry 49, 127
    advent of 196
    pitfalls in 51
Automated static threshold perimetry 93
Automated visual field
    interpretation of 130*t*
    test, selection of 121
Automatic pupil measurement 14

B

Berlin's edema 133
Biarcuate scotoma, incomplete 120*f*
Binary search, modified 162
Bipolar cells 4
Birdshot chorioretinopathy 134
Bivariate contour ellipse area 138
Bizarre peripheral defect 128*f*

Blind spot 3*f*, 38, 39*f*
    enlargement of 128*f*, 194
    sensitivity 92
Blindness
    night 137
    sea of 91
Bowl, light illumination of 192*f*
Bracketing 5
    threshold estimation 5*f*
Bruch's membrane
    invisible extensions of 105
    opening 109
Bulbs, changing 191

C

C3 field analyzer 186
Calibration 190
Campimetry 195
Cardinal spots, green and blue 37*f*
Carter's arc perimeter 194*f*
Cartridge, changing 191
Cataract 70*f*
    produce defects evident 55*f*
Central defects, detect early 93
Central field defects 133
Central retinal artery occlusion 133
Central ring scotomas, bilateral 150
Central serous chorioretinopathy 171
Central serous retinopathy 133
    presence of 146
Central visual field defects 121
Central visual function 121
Cerebral hemisphere, left 101
Chiasm 121*f*
Chiasmal and retro-chiasmal lesions,
      detect 120
Chiasmal compression 130*f*
Chiasmal disease 123
Chloroquine maculopathy 134
Chloroquine, screening for 134
Choosing test 132
Choosing test pattern 6
Choroidal neovascular membranes 148
Choroidal nevus 135
Clover leaf pattern, grayscale 9*f*
Clover-leaf pattern 34, 37
Cluster analysis
    and polar graph 42
    corrected 46*f*, 87, 89*t*

Cluster defects 88
Cluster progression analysis 88
Cluster trend analysis 87, 89*f*
    explanations used in 89*t*
Cognitive decline 12
Collaborative Initial Glaucoma Treatment
      Study 62
Conducting tests 17
Confocal scanning laser
      ophthalmoscope 105
Confounding factors and artifacts 8
Confrontation testing 132
Contact control 16
Coronavirus disease 2019 185, 192
    protocols for 188*f*
Corrected pattern standard deviation 96
Cranial nerve palsy 57*f*
Craniopharyngioma 122*f*, 123, 130*f*
Cup-to-disc 147
Cystoid macular edema 52*f*

D

Dart control 16
Defect classification systems 62
Defect curve 42, 45
Defect values 86
Dense centrocecal scotoma 140
Depressed central points 67
Detachments, long-standing 156
Deviation maps 37
Diabetic 126*f*
    macular ischemia 133
    papillopathy 126*f*
Diabetic retinopathy 133
    nonproliferative 141
    role of swap in 170
Diffuse defect 43, 46*f*, 87, 87*f*, 88
    change 88, 88*f*
Digital imaging and communications in
      medicine 24*f*
    compliance 178
Disc and retina, meticulous assessment
      of 132
Disc cleaning 191
Disease
    advanced stage of 110*f*
    progression, stages of 88
Dynamic test strategy 17

E

Electronic health records 173, 174
Electronic medical records 174
Epiretinal membrane 134
Equipment, proper care and maintenance 190
Ethambutol toxicity 123
Event analysis 62, 63
    detects 86
    with stable 73*f*
Eye
    left 53*f*, 111*f*
        fundus photography, 106*f*
    lid, dropping of 96
    monitor capability, remote video 14
    movements, voluntary 8
    right 53*f*, 111*f*, 152
        fundus image of visual fields 96
    sensitivity in 133
    tested 44, 49
    virtual fields, 96, 181, 187
Eyecatcher 183
Eyesi Surgical Trainer 180
EyeSuite perimetry 175
Eye-tracker, real-time 132

F

False depressions 54
False negative 10, 50, 64*f*, 69*f*, 78*f*, 79*f*, 81*f*, 82*f*, 83*f*, 95
    errors 34
False positive 10, 50, 64*f*, 69*f*, 78*f*, 79*f*, 81*f*, 82*f*, 83*f*
    errors 32, 33, 162
Fatigue 9, 55
Fixation
    errors 162
    instability 57
    losses 31, 50, 64*f*, 65*f*, 69*f*, 71*f*, 78*f*, 79*f*, 81*f*, 82*f*, 83*f*, 94
    monitor 94
    stability, real-time monitoring of 66*f*
    target 94
Flicker testing 13
Fluctuation
    higher long-term 86
    long-term 6, 62, 87
    short-term 6, 6*f*, 62
Fovea 3, 91
    sensitivity 36
Foveal threshold 95
    testing 14
Foveolar 3*f*
Frequency doubling illusion 159
Functional testing procedure, step-by-step 188
Fundus photography 106*f*, 107*f*, 108*f*, 109*f*, 112*f*, 114*f*, 117*f*
Fundus' brightness 29
Fuse, changing 190

G

Gamut 105
Ganglion cell inner plexiform layer 111*f*
Ganglion cell loss 52
Gaze tracking 8, 14, 31, 94*f*, 96
    method, using 66*f*
    records 17
Geniculate nucleus, lateral 169
Glaucoma 53*f*, 55, 105, 174
    advanced 13, 42, 44*f*, 45*f*, 46*f*, 47*f*
        intervention study 62
    atypical of 130*f*
    chronic primary angle closure 96
    clinical trials, large-scale 13
    damage 36*f*
    diagnosis 29, 52
    early manifest 13
    hemifield test 14, 30*f*, 32*f*, 40, 57*f*, 59*f*, 62, 64*f*, 65*f*, 67*f*, 69*f*, 71*f*, 72*f*, 73*f*, 74*f*, 75*f*, 76*f*, 78*f*, 81*f*, 82*f*, 84*f*,94*f*, 94, 95
    long-standing, 132
    management paradigm 174
    practice, clinical relevance in current 166
    primary open angle 110*f*
    progression analysis 63, 64*f*
        report, analysis of 63
    role of swap in 170
    staging system 62
    structural and functional 105, 111*f*
    vis-a-vis in neuro-ophthalmology 130*t*
    with right eye, open angle 96
    workplace, forum 175
Glaucomatous
    backward bowing 3
    change 62, 89*f*
    damage, severe 40*f*
    defect, early 96
    field defects 132
        typical 51*f*
    loss, functional 185
    progression, misdiagnosing 132
    visual field loss 3
Global indices 30*f*, 39, 42, 45, 94*f*, 95
Global progression analysis 87
Global trend analysis 87
    reflecting progression in 88*t*
Goldman's notation for stimulus size 92*t*
Goldmann
    bowl 196*f*
    kinetic 16
    perimeter 8*t*, 92, 93
Grays-cale
    graph 36, 37*f*
    presentation 42
    representation 43
Greenfield criteria 52
Guided progression analysis 14, 66, 67*f*, 68*f*, 69*f*, 71*f*, 72*f*, 73*f*, 74*f*, 75*f*, 76*f*, 83*f*, 119

H

Hallmark visual field defect 123
Hans Goldmann 196*f*

Harry Moss Traquair 195*f*
Head tracking 14
Head-mounted
    devices
        cons of 185
        pros of 185
    perimeter, inception of 185
    virtual reality perimeters, types of 185
    visual field analyzer 185
    use of 188*f*
Health systems 173
Healthcare institutions 173
Heidelberg retinal tomography 173, 174
Heijl-Krakau method 14, 94
    of monitoring fixation 50
Hemianopia 194
    bitemporal 121
    left incongruous 120*f*
Hemianopic visual fields 126
Hemifield glaucoma test 33
Henning Rønne 195*f*
Heru re: Vive visual field technology 187
HEYEX 2 178
Hodapp-Parrish classification 96*t*
Hodapp-Parrish-Anderson criteria 166
Homonymous hemianopia 126
    right 101
Humphrey's
    field analyzer 13, 13*f*, 29, 50, 62, 92, 93, 117*f*, 190
        decibels in 36*t*
        inside bowl of 192*f*
        test report, interpretation of 93
        using 180
    matrix frequency 165*f*
        doubling perimetry 163*f*
    models of 14*t*
    perimeter 8, 15, 24, 126
        background bulb 192*f*
        utilizes 94
    programs 6
    visual field 13, 17, 24*f*, 113*f*, 132, 180
        analyzer 190
            calibration 190
            changing cartridge 191
            changing fuse 190
            daily maintenance 190
            disc cleaning 191
            power supply 190
            printer head clogging 191
Hydroxychloroquine toxicity 134, 150

I

Idiopathic intracranial hypertension 128*f*
Incongruous hemianopia 123*f*
Infectious and inflammatory retinopathies 134
Inferior field loss (left) 51*f*
Inflammatory autoimmune retinal degenerative diseases 134
Inflammatory retinopathies 134
Instructions, cleaning 191, 192
Integrating technologies, current status 173

Internal limiting membrane 109
Intranet and medical records 174
Intraocular pressure 53f
Irvine-Gass syndrome 133
Ischemic optic neuropathy 130f
Isolated scotomata 134
Isopter 92

J

Jannik bjerrum 195f

K

Kinetic perimetry 92, 93

L

Lamina cribrosa 3
Learning
    curve 56f
    defect 54, 117f
    effect 9f, 9, 51
Lens artifact 10
Lens holder 191
    poorly cleaned 192f
Lens, contact 31
Lens rim
    artifact 12
    defects 60
Lesion, fundus image of 146
Lid artifact 10
Light intensity 4
Liquid trial lens 14
Local defect 43, 87, 87f, 88
    change 88f
Luminance 91
Luminous intensity 10

M

Macros, use of 175
Macula test 163
Macular disease 132
Macular drusen 134
Macular edema 144
    nondiabetic 133
Macular ganglion cell inner plexiform layer
    omplex 110f
Macular hole in left eye 149
Macular holes 134
Macular integrity
    assessment 132, 138
    index 150
Macular test 7
Macular threshold testing 7f
Maculopathies 134
Magnocellular cells 159
Magnocellular pathway 160, 169
Mask-induced artifacts 188f
Matrix frequency doubling technology,
    second generation 162
Mean defect 43, 45, 47, 86, 87, 87f, 88, 88f

Mean deviation 17, 30f, 39, 57f, 59f, 64f, 65f,
    69f, 72f, 73f, 74f, 75f, 76f, 78f, 79f,
    80f, 81f, 82f, 83f, 84f, 95, 162
    depressed 35f
    high 94
Mean sensitivity 43
Medical record system 119
Medmont automated perimeter 192
    cleaning instructions 192
Melanomas, anterior 135
Melbourne rapid fields 182
Merits and demerits 24
Microperimetry 132, 134
Microsoft HoloVision 180
Microsurgical procedures 180
Miotic pupil 12
Miotics, use of 56
Mobile virtual perimetry 181
Monocular field of vision 91
Monocular versus binocular testing 7
Moving perimeter 191
Multiple evanescent white dot
    syndrome 154
Myopic traction maculopathy 134

N

Near correction, improper 12
Nerve fiber layer, slit defects of 116f
Networking and compatibility 24
Neuroimaging pituitary macroadenoma 54f
Neurological causes 52
Neurological disease 51, 119
    management of 12
Neurological disorders 52
Neuro-ophthalmic diseases 9, 127f
Neuro-ophthalmic disorders 119
Neuro-ophthalmic visual field defects 120
Neuroretinal rim 109
    healthy 147
    thinning, bilateral superior 116f
    width, region-wise 109
    width, sectoral and regional 111
nGoggle 181
Notch in right disc, Superior 51f
Numeric plot 130f

O

Observer interpretation 60
Octopus 13, 17, 92
    different models of 16t
Octopus 300 15f
    basic 16
Octopus 600 15f
Octopus 900 15f
    EyeSuite with 24f
Octopus EyeSuite software 87, 88
    global progression analysis with
    progression analysis
        functions 86
        tools with 87f
    with polar trend analysis
        function of 89

Octopus perimeter 13, 42, 43f, 190, 191
    analyzing single field report 42
    cleaning instructions 191
    moving 191
    single visual field reports of 42
Octopus visual field report, single 47
Ocular hypertension treatment study 13
Oculus Easyfield 24
Oculus perimeters 24
Ophthalmic disorders 119
Optic disc 55f, 121, 121f
    dipping of 112f
    large
Optic nerve 4f, 159
    head 114f
        parameters 109f
        size of 111f
    tends 173
Optic neuritis, multiple episodes of
    postinfectious 129f
Optical coherence tomograph 46, 51, 105,
    109f, 111, 112f, 113f, 114f, 116f, 117f,
    152, 174
    retinal nerve fiber layer 96

P

Pallid optic disc edema 126f
Papilledema 123
Parafoveal telangiectasia 148
Pattern deviation map 38, 38f, 39f, 41f, 94f
Pattern standard deviation 17, 30f, 40, 57f,
    64f, 65f, 69f, 72f, 73f, 74f, 75f, 76f,
    78f, 79f, 81f, 82f, 83f, 84f, 95, 162
    high 95
Perimeters
    bowl disinfection 192
    care and maintenance of 190
    choice of 13
    comparison of 186t
Perimetric stimulus presentation 119
Perimetric tests 7
Perimetry 3
    development of 194
    devices, virtual reality 181t
    dynamic 190
    frequency doubling 159, 165, 166
        advantages of 164
        devices 160
        disadvantages of 165
        first generation 160
        principle 159
        printout 162
        target 160f
        technology 4, 105, 160, 169
        testing modes for 161
    fundus-correlated 138
    history of 194
    in diagnosis and management of
        neuro-ophthalmic disorders 119
        retinal or macular disorders 132
    in specific retinal diseases 133
    pearls and pitfalls in 49
    peristat online 182

recent advances in 180
standard automated 180
static 92
    threshold, advantages of 195
tablet 180
tendency oriented 17, 86
types of 132
virtual reality 180, 183
    procedure for 180
white-on-white 169
Peripheral field defects 152
Peripheral testing 132
Peripheral visual field 142
    loss, monitoring 132
    testing 121
Periscreener 181
Photoreceptor dysfunction 134
Pigmentary disturbance 133
Pituitary adenoma 121f, 123
Placoid pigment epitheliopathy, acute posterior multifocal 134
Polar graph 46
Polar trend analysis 87, 89f
Portable virtual reality 180
Power supply 190
Preretinal defects 52
Probability plot 94f
Program, test strategies and type of 93
Progression analysis
    methods 90
    rate of 81f, 82f
    selection of adequate visual fields for 86
Proliferative diabetic retinopathy 142
Pseudophakia 96
Psychophysical test 62
Ptosis 59f
    physiological/pathological 55
Pupil
    diameter 49
    perimetry 181
    position control 16
    size 8

Q

Quadravision 162
Qualitative techniques 132
Quality and threshold strategy, pay attention to 86
Quantitative techniques 132

R

Rapid
    counterphase flicker 160f
    efficiency binary search technique 162
    flickering 160
Raw data and grayscale 94f, 95
Raw numeric graph 36
Recording fields, practical pearls in 49
Red trend line, interpretation of 88
Refraction 44
Refractive
    blur, diopter of 9

errors 12, 55
status of eye 9
Reliability indices 31, 42, 50, 94f, 162
    low 56
Retina, inferior 145
Retinal
    defects 52
    detachment 134
    disease, develop 132
    disorders 132
    dystrophies 133
    ganglion cells 4, 29
        irreversible loss of 105
    locus 132
    nerve fiber layer 29, 89f, 108f, 109f, 113f, 174
        arrangement of 4f
        defect
            in left eye
            inferior 111f
        inferior wedge-shaped 106f
        segmental deviation 176
        wedge-shaped 107f
    pigment epithelium 141
    sensitivity 91, 92
        degree of 91
        mild central depression of 133
    vasculitis produces 133
    vein occlusion 53f
Retinitis pigmentosa 132, 133
    atypical 137
Retinochoroiditis 132
Rhegmatogenous retinal detachments 134
    inferior 156
Riddoch phenomenon 92
Rim artifact 10f, 71f, 101
Ring scotoma 194

S

Scanning laser
    ophthalmoscope 132
    polarimetry 105
    tomography 90
Scherk's bowl perimeter 195f
Sclerosis, multiple 127f
Scotoma 91, 96, 125f
    asymmetric bisuperotemporal 121f
    central 133, 134, 148
    large 132
    paracentral 133
    paracentral 134
    superior arcuate 107f
    typical ring 137
    white 33
Screening test 161
Sensitivity
    abnormal high 41, 94
    and glare, contrast 9
    and threshold maps 138
    general reduction of 41
    measuring range and scale of 13
Sensorama 180
Serial disc photography 175

Serpiginous choroiditis 134
Short-wavelength automated perimetry 4, 105, 113, 132, 169, 169, 170
    test, tips to increase reliability of 170b
Single field
    analysis printout 30f, 32f, 33f
    reports 42
SITA
    fast 16
    standard 16
Slit retinal nerve fiber layer 112f
Special perimetric methods 17
Spectacle prescription 49
Spectral domain optical coherence tomography 105, 133
Spectralis platform 178
Standard automated perimetry 4, 109f, 159, 160, 178, 180, 185
Stargardt disease 133
Stargardt's dystrophy 140
Statistical probability 40
Stereoscopic fundus photography 105
Stimulus
    and stimulus size 169
    generation 16
    type 44
    perceive 91
    duration 7, 14, 15
    size 7, 17, 16, 51, 92
Stress 12
Suprathreshold 93
    strategy 161
Swedish interactive threshold algorithm 5, 29, 105, 113f, 177f
    standard 180
    strategy 93

T

Tamoxifen toxicity 171
Telangiectatic vessels, superficial 126f
Telemedicine visual field test 181
Teleophthalmology and screening 185
Temporal field 91
Temporal quadrant, lower 37f
Temporal-superior-nasal-inferior-temporal graph 114f
    in left eye 115f
    of eyes 116f
    superior region of 112f
Test pattern and strategy 44
Test-retest variability 86
Threshold 4, 92, 93
    estimation, initial point of 5
    fluctuation 6
    perimetry 93
        analysis: single-field analysis 50
    strategy, full 161
    test 50
        library 14
    two-color increment 169
Topcon
    harmony health analytics 178f
    platform 178

Total deviation map 34*f*, 38, 38*f*, 39*f*, 41*f*, 41*f*
Toxic retinopathies 134
Trabeculectomy 78*f*
Traquair's normal visual field 3*f*
Trend analysis 62
Trigger happy 37
Tripod, hollow stem on 194*f*
Tübinger perimeter 196*f*
Tumor 130*f*, 135

V

Value table 43
Variance, square root of loss 43, 46, 87*f*, 87, 88
Vascular occlusions 133
Vertex monitoring 14
   uses 17
Video eye monitor 14, 17
Visibility, difficult 195
Vision
   analyser, advanced 181, 186, 187, 187*f*
   cellular basis for field of 4
   difficulty in left-sided 125*f*
   field of 91
   hill of 91
   island of 91, 195, 196
   related quality of life 86
   shape of normal hill of 169
   strategy, low 17
   sudden onset of blurring of 145
Visual acuity 29
   corrected 49
   stable 134
Visual field 10, 46*f*, 53*f*, 80*f*, 91, 119, 130*f*, 174
   abnormality 91
   analysis, single 29
   and OCT correlation 175
   artifact, causes of 10, 12
   assessment and measurement 91
   changes 55*f*
   concentric constriction of 194
   corrected comparison plot of 45*f*
   data 109*f*
   effect of miosis on 8*f*
   evaluation of 13
   grayscale representation of 44*f*
   improvement in 11*f*
   left 31*f*
   methods of assessment of 92
   normal 3, 23*f*
   polar graph of
   right eye 96
   severe constriction of 129*f*
   stable 74*f*
   testing of 180
   virtual reality 187
Visual field defects 54, 54*f*, 55, 60, 96, 126*f*, 130*f*, 134, 194
   altitudinal 123
   complex 50
   in glaucoma 120
   long-term 135
   pattern of 119m 121
   presence of 185
   scoring humphrey 166
   superior
   useful for assessing 109*f*
Visual field deficits 134
Visual field diagnose neuro-ophthalmic disorders 121
Visual field easy 181
   application screening test 182*f*
Visual field examination 3, 49, 42
Visual field function, diffuse depression of 134
Visual field index 14, 30*f*, 32*f*, 39, 68*f*, 69*f*, 70*f*, 71*f*, 72*f*, 73*f*, 74*f*, 75*f*, 76*f*, 77*f*, 78*f*, 79*f*, 81, 82*f*, 83*f*, 84*f*, 94*f*, 95, 175, 177*f*
   borderline visual field 40*f*
   trend 70*f*
Visual field interpretation 119
Visual field loss, detect early 105
Visual field of
   left eye 154
   right eye 122*f*, 128*f*
Visual field progression 62, 175
   analysis with octopus perimetry 86
   advantages 175
   assessment of 83
   challenges in assessing 62
   trend-based analyses of 67*t*
   on 10-2 protocol 83
Visual field report 42, 44*f*, 86
   seven-in-one 43*f*
   single 47
Visual field sensitivity, recovery of 134
Visual field testing 4, 36*f*, 46, 57, 57*f*, 62, 119, 133, 134, 137, 188*f*
   distance 14
   expectations of 119
   principles of 4
   program for 5*t*
   virtual 185
Visual function 91
   measure of 92
Visual pathway posterior 123
   lesions of 123
Visual stimuli 187*f*
   relies, detection of 4
Visual system assessed 170
VisuALL head-mounted perimetry 186
Vivid vision perimeter 181, 186
   advantages 186

W

White-dot syndrome, multiple evanescent 134, 154

Z

Zeiss machines 24
Zippy estimation of sequential testing 162

EU GSPR Authorised Reprsentative
Logos Europe, 9 rue Nicolas Poussin
1700, La Rochelle, France
Phone: +33 (0) 6 67 93 73 78
E-mail: contact@logoseurope.eu

www.ingramcontent.com/pod-product-compliance
Ingram Content Group UK Ltd.
Pitfield, Milton Keynes, MK11 3LW, UK
UKHW051829060825
461530UK00007B/84